A NEUROPSYCHIATRIC STUDY IN CHILDHOOD

Clinics in Developmental Medicine Nos. 35/36

A Neuropsychiatric Study in Childhood

MICHAEL RUTTER

PHILIP GRAHAM

WILLIAM YULE

LONDON: Spastics International Medical Publications
in association with William Heinemann Medical Books Ltd.
PHILADELPHIA: J. B. Lippincott Co.

SBN 433-28990-2

Printed in England at THE LAVENHAM PRESS LTD., Lavenham, Suffolk.

Contents

Preface

Over the past three decades physicians, psychologists and educators have become increasingly concerned with the possibility that certain of the child's prenatal and postnatal experiences result either in damage or in disorganization of his central nervous system, with disastrous consequences for development and adaptive capacity. When damage to the central nervous system either affects motor or sensory function or is manifested in episodic disturbances as in the epilepsies, little question exists as to the neurobiologic foundation of behavioural disturbance. The case is by no means as clear when children with apparently normal motor and sensory organization exhibit disturbances of control, specific learning disorders or a variety of other behavioural manifestations which may have their roots in structural or physiologic abnormalities of brain. In such children, studies of associated perinatal risk conditions together with the absence of a reasonable explanation for their dysfunction in the developmental environment has led increasingly to diagnoses of 'brain damage' on purely behavioural grounds. In these diagnoses the objective data are entirely behavioural or historical and the neurologic inference entirely hypothetical. To date, this unsatisfactory state of affairs has not been significantly improved by the use of electrophysiologic or other laboratory procedures.

What is most needed in the assessment of neurobehavioural associations is a detailed body of normative information on the neurologic and behavioural characteristics of a representative and age-specifically defined population of children. Most of our data to date derive from the experience of individual examiners in clinics, who in various ways have attempted to adapt either the techniques of adult neurologic assessment or items from developmental schedules to the task of paediatric neurologic diagnosis. We have little information on the reliability of the findings of such examiners and even less knowledge of the validity attaching to different aspects of the examination as predictors of behavioural and learning competence. In the absence of such data a variety of opinions exist with respect to the relative values of different features of neurologic assessment. In some circles, basing themselves upon the strength and undoubted value of the adult neurologic examination, workers have argued that only such 'hard' signs as reflex changes or abnormal reflexes should be seriously considered in defining a damaged brain. In other circles, considerable dependence is placed on the so-called 'soft' signs such as disturbances of language, speech, integrative activities and constructional abilities. Nowhere until the present volume has there been a careful consideration of the reliability of these individual signs in a representative sample of children. It will be surprising to some to find that in the assessment of children of school age, the so-called 'soft' signs are more reliably elicited upon repeated evaluation than are the 'hard' ones. Such signs as the authors state, are 'soft' not with regard to reliability but only because they are more difficult to interpret. They quite properly argue that these adjectives should be discarded.

In studying the children on the Isle of Wight and applying to all of them a systematic set of neurologic and behavioural measures, the authors have made a major contribution to our understanding of the prevalence and distribution of neurologic signs in school children, and of the relationship of such signs to important behavioural and educational outcomes. The study provides a model for neurobehavioural inquiry in populations of children and lays the basis for the further extension of our understanding through future studies of clinicopathologic associations in such groups.

HERBERT BIRCH

Introduction

In recent years physicians, psychologists and educationalists have been increasingly concerned with the problems of 'the brain-damaged child'. It has long been known that damage to the brain may have widespread effects on all aspects of development. However, there is a surprising absence of well-based knowledge about these effects in childhood. Lack of knowledge and a general conviction that brain damage affects mind functioning have given rise to a mire of tautological assumptions and assertions about presumed and hypothetical early injuries to the brain in the pathogenesis of child psychiatric disorder. This tendency has received impetus from the awareness that damage to the immature brain may lead to subtle distortions of development without any overt neurological condition of a textbook kind.

Our interest in these issues led to the present study which set out to investigate three related questions: how can mild neurological disorder be diagnosed in the clinic, how frequent are the common manifestations of neurological abnormality, and what influence has organic brain dysfunction on psychological development? As psychiatrists and psychologists, it was naturally the third question which first aroused our interest. In dealing with the neurological assessment, we are acutely aware of our limited neurological expertise*. Undoubtedly there are parts of the study which would benefit from replication by paediatric neurologists. Nevertheless, we believe that the questions raised by our findings are as relevant to neurological specialists as they are to psychiatrists.

It was obvious from the outset that any investigation of the psychological consequences of organic brain dysfunction should not be based on children attending any one clinic. Epileptic or cerebral palsied children may be cared for by family doctors without referral to hospital and those sent to specialists may attend neurological, paediatric or psychiatric clinics. Clearly, there are likely to be major differences between children who never go to hospital and those who go to different sorts of specialist clinics. If biases associated with referral policies to individual clinics are to be avoided, it is essential to obtain a total count of cases in the general population. A reliance on children attending hospital would be likely to bias findings in terms of an excess of children with multiple handicaps. It is not always appreciated that there are statistical reasons for the ratio of multiple to single diagnoses being higher in hospital patients than in the general population (Berkson 1946). This artifact is particularly marked in associations between conditions where only a small proportion of each is referred to hospital—a state of affairs which certainly applies to psychiatric disorder and in some measure to neuro-epileptic conditions.

*PG and MR have both had some post-graduate training in neurology and paediatrics, and both have a clinical practice which involves many children with neurological disorder. However, neither one is in any sense a practising neurologist.

Thus, the basis of our investigations had to be an epidemiological study of the general population. Because of the difficulties of case-identification among preschool children, the study was restricted to those of school age. This had the added advantage that psychological and behavioural assessments are easier and probably more valid in the older child.

The opportunity to carry out such a study arose through our involvement in a series of epidemiological enquiries concerning various forms of handicap in Isle of Wight children. Each of the studies used the same basic strategy. As a first stage, the total population of children (in the relevant age-group) whose homes were on the Isle of Wight were studied using multiple screening methods. Then a list was drawn up of all children who appeared from our information likely to have the condition in question. These possible cases were investigated intensively by a team of physicians, psychologists and social scientists, using methods which were based on ordinary clinical assessments but which had been modified in order to obtain a greater standardisation of approach, and so greater comparability. There is much to be said for greater standardisation of methods in ordinary clinical practice, but in an enquiry (such as this) which involved a large number of doctors, standardisation was essential.

The Isle of Wight studies of reading difficulties, intellectual retardation, psychiatric disorder and chronic physical handicap are reported in a companion volume.* The findings of these studies are referred to at several points in this book where comparisons between neurological and other handicaps are required. Sufficient detail is given here for the validity of the comparisons to be judged, but readers who wish for further information on the epidemiology of non-neurological handicap in school-age children are referred to the other volume. It will be appreciated that this attempt to avoid unnecessary cross reference has inevitably led to a certain amount of overlap.

*'Education, Health and Behaviour' (published by Longmans, Green & Co., 1970) edited by MR, Professor Jack Tizard and Dr. Kingsley Whitmore, who directed the enquiries.

Acknowledgements

A collaborative study such as this necessarily owes a great deal to the help of many people. The planning of the investigations was carried out jointly with Professor J. Tizard, Dr K. Whitmore, Dr I. B. Pless and Mr Leslie Rigley, and we are deeply indebted to them in many respects. Many of the ideas expressed in this volume arose from discussions with them during the planning, field-work, analysis and writing-up of the study.

At all stages of the work we have been especially fortunate in the willing collaboration we have received from the County Education Officer, Mr A. L. Hutchinson, the Medical Officer of Health and Principal School Medical Officer, Dr R. K. Machell, and from the teachers, parents and the children themselves on the Island. The County Education Officer arranged for the distribution of tests and questionnaires to the various schools on the Island. The Deputy Education Officer, Mr H. W. Barratt, who had a special responsibility for special services and who has since succeeded Mr Hutchinson as Education Officer, was closely involved in administrative aspects of the surveys. The teachers filled in behavioural rating scales on all children and completed questionnaires on physical disorder and handicap. They were also responsible for the distribution of rating scales for children to take home to their parents.

Dr Michael Ashley-Miller and Mr Ronald Davie, Senior School Medical Officer and Educational Psychologist respectively on the Isle of Wight, contributed greatly to the surveys in 1964 and were very helpful in the planning of the 1965 neurological study. Mrs Ann Chase gave invaluable assistance as Secretary to the survey. Throughout we have received the fullest co-operation from the Education and Health Committees of the Isle of Wight. Mr T. V. Pretty, Senior Welfare Officer to the Authority and his staff gave much help in numerous ways.

We were greatly assisted by Dr A. K. Miller, Consultant Physician on the Island Dr G. Knight, Consultant Child Psychiatrist, Mr J. Chisnell, Psychiatric Social Worker, Dr Gordon Browne, Consultant Psychiatrist, and Miss M. Godfrey, Children's Officer on the Island. The general practitioners on the Island and the Local Medical Committee, through its Secretary, Dr S. R. B. H. Kennedy, were kept informed of the progress of the work. The hospital and local authority records officers, in particular Mr W. H. Jay and Mr D. Rhodes, gave us access to their records, as did Dr C. Haffner, Consultant Psychiatrist to the City of Portsmouth Child Guidance Service. The speech therapists, Miss I. Haddock and Miss C. Ronalds, were most helpful in providing information on the children they had seen.

Much of the field work was carried out by psychiatrists, psychologists and social scientists who came from London to the Island for this purpose. They are too many to name individually. The Institute of Psychiatry and the Bethlem Royal and Maudsley Hospitals generously allowed staff to be released to take part in the fieldwork, as did a number of other authorities. Mr T. Cleaton and Miss M. Hemming were responsible for much of the computer work, which was carried out by the University of London Atlas Computer and on the Imperial College IBM 1900. We are also grateful to Mr Harvey Goldstein of the Institute of Child Health for providing some of the computer programmes. The University of London Examinations Department punched the IBM and Hollerith cards with great accuracy and speed.

Grants for the study were provided by the Department of Education and Science, the Nuffield Foundation, the Medical Research Council, the American Association for the Aid of Crippled Children, and the Social Science Research Council. They were administered by the University of London Institute of Education which also generously provided room for the work. Mr G. Nichols, Deputy Accountant to the Institute, was responsible for most of the financial transactions.

Much administrative and clerical work was carried out at the Institutes of Psychiatry and Education in London. A heavy responsibility was taken by the secretaries—Miss Olwen Davies at the Institute of Education, and Miss Cherry Hambrook, Miss Gudrun Hanson and Miss Catherine Greenwood at the Institute of Psychiatry. We are grateful to Miss Bridget Osborn for help with the data analysis and for checking the bibliography. Dr T. T. S. Ingram and Dr Martin Bax provided many invaluable suggestions and comments on the manuscript, as did our collaborators on the study, Professor J. Tizard, Dr K. Whitmore and Mr Leslie Rigley.

Finally, most of all we are deeply indebted to the many parents and children on the Isle of Wight whose outstanding co-operation made the research possible.

PART I

Organic Brain Dysfunction and Child Psychiatric Disorder: Overview

CHAPTER 1

Review of the Literature and Consideration of Issues

There is now a very large literature on the associations between organic brain dysfunction and child psychiatric disorder. This has already been reviewed in relation to cerebral palsy (Cruickshank and Bice 1955, Nielsen 1966, Oswin 1967), epilepsy (Bridge 1949, Keating 1961, Pond 1961), 'brain damage' (Benton 1962, Birch 1964, Schulman *et al.* 1965), 'minimal cerebral dysfunction' (Bax and Mac Keith 1963) and psychological test findings (Graham and Berman 1961, Herbert 1964). No attempt, therefore, will be made to provide a comprehensive survey; instead, selected papers will be discussed briefly in order to summarise the main findings for which there is sound support and to consider the basic questions in this field which still require an answer. Associations between organic brain dysfunction and child psychiatric disorder have sometimes been considered in relation to broad concepts of 'brain damage' and sometimes in relation to specific syndromes or diseases. While there is considerable overlap between these different approaches, it is convenient to deal with them separately.

Cerebral Palsy

The term 'cerebral palsy' does not describe any discrete disease entity, nor even a homogeneous clinical grouping (Cruickshank and Raus 1955). The disorders it comprises differ widely in aetiology, pathology and associated clinical findings (Courville 1958, Ingram 1964, Illingworth 1958) and they should perhaps be properly regarded as motor manifestations of a much wider group of syndromes of brain damage or defect which may also include epilepsy and mental retardation and which are often, but not always, due to obstetric disorders (Denhoff and Robinault 1960, Mitchell 1961). Nevertheless, although the definition of cerebral palsy is necessarily arbitrary, the category has a certain usefulness and has been very widely employed throughout the literature.

Unfortunately, despite a large number of papers on the personality and behavioural characteristics of cerebral palsied children, very few conclusions can be drawn. The best studies contain very little information on the children's psychiatric state (Henderson 1961, Ingram 1964) and the systematic psychological studies have been more concerned with cognitive, perceptual and visuo-motor disturbances than with emotional or behavioural attributes (Nielsen 1966). Numerous statements in the literature regarding the personality characteristics of cerebral palsied children have never received corroboration through controlled studies (Cruickshank and Bice 1955). Most writers on the subject have noted the frequency with which psychiatric problems occur in association with cerebral palsy (Cockburn 1961, Dunsdon 1952, Floyer 1955, Gardner 1961, Oswin 1967, Woods 1957) but none has made a systematic comparison of the psychiatric state of children with cerebral palsy and children with other conditions (particularly physical handicap) or children in the general population. Until these studies have been made (Hersov 1963) the conclusion that psychiatric disorder is more common among cerebral palsied children must remain tentative.

Only Nielsen (1966) has studied matched groups of cerebral palsied children of normal intelligence and children of the same age, sex, IQ and social class without evidence of any kind of cerebral damage. This study provides much useful information and the conclusions are well considered. Unfortunately the only organised information on emotions and behaviour was derived from three projective tests of dubious validity (the Duss Fable test, the Handicap Thematic Apperception test and the Rorschach test). The agreement between the projective tests was poor, but it was found that significantly more cerebral palsied children than controls showed signs of moderate or severe personality disorder, in a ratio of between $1\frac{1}{2}$ to 1 and 4 to 1 according to which measure was taken. The kind of disturbances found varied greatly.

What factors lead to the development of psychiatric disorder in cerebral palsied children? The presence of a visible disability, the frustrations inherent in physical restrictions, adverse parental reactions to the child's handicap, perceptual abnormalities, poor speech and language resulting in the child not being able to express his wants adequately, visual defects, low intelligence, the effect of drugs, community prejudices in relation to the disorder, the child's reactions to his disability and impaired emotional control produced by direct brain dysfunction have all been suggested as possible causes (Bradley 1955, Cruickshank and Raus 1955, Floyer 1955, Garrard and Richmond 1957, Gibbs 1958, Oswin 1967). There is some suggestion that emotional disturbance may be more common in children of low IQ (Bradway 1937, Dunsdon 1952) but there is no evidence which allows an evaluation of the relative importance of these factors, most of which have never been systematically studied.

Epilepsy

The literature on emotional and behavioural disturbances in epileptic children is large (Keating 1961) but for the most part the studies have been remarkably unsystematic. Estimates of the frequency of psychiatric disorder in epileptic children vary widely. Henderson (1953) found that 12 per cent of a representative sample of epileptic school children were emotionally disturbed or badly behaved, whereas Pond and Bidwell in their general practice survey (1960) found that 25 per cent of school age epileptic children showed psychological difficulties. Bridge (1949) reported that of 742 children attending the epilepsy clinic, 9 per cent showed severe personality disorder and 37 per cent exhibited mild or moderate disorders. Price (1950) noted disturbances through behaviour or mental impairment in 56 per cent of 50 epileptic children at school. However, these estimates from some of the best reported studies mean little without a specification of the criteria which have been employed and an investigation to determine the rate of disorder in the general population when the same criteria are used. Although it seems likely that the rate of psychiatric disorder in epileptic children may be higher than that in the general population, further studies are required to determine if this is the case and, if so, by how much the rate exceeds that in the general population.

More is known of the types of psychiatric disorder shown by epileptic children. It is quite evident from the studies mentioned above and from others (Keating 1961) that the types of disorder shown include all the disorders shown by non-epileptic children (Pond 1961). For the most part there seems to be nothing characteristic about the emotional and behavioural problems of the epileptic child. The concept of the typical 'epileptic personality' is no more applicable to the child with epilepsy than it is to the adult (Tizard 1962).

On the other hand, the hyperkinetic syndrome, although only present in a minority of epileptics, does seem to be particularly associated with epilepsy or brain damage (Ingram 1956, Ounsted 1955, Pond 1961, see also page 10).

Many factors have been suggested as significant in the development of psychiatric disorder in epileptic children. There are factors which may be relevant in any child with psychiatric disorder, whether epileptic or not. With epileptic children, there are also the problems of altered brain function associated with epileptic discharge, the family attitudes to epilepsy and the effect these have on their relationship with the epileptic child, the problems of post-convulsive symptoms, the child's reactions to his fits, the effects of limited intelligence and the consequences of community prejudices to epilepsy (Bradley 1951, Bridge 1949). In addition, there is the possible effect of drugs (Pond 1961). Pond and his associates have made considerable progress in attempting to determine the relative importance of each of these possible pathogenic factors.

It is well known that phenobarbitone tends to make children irritable, but it seems that drugs play little part in the more serious intellectual and social deterioration occasionally seen in epileptics (Chaudhry and Pond 1961). What role drugs play in the more common psychiatric disorders shown by epileptic children is not known.

Grünberg and Pond (1957) have shown the importance of family disturbance in the development of antisocial and aggressive behaviour in epileptic children by comparing the family background of epileptic children with conduct disorders, epileptic children without conduct disorders and non-epileptic children with conduct disorders. The relevance of 'organic' factors could not be determined as the non-epileptic children had all had an EEG for clinical reasons and so showed a relatively high rate of possible 'organic' background factors. The importance of environmental influences in the development of psychiatric disorder is well-supported by Grünberg and Pond's findings and is consistent with the conclusions of other less systematic investigations. However, it should be noted that the children studied all attended a psychiatric clinic and that the children and their family backgrounds were not studied independently, so leaving the opportunity for possible bias in the results.

Epileptic children attending Pond's clinic were also studied by Nuffield (1961) who showed that physiological as well as psychological factors played a part in the development of psychiatric disorder. Temporal lobe foci on the EEG were significantly associated with aggressive behaviour, and 3 cycles per second spike and wave were associated with neurotic manifestations. These results are in keeping with most other studies.

Ounsted found that the hyperkinetic syndrome was more common in children with temporal lobe epilepsy than in children with other varieties of epilepsy (Ounsted

1955, Ounsted *et al.* 1966). The latter is undoubtedly the fullest and most systematic study of temporal lobe epilepsy in children which has so far been undertaken but, in relation to the significance of the behavioural associations reported, it should be noted that the groups of children with different types of epilepsy were not matched for age, sex and IQ. In keeping with Ounsted's findings, Glaser and Dixon (1956) reported that the majority of a group of 25 children with psychomotor fits showed inter-seizure personality disturbances characterised by overactive aggressive behaviour. However, no control group was used. A high rate of aggression and hyperactivity is typical of most reports of temporal lobe epilepsy in children. On the other hand, Wilson and Harris (1966) found no difference in the frequency of psychiatric problems in epileptic children whose EEG's showed temporal lobe foci compared with that in children with frontal lobe and Rolandic spike foci. It is hard to know how much emphasis to place on this negative finding as there were substantial age differences between their groups. In addition, there needs to be considerable caution in the interpretation of spikes, especially posterior temporal spikes, in view of the findings on the migration and disappearance of spike foci in children (Gibbs *et al.* 1954). There is only a weak relationship between EEG findings and clinical fit pattern (Glaser and Golub 1955); many children with psychomotor seizures have a normal EEG and when an abnormality occurs it is more frequently bilateral atypical $1\frac{1}{2}$ to 3 cycles per second spike and wave rather than temporal lobe spikes.

Although temporal lobe abnormalities probably have a particular association with behaviour disorders, several studies have shown that there is a complex relationship between EEG findings and psychiatric findings. Aird and Yamamoto (1966) found that temporal lobe foci were those most strongly associated with psychiatric disorder, but within a group of children all of whom had behavioural disorders, there was no relationship between EEG findings and the type of behaviour disorder (except that learning difficulties tended to be more common in children with occipital and possibly temporal lobe foci). Similarly, Stevens *et al.* (1968) found that among children attending a psychiatric clinic there were scarcely any clinical differences between those with a normal EEG and those with EEG abnormalities. Complicated associations were found between psychiatric findings and different types of EEG phenomena: temporal lobe abnormalities were associated with defective memory, poor arithmetic and social withdrawal rather than aggression, whereas occipital abnormalities were associated with hyperactivity.

In adults, too, individuals with temporal lobe epilepsy have generally been found to have an increased rate of psychiatric disorder and to constitute a disproportionate percentage of inmates of long stay mental institutions (Gibbs 1951, Margerison and Corsellis 1966, Margerison and Liddell 1961, Pond and Bidwell 1960). Small and her colleagues (1962, 1966) reported no difference in the psychiatric disorders of adults with temporal and non-temporal lobe epilepsy but the interpretation of this finding is made difficult by the fact that nearly everyone in all their groups showed psychiatric disorder. Furthermore, they studied clinic samples which showed considerable age and sex differences between temporal and non-temporal groups.

The findings are not entirely conclusive but it seems that temporal lobe abnormalities and deviant family situations both play a part in the development of psychiatric disorder in epileptics. The relative importance of each and the role of other factors is not known, nor has the frequency of psychiatric disorder in epileptics been determined.

Behavioural Consequences of Organic Brain Disorders other than Cerebral Palsy

Psychiatric disorder has also been noted in relation to a wide variety of organic brain disorders other than cerebral palsy and epilepsy. Some of the chief issues were outlined clearly in a key paper by Still in 1902. He noted that various forms of aggressive and disinhibited behaviour were particularly common in children with a general impairment of intellect but that there was no direct relationship between the degree of behavioural disturbance and the degree of intellectual impairment. This lack of relationship suggested that physical changes in the brain, rather than the intellectual level itself, might be responsible for the psychiatric disorder. Consequently, Still went on to examine cases of organic brain disorder in which there was no intellectual impairment and found the same problems in what he termed 'moral control'. Less commonly, the psychiatric difficulties occurred in relation to non-cerebral physical disease and also in the absence of any known physical disability. However, circumstantial evidence suggested that in these children, too, a physical defect might play some part in the development of the disorder. Still also noted the importance of the age in the child's life at which the cerebral trauma occurred, the influence of the family situation and the improvement which might occur when the surroundings were changed.

Apart from those concerned with cerebral palsied or epileptic children, most subsequent investigations have been of very heterogeneous groups of cases. The rationale for doing this has generally been as follows: (*a*) general damage to the brain may have important consequences for behavioural development, quite apart from the specific effects of focal lesions; (*b*) the same diagnostic label may include children with very different kinds of cerebral pathology and physical handicaps, as in most studies of cerebral palsy; and (*c*) different diagnostic groups (*e.g.* cerebral palsy, mental deficiency and some cases of epilepsy) may share similar pathology (Denhoff 1955).

The rate of psychiatric disorder in children with organic brain dysfunction compared with the general population is unknown, but most studies have tended to find quite high rates of disorder. As with cerebral palsy and epilepsy, the great variety of psychiatric disorders found in association with organic brain disorders has been striking. Small (1962) found that a third of the children attending a clinic for cerebral palsy and language disorder, the majority of whom had some variety of organic brain condition, showed psychiatric disorder. A quarter of those with psychiatric disorder showed the hyperkinetic syndrome but most exhibited other types of disorder including transient adjustment problems, neurosis, psychosis and behavioural problems. Psychiatric disorder was associated with both severe visual or hearing impairment in the child and severe emotional difficulties in the parents and, as with epilepsy, it seemed to be associated with both organic factors in the child and environmental influences. Pond's survey of brain-damaged children attending a psychiatric clinic also showed that the psychiatric disorders were very varied in type (Pond 1961).

Hyperkinesis was most frequent in young boys of low IQ whereas neurotic symptoms were more common in older children of average intelligence or above. No association was found between the presence of hyperkinesis and abnormal parental attitudes, but it was said that none of the hyperkinetic children came from normal homes.

In a well controlled clinical-experimental study of children with neurological disorder, Shaffer (1969) showed that although brain damage was associated with a higher rate of psychiatric disorder, it was not associated with a specific type of disorder. Aggressive children tended to be overactive and impulsive but this was equally true of children with no detectable neurological abnormalities.

Follow-up studies of children with proven or suspected cerebral injury have also shown the very variable outcome, for example, in relation to very low birth weight and pregnancy complications (Drillien 1964, Preston 1945), lead poisoning (Byers and Lord 1943), meningitis (Lawson *et al.* 1965, Lorber 1961, Nyhan and Richardson 1963), encephalitis (Finley 1958, Meyer and Byers 1952) and head injury (Harrington and Letemendia 1958, Hjern and Nylander 1962). However, comparisons between groups are hazardous in view of the uncertainties about the presence or extent of brain damage and the variability in the type and quality of the behavioural examinations. There has been a much greater concern in the literature with the perceptual and cognitive disturbances associated with brain damage than with the psychiatric disorders.

The Hyperkinetic Syndrome

Is hyperkinesis particularly associated with brain damage? Early statements that hyperkinesis was the usual behaviour associated with brain damage (Strauss and Kephart 1940, 1955; Strauss and Lehtinen 1947) have not been supported by the evidence of systematic studies (Ernhardt *et al.* 1963, Gallagher 1957, Schulman *et al.* 1965).

Strauss' claim that all types of brain lesions usually lead to the hyperkinetic syndrome appears to rest largely on the results of his early study with Kephart (1940), in which the behavioural ratings of brain-injured and non-brain-injured retarded adolescents were compared. Hyperkinesis was significantly associated with brain injury but there was considerable overlap between the groups. The study is open to serious methodological criticisms (Gallagher 1957, Nielsen 1966) and, as Nielsen concluded, '... this investigation would hardly be regarded today as particularly important, on account of the serious objections which can be made both to the selection of subjects, to the test constructions, and to the instruction of the raters'. More recent studies have consistently produced findings which are against the view that most brain-injured children are hyperkinetic. Gallagher (1957) found significant differences between brain-injured and non-brain-injured mentally retarded children as regards hyperactivity, but the overlap was great; many brain-injured children were not hyperkinetic and many children without brain injury were hyperkinetic. Ernhart *et al.* (1963) produced even more negative results. Brain-injured children were found to have an increased frequency of maladjustment, but the types of problems were the same as in other children. The hyperkinetic syndrome was not at all typical of the brain-injured and inactivity was at least as common as overactivity. Schulman *et al.* (1965) also found that hyperactivity was not associated with neurological abnormality as measured in a variety of ways.

The results of these and other studies make it quite clear that most children with organic brain disorders are not hyperkinetic, although it is quite possible that hyperkinesis is found more often in brain-injured children than in other children. Hyperkinesis is most characteristic of the young child of low IQ (Pond 1961) and there are important developmental changes with increasing age. Overactivity diminishes in later childhood and is often even replaced by underactivity in adolescence (Eisenberg 1966, Pond 1961, Rutter *et al.* 1967*a*). Accordingly, age differences between the studies (a mean of nearly 17 years in Strauss and Kephart 1940, a range of 11 to 15 years in Schulman *et al.* 1965 and of 3 to 5 years in Ernhart *et al.* 1963) vitiate any comparisons. Furthermore, most studies showing an association between hyperkinesis and brain damage have been concerned with mentally retarded children in institutions and, as the authors themselves point out, the results cannot be generalised to mentally retarded children in the community and even less to children of normal intelligence.

Although there can be no doubt that the hyperkinetic syndrome is not the usual behaviour of the child with brain damage, it might still be the case that when the syndrome occurs, it does so only in relation to structural brain disease. The examination of this issue is complicated by the difficulties in deciding how active a child must be before he is 'overactive' or 'hyperkinetic', and whether or not the overactivity must be linked with other features such as impulsiveness, disinhibition and distractibility before the hyperkinetic syndrome can be diagnosed. A further difficulty is that reports and observations of overactivity do not agree particularly well with objective measures of the amount of movement (Schulman and Reisman 1959, Schulman *et al.* 1965, Shaffer 1969). The appearance of overactivity is probably partly due to the short attention span and the inappropriateness and lack of control over activity rather than to an absolute increase in the tempo or the amount of movement.

Ounsted has linked the hyperkinetic syndrome specifically with temporal lobe dysfunction (Ounsted *et al.* 1966). He found that the frequency of the hyperkinetic syndrome in children with temporal lobe epilepsy was higher than in children with other types of epilepsy (Ounsted 1955), but as comparable information was not given for matched groups the interpretation of his findings remains uncertain. In particular, since Pond (1961) has pointed out that hyperkinesis is associated with low IQ, it is not clear how far Ounsted's findings are explicable in terms of the low IQ of the children with temporal lobe epilepsy. Ounsted has suggested that hyperkinesis *causes* low IQ through impairment of learning opportunities (Ounsted *et al.* 1966; Ounsted 1968, 1970), while Pond (1961) has considered that mental immaturity is a factor in the causation of the hyperkinesis. At present there are no data which allow a firm choice between these two alternatives. Ingram (1956, 1963*b*) has pointed to other evidence linking the hyperkinetic syndrome with temporal lobe dysfunction. Undoubtedly, hyperactivity sometimes arises on the basis of temporal lobe abnormality, but how often it does so is as yet unknown.

Hyperkinesis has also been found to be associated with poor speech, poor co-ordination, strabismus, EEG abnormalities and a history of incidents which could have caused brain damage (Stewart *et al.* 1966, Werry *et al.* 1964, Werry 1968). Nevertheless, the evidence did not suggest that all cases of hyperkinesis were due to brain damage and Knobel *et al.* (1959) found that hyperkinetic children had no more evidence of organic brain dysfunction than any other children attending a psychiatric clinic. It should be noted, however, that these workers employed a wider definition of the hyperkinetic syndrome than that put forward by Ounsted (1955), Ingram (1956) and Laufer *et al.* (1957). Ounsted's excellent description of the hyperkinetic syndrome made it quite clear that this was an uncommon disorder involving more than mere overactivity. This view has been reiterated in more recent papers (Hutt and Hutt 1964, Ounsted *et al.* 1966), in which features other than the activity level (especially the short, relatively fixed attention span) have also been emphasised.

We believe, therefore, that there is a significant association between the hyperkinetic syndrome and evidence of neurological abnormality or brain damage. On the other hand, most brain-damaged children are not overactive and many overactive children show no evidence of brain damage. The milder and less specific types of overactivity may or may not represent the same phenomenon as the hyperkinetic syndrome described by Ounsted and others. The 'classical' type of hyperkinetic syndrome may usually be associated with organic brain dysfunction but the existing evidence is inconclusive.

'Brain Damage' and 'Brain Dysfunction' as Behavioural Concepts

On the face of it, the terms 'brain damage' and 'brain dysfunction' appear to be quite explicit and unambiguous. However, even a cursory glance at the literature is enough to demonstrate the confusion surrounding the concept of brain damage or dysfunction. The terms have been used in astonishingly divergent ways by different people; in particular, some have used them to describe a neurological pattern, others to describe a psychological or cognitive or perceptual pattern and yet others to define a behavioural syndrome.

Pond (1960) has questioned whether there is such a thing as a syndrome of brain damage in children, and Wigglesworth (quoted by Mac Keith 1963) has said that 'it cannot be a syndrome, any more than it would be logical to have a heart damage syndrome'. On the other hand, Hatton (1966) has accepted both the concept and the term 'minimal cerebral dysfunction' as a clinically definable and useful category. Birch (1964) also recognised the existence of the syndrome but said that 'it is not a neurologic designation but a behavior pattern'. In contrast, Sandifer (quoted by Mac Keith 1963) took it to mean cerebral palsy in which the abnormalities were hard to find; that is, cerebral palsy which was difficult to diagnose. Masland (quoted by Mac Keith 1963) put forward yet another view of the term in which it was used to cover 'children who have specific learning difficulties, and/or an irregular profile in the WISC test and/or certain patterns of reaction to visuo-motor tests such as the Bender-Gestalt'. Illingworth (quoted by Mac Keith 1963), however, 'would not include the so-called psycho-neurological learning difficulties'. It seems that unless some order can be introduced, it would be better, as Brodal (quoted by Mac

Keith 1963) suggested 'to avoid any grouping of morbid conditions ... as brain damage'.

Before discussing these concepts it may be appropriate briefly to consider the ways in which the concept came to be used so widely but in so variable a fashion.

At the beginning of the century there were a few isolated accounts of the behavioural consequences of brain damage (Still 1902), but there was a marked upsurge of interest in the 1920's when behaviour disorders were reported to occur frequently as an aftermath of encephalitis (Bond and Partridge 1926, Ebaugh 1923). Various types of behavioural changes were noted, especially antisocial traits and emotional instability. Both hyperkinesis and hypokinesis were found, but most emphasis came to be laid on the former, so that, for example, Bond and Partridge concluded that 'the intensively hyperkinetic form of reaction ... seems the most conclusively organic'. A few years later, Kahn and Cohen (1934), in a seminal paper, coined the term 'organic drivenness' to describe a syndrome of hyperkinesis associated with neurological disorder. Restlessness, clumsiness and disinhibited explosive motor activity were the characteristic features. Bradley (1937) found that the overactivity often responded to the administration of amphetamine sulphate.

The view that hyperkinesis might be taken as an indication of damage to the brain gained ground; it received considerable force from Strauss' very influential reports of his studies of 'brain-injured' children (Strauss and Kephart 1940, 1955; Strauss and Lehtinen 1947). In these, the brain-injured child was characterised as hyperactive, disinhibited and distractible, as well as showing perseveration and an increased intensity of response. The assertion (not based on any sound evidence) was made that all brain lesions, wherever localised, are followed by a similar kind of disordered behaviour. The 'Strauss syndrome' rapidly came to be accepted as the response to organic brain dysfunction (Bradley 1955). This view was given further impetus by reports of the frequent occurrence of the syndrome in children with epilepsy and various forms of brain disorder (Bakwin 1949, Ingram 1956, Ounsted 1955). At about the same time, Laufer *et al.* (1957) described a series of cases of 'hyperkinetic impulse disorder' in which organic background factors were found more frequently than with other behaviour disorders. Also, Pasamanick and his colleagues reported that obstetric complications were frequently associated with disorders characterised by hyperactive, confused and disorganised behaviour (Rogers *et al.* 1955)

Several leading psychiatrists at this time were emphasising that the hyperkinetic syndrome was but one of the reactions to brain damage and that many of the psychiatric disorders of brain-damaged children were very similar to those of other children attending psychiatric clinics (Bender 1956, Pond 1961). Despite this, the view that hyperkinesis was always an indication of brain damage and that all brain damaged children were hyperkinetic was becoming widely accepted, although it bore no relationship to the relevant evidence. Hyperkinesis, impulsivity, emotional lability, short attention span and distractibility were taken as evidence of 'minimal brain dysfunction' (Clements and Peters 1962) and the term 'brain damage' itself came to be regarded as a behavioural syndrome (Birch 1964). One of the best modern textbooks on child psychiatry (Bakwin and Bakwin 1966) now states without qualification, 'The behavioural manifestations of cerebral damage, whatever the aetiology, are fairly uniform and characteristic'.

This statement is clearly false. The development of the behavioural stereotype of 'the brain damaged child' is of little importance in its own right as it runs counter to the available facts. However, it is of considerable interest as an example of how scientific myths can arise on the basis of equivocal findings and persist in the face of results which contradict them. O'Connor (1968) has pointed out how, in the same way, the permanent ill-effects of temporary maternal separation came to be generally accepted in spite of a lack of adequate supporting evidence and, indeed, an increasing amount of evidence to the contrary. Initially, tentative conclusions came to be stated as facts although no new findings had arisen to support this change (Wootton 1959). Spitz's study of 'hospitalism' (1945) is still frequently quoted in support of the ill-effects of separation, although the institutional infants that he studied had had all sorts of maladaptive experiences apart from the separation from their mothers and in spite of many devastating criticisms of the studys' several weaknesses (O'Connor 1956, Orlansky 1949, Pinneau 1955). Similarly, the Hawthorne studies (Roethlisberger and Dickson 1939) rapidly came to be regarded as a classic in the history of social science and the term 'Hawthorne effect' entered the English language. Yet a detailed comparison between the Hawthorne conclusions and the Hawthorne evidence shows the conclusions to be almost wholly unsupported (Carey 1967), so that the question has been put as to how it was possible for studies so nearly devoid of scientific merit to gain so influential and respected a place within scientific disciplines and to hold this place for so long.*

Although there is reason to believe that hyperkinesis may be significantly associated with brain damage, the concept of hyperkinesis as the usual response to brain damage (as *the* 'brain damage syndrome') is another example of such a scientific myth. In any case, whatever the evidence linking the hyperkinetic syndrome with abnormalities in brain function, it is quite misleading to use a term which seems to define an injury to an organ as a means of describing a type of behaviour. The resulting confusion was described very clearly by Birch (1964), who regrettably went on to retain the term because some name was needed to describe the clinical problem. Other workers have preferred terms which simply describe the disorder in behavioural terms such as the 'hyperactive child syndrome' (Stewart *et al.* 1966, Werry *et al.* 1964) or the 'hyperkinetic syndrome' (Eisenberg 1966). This seems much preferable, in that it describes the problem and involves no unwarranted assumptions. In considering possible associations between organic brain dysfunction and psychiatric disorder in

*The use of the term 'scientific myth' in the context of these three areas should not be taken as implying that hyperkinesis is unrelated to brain damage, or that maternal separation may not lead to distortion of personality development, or that social and attitudinal factors play no part in the response of factory workers to a change in work routine or work conditions. Nor is it the intention to imply that the originators of the ideas that led to these myths meant that what they wrote should be extended in so wide and uncritical a fashion. On the contrary, there is good evidence in favour of all three views and some of the original expressions of the views were put in cautious terms. What constitutes the 'myth' is the gross over-generalisation of the views which has come to receive surprisingly widespread acceptance in spite of contrary evidence.

this volume, the term 'hyperkinetic syndrome' will be used to describe a behavioural syndrome and the term 'brain damage' will be used only in its literal sense.

Other Definitions of 'Brain Dysfunction' or 'Brain Damage'

Alternatively, and perhaps most commonly, 'brain damage' or 'brain dysfunction' have been used as general terms to include a number of different syndromes which are the result of some kind of impaired functioning of the brain (Bax and Mac Keith 1963). This use of the term would certainly include children with cerebral palsy, but it would also include many other children with less severe and more subtle handicaps such as defects in co-ordination, perception or language (Rutter 1968). However, although this group of disorders is associated with abnormal development or abnormal functioning of the brain, the abnormality is only sometimes associated with actual disease or damage. To this extent, 'brain dysfunction' is more accurate a term than 'brain damage'. There is much to be said for retaining some general term of this kind to include the variety of disorders not covered by the classical textbook neurological diseases. This issue is discussed more fully in chapter 4, but in considering relationships between organic brain dysfunction and psychiatric disorder, this group of less well defined 'border-line' neurological disorders will be excluded. This is not, of course, to suggest that the psychiatric aspects are unimportant; on the contrary, they are probably rather more important than in cerebral palsy and like disorders. Rather, the issue is that in these disorders the association between psychiatric and neurological aspects is probably more complicated and certainly less well understood, so that in trying to disentangle the relationships between organic brain dysfunction and child psychiatric disorder, more clear-cut conclusions are likely to emerge from a study of better defined conditions like cerebral palsy and epilepsy.

Age, Localisation of Lesion and Nature of Pathology in Relation to Psychiatric Disorder

The lack of knowledge on general associations between organic brain dysfunction and psychiatric disorder in childhood is accompanied by even greater ignorance on the ways in which the effects of organic brain dysfunction on behaviour and emotions are influenced by the age at which the insult is sustained and by the locus, the extent and the nature of the lesion both in pathological and electrophysiological terms. However, in view of the evident importance of these factors in relation to the effects of injury on cognitive and other aspects of development, it is important to consider how they might influence the behavioural consequences of damage to the brain.

Age of the Child at the Time of Brain Injury

The developmental stage at which the brain injury is sustained has a major influence on both the short-term and long term consequences of brain damage. However, the effect is by no means straightforward in that developmental maturity influences both the biological susceptibility of the organ to damage and the plasticity of the organ in its ability to transfer functions from one side to the other or from one part to another. As will be seen, to some extent these lead to contradictory expectations.

Different abilities may be required in the development of functions from those needed in the retention of functions (Hebb 1942).

In general, immature organs are more susceptible to injury than are mature ones; furthermore, organs are most susceptible to damage at the time of their most rapid growth (Dobbing 1968). This is evident, for example, in relation to the effects on growth of severe malnutrition occurring at different stages in the development of animals. As far as the brain is concerned, it is still a relatively immature organ at the time of birth and there is a period of particularly rapid growth during the first two years of life (Falkner 1966, Marshall 1968, Minkowski 1967). This period of rapid growth is accompanied by an extensive growth of cell dendrites (Conel 1952, 1939-63), by changes in the chemical composition of the brain (Brante 1949; Folch-Pi 1952, 1955; Sperry 1962), and by changes in the electrical activity (Gibbs and Knott 1949, Smith 1941). Unlike other organs a marked slowing down in the rate of brain growth and development occurs after the age of two or three years.

Accordingly, the effects of infections or other traumata should be most marked during the infancy period. This has been clearly shown in relation to encephalitis where the rate of neurological sequelae is highest in the first months of life, with the incidence and severity of sequelae showing a progressive decline thereafter (Finley 1958). Both the death rate (Nyhan and Richardson 1963) and the sequelae (Lawson *et al.* 1965, Nyhan and Richardson 1963, Wolff and Smallwood 1952) of meningitis are also greatest in early infancy. These findings strongly suggest that the brain of the newborn infant is more susceptible to damage than that of the older child, but it should be realised that the findings also reflect the greater difficulties in diagnosing meningitis in very young children and the individual's total resistance to infection as well as the vulnerability of the brain (Nyhan and Richardson 1963, Swinyard *et al.* 1963).

It is not known whether the vulnerability of the brain continues to decline after the infancy period, but data on its growth and maturation suggest that little change would be expected after the age of three years. D'Avignon (1963) found that acquired cerebral palsy was more often associated with severe mental impairment if the onset was between the ages of 7 and 11 years rather than before 7 years. However, this may reflect the plasticity of brain function (see below) rather than the vulnerability of the tissue to the effects of infection or trauma. The prognosis for herpes encephalitis also appears to be worse for adults than children (Miller and Ross 1968), but again, this may be less a function of brain vulnerability than of age differences in response to the virus. It should be added that it is not known if the vulnerability to mechanical injury or anoxia follows the same pattern as that to infection. There is some suggestion that the visual cortex of the infant brain may be more resistant to the effects of anoxia than that of the mature brain (Weinberger *et al.* 1962) but this requires confirmation and it is not known if the same is true for other parts of the brain.

Thus, the vulnerability of the brain, at least in some respects, is at its height in infancy, so that the effects of generalised damage are greatest in the first few months of life. However, this general vulnerability, which is related to physiological immaturity, is counterbalanced by the greater plasticity of the immature brain, so that functions are readily transferred from one hemisphere to the other in the case of severe unilateral damage. To a lesser extent, also, functions may be transferred from one part of the brain to another in the case of localised bilateral damage. This was beautifully demonstrated in the monkey in the important early studies of Kennard (1936, 1938). She showed that the young and immature monkey recovered motor function much more quickly after ablations of precentral cortex than did the adult monkey. In the infant there was virtually complete motor recovery after unilateral lesions and even after bilateral lesions good voluntary movements were possible, in spite of some permanent deficit of motor function. The effects of similar lesions in the adult animal were much more devastating and much more persistent. There were, however, definite limits to the plasticity of the brain in infancy in that the size of the lesion was related to recovery and the defect in bilateral lesions was worse than in unilateral lesions.

These results have been amply confirmed in more recent studies utilising precise quantitative measures rather than the more naturalistic approach of Kennard. It has also been clearly demonstrated that the plasticity of brain function applies to learning skills as well as to motor function. For example, Scharlock *et al.* (1963) showed that auditory discriminations in the cat were prevented by ablation of temporal cortex at maturity, but not in infancy. In the same way, Benjamin and Thompson (1959) found that adult cats subjected to ablations of sensorimotor cortex showed very gross impairment or total loss of the ability to make roughness discriminations, whereas the same lesion in very young cats produced only slight impairment. A wider range of learning was examined by Akert *et al.* (1960) and by Harlow *et al.* (1964) in their studies of extensive bilateral prefrontal lesions in infant Rhesus monkeys. Lesions made at 5 days and at 150 days had no effects on later learning capacity as measured by an extensive battery of tests.

Similarly, Beach (1938), in some early studies of the rat, found that maternal behaviour was less affected by cortical lesions made in infancy than by similar lesions made in adult life. Furthermore, as the size of the lesion increased, so the degree of superiority of the infant operated rats over the adult rats grew larger. However, animals operated in infancy still tended to be inferior to normal females on tests of maternal behaviour and the inferiority was greatest with the largest lesions. The loss of function following cortical ablations was largely in the ability to integrate discrete behaviour units into a unified whole.

Hippocampal destruction in the neonate cat generally produces less behavioural deficit than similar damage at later ages, but at any age it produces some impairment (Isaacson *et al.* 1968). Similarly, topectomy and bilateral frontal lobectomy produce greater handicaps in older Rhesus monkeys than in infants, but even in infancy lobectomy has some effect on later discrimination learning (Harlow *et al.* 1968). There is some evidence that the integrity of subcortical systems is more important than an intact cerebral cortex for the survival of neonate monkeys (Kling and Tucker 1968). In examining the effects of brain lesions in animals of different ages, it is also important to realise that some sequelae may only develop later, long after the initial lesion. Kennard (1942) found delayed progressive deterioration in some animals who had

had motor cortex lesions made in the neonatal period, and Kling and Tucker (1968) noted that hyperactivity and circling did not develop until eighteen months in monkeys who had received frontal lesions in the neonatal period.

Thus, in animals, cortical lesions acquired in infancy have generally been shown to have remarkably little effect on behaviour whereas similar lesions in the adult leave permanent defects in function. Nevertheless, lesions in the infants do lead to partial loss of some functions and there is a suggestion that impairment may be most marked with the most complex forms of integrated behaviour. Whether the marked differences between early and late brain injury are due to less specific localisations of function in the infant brain or to a reorganisation of function made possible by greater plasticity is still a matter of dispute.

To a considerable extent the results of these animal studies are paralleled by the findings in relation to brain lesions in the human. The clearest illustration is seen in the effects of unilateral aphasia-producing lesions, when the sequelae in terms of language deficits are very much greater in adults than in children (Alajouanine and Lhermitte 1965, Basser 1962, Guttman 1942, Lenneberg 1967). Up to the age of about three years, unilateral cerebral trauma causes temporary loss of language or delay in language development, but not the aphasic disturbances seen in adults. After the age of four years, the clinical picture is generally similar to that in adults, but in sharp contrast to the adult situation, up to the age of nine years the aphasic handicap is almost always transient and followed by complete recovery. It seems that in infancy the two hemispheres are more or less equipotential and if one side is damaged its functions as regards language and intellect are readily assumed by the other side. The transfer appears to be virtually complete with respect to language but it may not be so for some intellectual functions (Alajouanine and Lhermitte 1965, McFie 1961*a*).

The same pattern is reflected in the results of left hemispherectomy (Basser 1962, Lenneberg 1967), where the consequences of aphasia depend upon the age at which the original insult was incurred. If the child has had a lesion on either side in infancy, speech function is eventually confined to the healthy hemisphere; thus, when the diseased hemisphere is removed later in life it causes no aphasia (Lenneberg 1967). On the other hand, patients who have acquired their lesions in later life and who subsequently have a hemispherectomy have permanent aphasic symptoms if the operation is done on the left side and no aphasia if it is done on the right side.

Therefore, interference with language from a unilateral lesion in childhood is not permanent because the two sides retain versatility of function. Damage to the left hemisphere will interfere with language, but only temporarily, because the right hemisphere is still involved with language and language learning can continue to take place between the ages of 2 years and about 13 years (Lenneberg 1967). This difference in the effects of lesions at different ages can be related to the process of physiological maturation of the brain. Similar effects can be seen with respect to the effects of age in relation to damage to other areas and other specialised functions (Lenneberg 1967, Solomons *et al.* 1963). Damage in early life leaves little or no deficit, whereas comparable damage at a later stage of development results in irreversible symptoms.

This might lead one to suppose that persisting language defects are never seen in childhood, but this is not the case. Persistent aphasia is never seen after unilateral lesions arising in early childhood, but long-lasting language abnormalities are still known to occur. Delays in the development of language are well recognised (Ingram 1959 *a* and *b*, Morley *et al.* 1955). They usually occur in the absence of known structural disease of the brain; the disorder is very much more common in boys and is often familial in origin. It is usually regarded as a genetically determined simple delay in the maturation of a specific function and the features of the condition are nothing like aphasia in adults. Although the children with delayed speech go through similar stages in language development to normal children (but at an unusually late age), there is some evidence to suggest that their use of grammar is not exactly comparable to that of the normal younger child (Menyuk 1964); that is, the language may to some extent be deviant as well as delayed. Whether or not that is so, the great majority of the children with specific delays of speech and language do go on to develop normal language although there may be continuing difficulties in reading (Ingram 1963*a*, Mason 1967) and the findings are still consistent with the view that persistent language defects are rarely found in childhood.

On the other hand, cases of children with severe global defects of language involving profound difficulties in comprehension existing from infancy are well documented (Benton 1964, Gordon and Taylor 1964, Worster-Drought and Allen 1929). These cases are not consistent with the above view, in that most of them do not eventually gain normal language. The brain pathology in such cases is unknown. Only one case has come to post-mortem and that was atypical in that the child was also diplegic (Landau *et al.* 1960). It cannot be assumed that the extensive bilateral loss of cortical substance extending from the inferior and posterior margin of the central sulcus to the occipital lobe found in that case would apply to others. Nevertheless, in view of the highly consistent and well established findings in relation to unilateral lesions in childhood, it does appear that whatever the nature and locus of the pathology it is very probably bilateral.

This also applies to the rare cases in which children entirely lose their speech after a period of normal development (Worster-Drought 1964). The loss of speech is often associated with gross but transient (usually bilateral) EEG abnormalities and epileptic fits occurring only for a short while after the onset. There are no motor abnormalities and the intellect is usually unimpaired on non-verbal tasks. These children also usually remain permanently handicapped in their language although their development in other respects is normal. Again the pathology is not known.

These findings may be integrated with the results in relation to unilateral aphasia-producing lesions if it is assumed that the lesion is bilateral. If that is the case (and at the moment that is purely speculative) then it may be concluded that as far as language is concerned, transfer of the function from one hemisphere to the other is readily accomplished in childhood, but that transfer from one part of the brain to another (as from one lobe to another on the same side) in the case of bilateral lesions is much more difficult. The ultimate development of speech (but not normal speech) in Landau's case, in spite of widespread bilateral damage, suggests that some intra-hemispheric transfer of functions may be possible (although it is also possible that speech may develop on the basis of a few remnants of tissue which normally subserves language function). Further research is required to elucidate this issue. In general, however, early brain lesions have a lesser effect on function than do similar lesions at maturity.

Somewhat different views have been expressed by Birch and Belmont (Belmont and Birch 1960, Birch and Belmont 1960) and by Teuber and Rudel (1962). Birch and Belmont compared the perceptual-motor performance of hemiplegic adults with that of brain-damaged children studied earlier by Werner and Strauss, and concluded that in some respects the performance of the children was worse than that of the adults. Teuber and Rudel studied the behaviour of cerebral palsied children at different ages and found that the results differed according to the type of task involved and the age at which the child was tested. These studies illustrate the much greater problems in human research into developmental neurology compared with animal research, because one cannot control experimentally the size and location of the lesions. As Belmont and Birch pointed out, their study made no direct comparisons between brain-injured adults and children, rather there was an indirect 'pseudo-comparison' (as they termed it) which raises many methodological questions. Their procedure entirely relies on the assumption that brain injuries at all ages are similar with respect to locus, extent and type of pathology and whether this is so is quite unknown. If the effects of cerebral lesions in the human are less in infancy, as seems likely from the results of animal experiments and from the studies of aphasia in children, it is quite probable that larger lesions are needed in children to produce comparable motor handicaps. If this is so, what Birch and Belmont, and Teuber and Rudel have done is to compare the effects of large lesions in children with those of small lesions in adults; in the absence of information on the size and location of the lesions in their subjects the findings are therefore inevitably inconclusive.

One cannot assume that the results of animal studies will necessarily apply to humans, nor that the findings with respect to simple discriminations in the animal will necessarily apply to higher intellectual functions in the human. In addition, it is important to note that the ability to transfer functions from one part of the brain to another in the case of bilateral lesions may not be as great as the ability to transfer functions from one side to the other in the case of unilateral lesions. This needs to be borne in mind when considering the effects of bilateral damage to the frontal lobes.

In 1942, Hebb wrote a stimulating and influential paper in which he noted that brain injury in adults tends to lead to rather specific defects in cognitive function, whereas injuries to the brain at birth more usually led to a general depression of intelligence. He suggested that the abilities needed for the development of intelligence in childhood may be different from those needed for the retention of intelligence in the adult, and that for this reason early injuries to the brain may have a less selective and more widespread and profound effect than late injuries. This argument was taken up by Russell (1948, 1959) and applied specifically to the frontal lobes in his postulation that the effects of frontal lobe damage may be more devastating in children than in adults. In adults, frontal lobe damage is characterised by little change in IQ but profoundly disturbed intellectual activity (Luria 1966). In children whose intelligence is still developing, the disturbed cognitive function may also lower IQ.

Russell put forward the hypothesis that the frontal lobes play an important part in conditioning and moulding the behaviour responses of the rest of the brain in early childhood but that this effect is no longer as important in adult life. If this were true it would prove a very important exception to the general rule that the effects of early injury are much less than those of later injury and it might also shed valuable light on the question of the development of intelligence.

Unfortunately, there is very little relevant information from human studies, and what there is is contradictory. It is necessary here to refer to isolated case reports of varying quality; few firm conclusions can be drawn from them but they are useful in highlighting the issues. Apparently in support of Hebb and Russell's hypothesis is Norman's case (1945) of a girl who sustained gross destruction of both prefrontal lobes (but no other part of the brain), probably at about the age of 13 months. No locomotor defect was detected but there was severe intellectual impairment and a behavioural disturbance. As the extent of the lesion was confirmed at post-mortem, the findings stand in striking contrast to the minor effects on intelligence of prefrontal lesions in adults as judged by the effects of head injury and of the operation of prefrontal leucotomy (Lishman 1968, Miller 1964, Piercy 1964). Although confusion and hypokinesis are quite common in relation to frontal lobe tumours (Hecaen 1962), other disturbances of behaviour are not particularly striking in adult frontal lobe lesions (Lishman 1968).

Also in keeping with Hebb and Russell's hypothesis is Oldfield and Williams' case (1961) of a child who sustained a penetrating head wound at $5\frac{1}{2}$ months in which the damage, although extensive in the right frontal lobe, appeared to be confined to the one side. Unfortunately this could not be confirmed by histological examination of the brain as permission for post-mortem examination was withheld. The child showed no abnormality on neurological examination when seen between the ages of 6 and 19 years but there was some intellectual retardation (WAIS verbal IQ of 79 and performance IQ of 59) and behavioural disturbance. This child was not as handicapped as Norman's case but the findings are as impressive in that the lesion was apparently unilateral.

Against these cases, however, must be placed Ackerley's well documented case (1964) of a man with extensive cystic degeneration of the left frontal lobe and absence of the right prefrontal lobe. The age of onset of the lesion was not known directly but the history strongly suggested that it had been present from birth. There had been a prolonged labour and difficult birth followed by considerable neonatal difficulties, convulsions following a fall on the head at 4 years, and a life-long history of behavioural disturbances. The extent of the frontal lobe damage was demonstrated by pneumoencephelography and craniotomy at the age of 19 years. The patient's IQ was 92 on the Stanford-Binet test and 100 on the Army Alpha. However, in spite of these normal scores there was evidence of considerable defect in conative and some types of cognitive function. In addition, Ackerley reported a case of McLaurin's of a child with bilateral frontal lobe lesions from toxoplasmosis cysts, documented by operation at 2 months of age. This child had an above average IQ at 7 years (score not reported) which, taken in conjunction with the case of the porencephalic cyst, suggests that severe bilateral damage to the frontal lobe does not necessarily lead to general intellectual impairment. Why it did so in the other two cases remains uncertain and more studies are required before one can accept or reject Hebb and Russell's suggestion that early lesions of the frontal lobes have more severe and more permanent effects on intelligence than do lesions in adult life.

In summary, the neonatal brain is more susceptible to injury by virtue of its immaturity and rapid rate of growth, but the effects of unilateral lesions in childhood tend to be transient because of the ability of the immature brain to transfer functions from one side to the other. To some extent the sequelae of bilateral lesions in infancy are also less than the sequelae of similar lesions acquired in adult life, but the differences in the human are less clear-cut than in animals. There is some suggestion (still requiring confirmation) that in humans, but not in animals, higher intellectual functions may be more dependent on the frontal lobe in infancy than they are in adult life. The importance in relation to behaviour and personality development of the age of the child at the time of brain injury has not been systematically studied. Nevertheless, a detailed consideration of its importance in relation to cognition has been undertaken in the belief that the study of the psychiatric aspects of brain damage must take place in a developmental context.

Locus of Lesion

The locus of the lesion has well known and obvious effects on the nature of motor and sensory deficits following brain injury. In the adult, the locus also has important associations with the nature of cognitive, perceptual, behavioural and emotional defects following brain damage. The findings have been considered in detail by Hecaen (1962), Lishman (1968), Milner (1962), Piercy (1964) Teuber (1962) and others, and are too complex to recount in detail here. It may be said that posterior lesions generally produce greater intellectual deficit than anterior lesions and that the left hemisphere is particularly concerned with verbal functions and the right hemisphere with visuo-spatial functions. This distinction is certainly not absolute and there are some ostensibly non-verbal deficits (particularly ideo-motor apraxia) which are uniquely associated with left hemisphere damage. The temporal lobe (and especially the hippocampus) is specifically concerned with memory functions so that bilateral damage leads to a characteristic hippocampal memory defect. Language functions are not sharply localised but deficits following injury are greatest in the case of posterior lesions in the region of the Sylvian fissure. Apraxic and agnosic defects tend to be associated with the parietal lobe, as does route-finding.

Lesions of the temporal lobe, particularly the left temporal lobe, are more closely associated with psychiatric disability than are lesions in the frontal, parietal or occipital lobes. This is only partly explicable in terms of the association between psychiatric disability and visual field or dysphasic defects. To a lesser extent psychiatric disability seems to be associated with left parietal and right frontal lobe lesions. Intellectual disorders occur more commonly after left hemisphere damage, while affective disorders, behaviour disorders and somatic complaints are more frequent after right hemisphere damage. Intellectual disorders are especially associated with parietal and temporal lobe damage and are infrequent after frontal lobe injury. In contrast, affective disorders, behavioural disorders and somatic complaints are more frequent after frontal lobe damage. Sexual abnormalities and criminal behaviour are particularly closely associated with frontal lobe injury.

Much less is known about the effects on cognitive, perceptual, behavioural and emotional functions of lesions occurring in childhood in different loci or on different sides of the brain. From the few studies that have been undertaken it appears that the pattern is broadly similar to that in adults but the differences according to the locus of injury are less clear-cut (McFie 1963). Wedell (1960) compared the performance of children with left and right hemiplegia on visuo-spatial tasks. Those with left hemiplegia performed less well, suggesting the association of these functions with the right hemisphere. In a study of intellectual impairment in 40 children with postnatal lesions occurring after the age of one year, McFie (1961*b*) found a pattern similar to that in adults but with the difference less marked in relation to verbal tasks, where the performance was impaired with lesions on either side. However, only tentative conclusions can be drawn as all but five of the children were at least five years of age at the time of onset of the lesion, the type of lesion was very varied (10 of the 40 showing only an EEG focus) and the number of children with a lesion in each locus was too small for anything but laterality comparisons. Annett *et al.* (1961) have shown a greater deficit on performance tests in children with unilateral EEG foci on the same side as the 'dominant' hand than in children with foci on the opposite side to the dominant or preferred hand.

Even less is known about the behavioural differences in childhood associated with lesions in different loci. The association between temporal lobe lesions and psychiatric disorder, particularly the hyperkinetic syndrome, has already been mentioned in the discussion of epilepsy, and the effects of frontal lobe lesions have also been previously considered. The results of studies in adults suggest that this is likely to be a fruitful area for investigation.

Extent of Lesion

It is well established that the IQ of quadriplegic cerebral palsied children is lower than that of hemiplegic children (Asher and Schonell 1950, Floyer 1955, Ingram 1955, Woods 1957), reflecting the general finding that widespread brain damage is more likely to lead to intellectual impairment than is localised damage. More relevant to the issue discussed in this chapter is Lishman's very important finding (1968) that in adults who have had a penetrating head injury, subsequent psychiatric disorder is more likely the greater the depth of penetration of the wound and also (independently) the larger the total amount of brain tissue destroyed, even after controlling for the effects on intellectual function. Psychiatric disorder was thus associated with both the quantity of focal brain destruction in different parts of the brain and the extent of coincident diffuse brain damage. This finding strongly suggests that the brain damage itself was important in the aetiology of psychiatric disorder, rather than the associated physical disability which did not relate to psychiatric disorder and rather than the psychological reactions to the accident and the consequences. No comparable data are available for children.

Nature of Lesion

Virtually nothing is known about behavioural differences in relation to differences in the pathology causing cerebral lesions. There is some evidence to suggest that psychiatric problems are associated with a physiological disturbance more often than with a loss of cerebral function. For example, psychiatric disability in adults is more liable to follow head injury when epileptic fits occur (Lishman 1968). Also, differences have been found between the effects of epileptogenic and non-epileptogenic temporal lobe lesions (Bingley 1958). In childhood, the fact that active disturbance has a greater effect than loss of function may be more strikingly seen in the improvements in behaviour, and sometimes in intelligence, which may follow the operation of hemispherectomy (Griffith and Davidson 1966). The children are often behaviourally much better off with only one hemisphere than with two hemispheres, one of which is producing active electrical disturbance.

Further evidence that, at least in adults, epileptogenic lesions may have effects due to electrical discharge apart from that occurring in overt fits and apart from any effects of loss of brain function, stems from studies of temporal lobectomy where there is a close relationship between a reduction in the number of fits and a decrease in aggressive behaviour (Falconer and Serafetinides 1963, James 1960).

Although further studies are needed on the different effects of disturbance of function and loss of function, especially in children, the behavioural consequences of abnormal brain function appear to be often greater than those of loss of brain function.

Summary of the Issues

In spite of a considerable literature on various aspects of the association between organic brain dysfunction and child psychiatric disorder, it remains a largely uncharted territory with most of the basic questions still unanswered. Important advances have been made in understanding the emotional and behavioural correlates of epilepsy. Yet, from the studies which have been reviewed it is not possible to draw any conclusions about the prevalence of psychiatric disorder in children with epilepsy, cerebral palsy or any other variety of organic brain dysfunction. Most studies suggest that children with an organic brain disorder may have rather more behavioural and emotional problems than children in the general population. In the absence of properly controlled comparative studies, however, it remains unknown whether the supposed increase in psychiatric disorder is slight or great. There can be no doubt that many children with organic brain dysfunction show no psychiatric disorder and, furthermore, that the disorders found in association with brain disease or brain damage vary considerably in type; whether some disorders are more characteristic of the difficulties of the brain damaged child than others is still a matter of dispute.

Some important clues have emerged as to the factors leading to psychiatric disorder in relation to brain damage or epilepsy but this, too, still remains an area of great controversy and disagreement. Pond (1960) has claimed that 'apart from the symptoms that arise directly from the loss of brain function, chronic disorders following brain damage are largely the result of the handling or mishandling of the handicapped child by parents and society generally'. In contrast, Stone (1960), while accepting that environmental factors play some part, has agreed that the presence of brain damage leads to an impairment of ego control which causes the brain-damaged child to react to stress in an extreme and characteristic fashion. Furthermore, gross perceptual defects which are often part of organic brain conditions lead to subsequent distortions in personality development. There is a continuing disagreement between those who view the brain damaged child's psychiatric problems as arising largely or entirely from environmental circumstances and those who regard the problems as due in large part to factors within the child associated with organic brain dysfunction.

This unsatisfactory state of affairs is in no way different from that existing with respect to the emotional and behavioural problems of children with other varieties of physical handicap. The authors of a recent survey of the literature on the physically handicapped child judged that 'no clear-cut conclusions emerge from the various studies which have been reviewed' (Pringle 1964). To a considerable extent the reasons why so few certainties have emerged from so much work are the same in relation to organic brain dysfunction as those in relation to physical handicap (Barker *et al.* 1953, Pringle 1964). The problem is a complex one so that simple conclusions are unlikely, and its complexity demands the control and comparison of many variables which are only possible in well chosen and fairly large samples. Many of the studies have been concerned with highly selected groups of children attending hospitals or clinics. Because different clinics have different sorts of children referred (the cerebral palsied or epileptic children attending a neurological clinic are likely to be very different from those seen by a psychiatrist), the findings have necessarily been subject to considerable bias (Rutter *et al.* 1967*b*). Barker *et al.* (1953) pointed out that, with respect to studies of physical handicap, many investigations have failed to provide control groups or have used inappropriate controls not matched on variables known to affect the development of psychiatric disorder.

A further major difficulty has arisen from the lack in the past of reliable and valid instruments with which to measure psychiatric disorder. There has often been a reliance on paper and pencil tests which may not be as suitable for physically disabled children as for normal children (Pringle 1964). Often, too, psychiatric disorder has been judged from the results of projective tests which, whatever their merit in other respects, are very poor tools for determining the presence or absence of disorder. Different studies have used different measures such as interviews, questionnaires, projective tests or laboratory measures (often of dubious or untested reliability and validity) and no meaningful comparisons can be made between their findings.

Additional problems have sometimes arisen from a failure to define the neurological groups being studied or from defining them tautologically in psychological or behavioural terms. Lastly, almost no attention has been paid to the behavioural differences associated with damage to an immature and developing brain and damage to a mature adult brain.

The basic questions still requiring answers may be summarised as follows:

1. Is the rate of psychiatric disorder increased in children with organic brain dysfunction?

2. If it is increased, is the high rate of psychiatric disorder due to the presence of physical handicap or to the presence of a disorder specifically of the brain?
3. Is there a specific type of psychiatric disorder which is associated with organic brain dysfunction?
4. As it is abundantly clear that not all children with disorders of the brain have psychiatric abnormality, what features of the child, his brain disorder or his environment determine the development of emotional or behavioural problems?

As particular issues arising as part of the last question we may add:
(*a*) Are the different types of psychiatric disorder associated with different aetiological factors?
(*b*) Is the locus of brain injury associated with differences in the frequency or type of psychiatric disorder?
(*c*) Is the extent of brain injury associated with differences in the frequency or type of psychiatric disorder?
(*d*) Are there differences in the disorders of behaviour or emotions which are associated with loss of brain function and those which are associated with distortion of brain function?
(*e*) Are the psychiatric correlates of damage to the immature brain different from those of damage to the mature brain?

These are the main psychiatric issues to be considered in subsequent chapters of this book when the findings from the Isle of Wight survey of neurological disorders in school age children are described. Tentative conclusions will be drawn in relation to the four main questions but it will not be possible to say much about the five subsidiary questions. These are important issues in relation to developmental theory and further research is much required.

Before we can proceed to a consideration of these issues, however, it is necessary to examine the reliability and validity of neurological assessment and the epidemiology of neuro-epileptic disorders; these are the topics considered in the next two sections.

PART II

Neurological Assessment

CHAPTER 2

The Neurological Examination: Description

Comprehensive assessment and good management of a child with neurological disease is impossible without a full history. As Paine and Oppé (1966) point out, the history is often a better signpost to a correct diagnosis than the physical examination or special investigations. A careful history was taken of all the children with neuro-epileptic disorder considered in this study; the diagnosis of epilepsy, of course, was entirely based on this history. Much the most common of the other neurological disorders was cerebral palsy, the diagnosis of which rested largely on the findings of the examination of the child.

The children included in this study had to have a current handicap which could be demonstrated by ordinary clinical examination; children with neurological disorder in early childhood which had cleared up without neurological sequelae at the time of examination were excluded. As part of the method of selection of children with neurological disorder, a neurological examination for screening purposes was devised. Its purpose was to detect the presence of a neurological disorder rather than to diagnose its nature or pathogenesis or to form part of an assessment for treatment purposes. If a neurological abnormality was found, the examining physician was instructed to proceed to a fuller assessment along whatever lines were necessary to decide upon diagnosis. This chapter and the other chapters in this section of the book, however, are only concerned with that part of the neurological examination used for screening purposes.

In deciding which items to include, we concentrated on those signs which have the greatest validity in the age-group with which we were concerned (5 to 15 years) and omitted those which were relevant only to very rare disorders or which were superfluous to other more pathognomonic signs. This necessarily meant the omission of some items which should certainly be included in the examination of a child known to have some neurological disorder. Those signs that were included, some of which were selected because of their possible educational significance, were intended to be examined for thoroughly and rigorously. The examination, therefore, is one which might be used in a psychiatric clinic to detect those children requiring further neurological study.

In order to gain the co-operation, particularly of young, unintelligent or disturbed children, it is necessary to plan the examination so that it appears informal and leisurely and is interesting to the child. This does demand that time be spent in establishing a good relationship with the child and that the ordering of the examination be such that it progresses smoothly from one part to the next. Wherever possible, tests should be devised to allow the assessment of several functions simultaneously in order to avoid duplication. Parts of the examination which might distress the child (such as examination of plantar responses) should be left until the end of the interview, though every attempt should be made to finish on a neutral or happy note.

The children in this study were all examined in schools which varied greatly as to the facilities they could offer. The examination was planned so that it could be performed in its entirety with the child sitting or standing; no couch was required and the only undressing needed was the removal of shoes and socks. The neurological examination took about twenty minutes and it always followed a half-hour interview with the child for the purpose of psychiatric assessment. This meant that the child was usually well at ease before physical examination began. The preceding interview, however, was also utilised for some aspects of the neurological examination itself, particularly the evaluation of speech and language.

The neurological examination was demonstrated to all physicians participating in the study, and they were instructed on how the tests were to be carried out and how abnormalities were to be rated. This chapter is based on those instructions.

Cranial Nerves

Eyes

Ptosis was noted by careful observation of the face at rest, during spontaneous movement and during movements on command (see page 29). The pupils were examined for shape and for equality of size but pupillary reflexes were not tested routinely. External ocular movements were tested for each eye separately and the presence or absence of nystagmus was noted. Nystagmus was regarded as present only if there were four or more beats occurring after the eye had reached a position of rest when fixating a finger 18 inches away and 60° from the midline. It was coded as 'none', 'slight' or 'marked', but a full description was recorded whenever it was present.

Overt strabismus was noted by observing the position of the eyes throughout gaze in all directions, both spontaneously and in response to command. Latent strabismus was looked for by getting the child to fixate on a finger with both eyes open. Each eye in turn was then covered for a few moments. On removing the cover, the position and any movement of the covered eye were noted.

As all the school children had had visual testing during the routine school medical examination, it was not repeated during the neurological examination. In retrospect this was seen to be a mistake, as the visual testing of handicapped children at home, at junior training centres or in mental subnormality hospitals was found to be sometimes inadequate or incomplete.

The examination of visual fields (as described by Paine and Oppé 1966) can be a most informative part of the neurological examination, but it is of very limited use as a screening test for neurological disorder in that very few children have a visual field defect without other signs of neurological significance. Accordingly, it was omitted from the screening examination, as was a routine examination of the fundi.

Face

Facial symmetry was noted and coded separately according to the state of the face at rest, during spontaneous emotional movements and on movements to command. Asymmetry at rest and during spontaneous movements is best examined when the child does not know he is being closely observed, and this was studied during the interview preceding the physical examination proper. To assess asymmetry during movements to command and to assess facial weakness the child was asked to open his eyes wide, to screw up his eyes tightly, to show his teeth, to blow out a match, to frown and to raise his eyebrows. Where necessary these movements were demonstrated by the examiner

Tongue (Figs 1-5)

The position of the tongue at rest with the mouth open was noted and examined for atrophy or fasciculation. The child was asked to protrude the tongue and its position in the midline was noted. He was asked to waggle his tongue quickly from side to side so that it touched the corners of the mouth and then to lick his upper lip pretending there was jam on it. As well as coding 'possible' and 'definite' tongue weakness, separate codings were made for the co-ordination of side to side and upward tongue movements. To score '0' (normal) on licking the top lip, the child's tongue had to perform an upward curl; to score '0' on side to side movements the movements had to be fairly brisk and well co-ordinated. As on all co-ordination items, 'slight' and 'marked' abnormalities were differentiated in the coding.

Defects in tongue co-ordination are of little value in detecting general neurological disorder but were included because of their interest and probable importance in speech and language disorders.

Other Cranial Nerves

No routine sensory testing or testing of other cranial nerves was done, but a full examination of the cranial nerves (except the first which is of little diagnostic value) was asked for if any abnormalities of the eyes, face or tongue were found.

Fine Motor Co-ordination

Limb co-ordination involves (a) fine co-ordination such as is necessary in finger movements and (b) large muscle co-ordination such as is used in throwing and walking. These need to be differentiated conceptually but it is also convenient to examine for them at different stages, since fine co-ordination is best tested for with the child sitting whereas gross co-ordination needs the child to be up and about. In testing co-ordination, of course, it is appropriate to look for abnormal movements and true ataxia at the same time. Two 'classical' tests of fine co-ordination were included (touching fingers in turn with the thumb and the finger-nose test) but both these tests are sometimes difficult to evaluate because young or retarded children may have difficulty in understanding what is required of them. For this reason a number of tests involving more everyday actions were added.

During the preceding interview children were asked to draw a picture of a man. This served several purposes: it constituted a task which allowed the assessment of attention span and distractibility (see chapter 13); it was one of the three tests of handedness; it provided evidence of the child's constructional skills; and by observing the way the child picked up, held and used the pencil, it allowed the assessment of fine co-ordination.

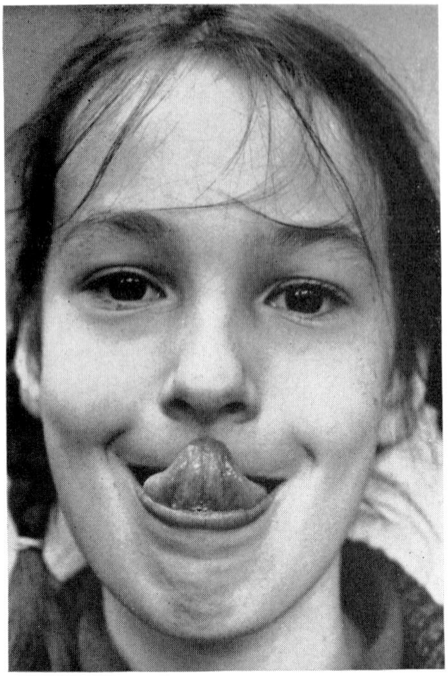
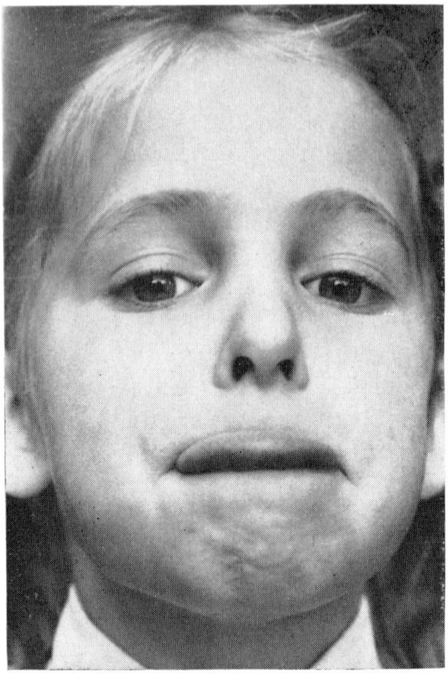
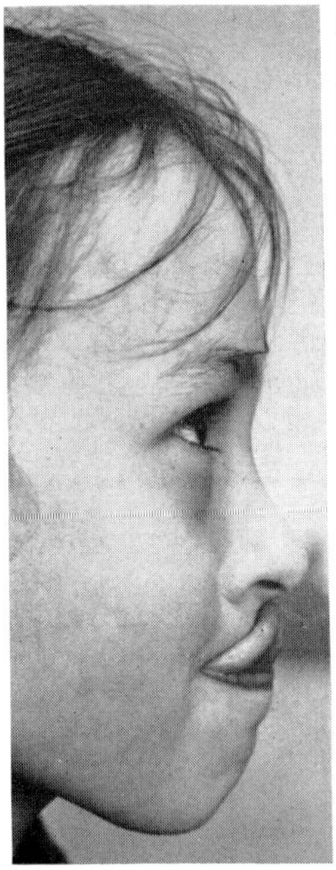
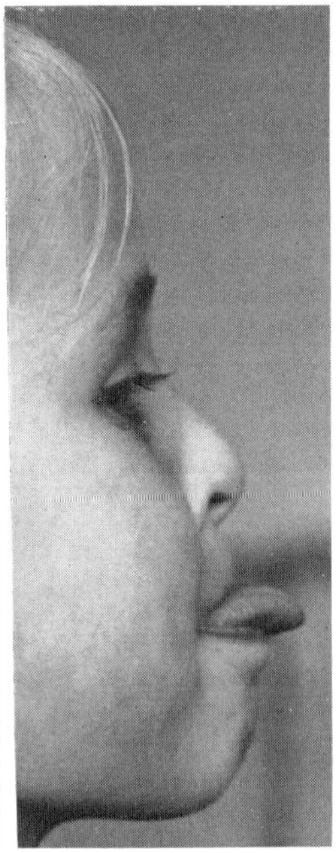
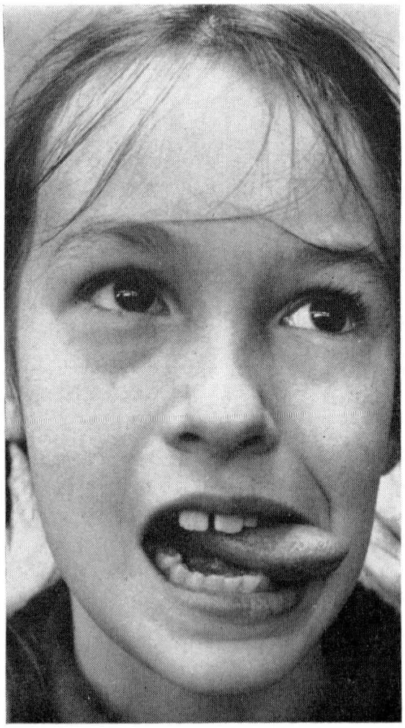

Fig. 1 (top left). Licking upper lip (normal). **Fig. 2** (top right). Licking upper lip (abnormal). **Fig. 3** (bottom left). Licking upper lip (normal.) **Fig. 4** (bottom centre). Licking upper lip (abnormal). **Fig. 5** (bottom right). Moving tongue from side to side.

Later in the interview (see page 36) it was necessary for the child's shoes and socks to be removed. Each child was asked to do this himself, and to put them on again at the end of the examination. This, again, gave the examiner the chance to observe fine co-ordination. Tying shoe-laces used to be a very good test of fine co-ordination but, with the advent of elastic-top shoes and buckles, children vary greatly in their experience of laces and this factor must be taken into account.

Threading beads was used as a test of co-ordination, intention tremor and other involuntary movements. The child was given a shoe-lace knotted at one end and then asked to place on it a round bead of standard size, first holding the two wide apart and then slowly approximating them (Figs 6 and 7). Intention tremor is best observed as the child brings together the bead and the shoe-lace, while his co-ordination is evident in the way he threads the bead on the lace. This was repeated using the other hand to hold the bead, and then with two oval beads (which were more difficult to thread). Young children, especially, found this an interesting task.

The finger-nose test required the child to place the tip of the palmar surface of his index finger first on his nose and then on the palmar tip of the examiner's index finger, held about 12 to 18 inches away. This movement from nose to finger to nose was repeated while the examiner slowly moved his finger from side to side and nearer to and further from the child's nose (to test for intention tremor).

In touching fingers with the thumb, the child had to touch the tip of each finger in turn with the thumb of the same hand. This was repeated with the other hand.

Codings were made for each of the tests of co-ordination and there was an overall rating of limb 'dyspraxia'. This referred to clumsiness thought to be due to a central defect in co-ordination separate from or additional to that caused by weakness, abnormal tone, local mechanical defect, abnormal movements, limb tremor or cerebellar dysfunction. In rating abnormality, the examiner was asked to rate the performance of the worse hand, but to take into account the usual preferred/non-preferred hand difference.

Fig. 6.

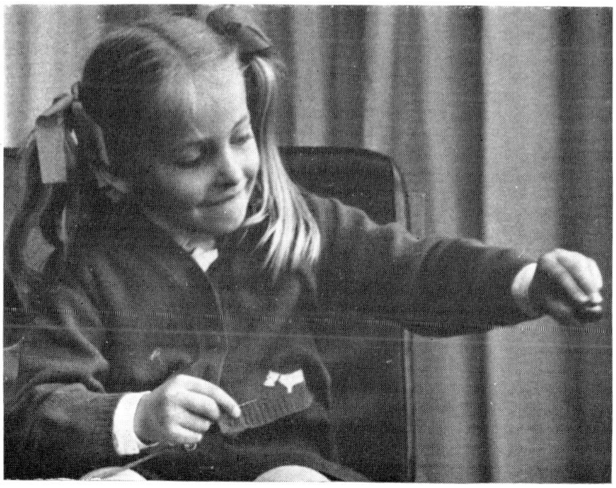

Fig. 7.

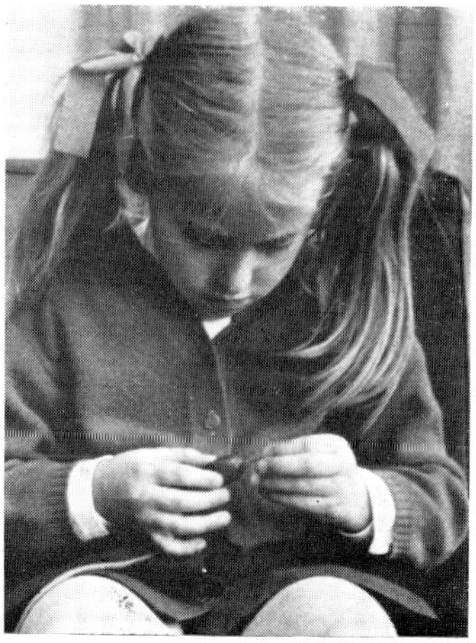

Constructional Abilities

The skills involved in perception and visuo-motor co-ordination are complex and a thorough examination is very time-consuming. For example, a child's inability to draw a diamond may be due to his inability to perceive different shapes, to difficulties in recognition or reproduction of shapes, or to problems in motor co-ordination. In planning treatment for a child with such difficulties, it is helpful to know precisely in which aspects of perception and visuo-motor co-ordination he shows abnormalities. Fortunately, for screening purposes it is sufficient to determine if a child can reproduce shapes accurately, as this involves perception, recognition and reproduction. However, it is important that this should be assessed in such a way that the child is not handicapped by clumsiness, weakness, tremor or abnormal tone. For this reason drawing is not a good test.

Five matchstick shapes (Fig. 8) were provided on cards. The child was given one card at a time in the order illustrated, and asked to make the same shape with matches from a large pile provided. It was important to ensure that the child was sitting squarely in relation to the test card when performing the task (Fig. 9).

Scoring was based on the accurate reproduction of the appropriate shape, and not on speed or neatness. A score of '0' was given for correct reproduction, '1' if there were only minor errors in shape or if the child failed to join up the matches by 1 cm or more, and '2' was scored if the shape was severely distorted. The child was not penalised if the heads of the matches did not point in the same direction as on the pattern cards; rotation was only penalised if the shape was also affected (*e.g.* a diamond to a square or a rhomboid). If '1' or '2' were rated, the examiner was asked to draw on the schedule a copy of the child's shape so that the scoring could be rechecked later and comparability ensured. If the child failed completely on two consecutive tasks, the rest of the shapes were omitted but were scored as '2'. The sum of the scores on the five individual shapes gave a total within the range of 0 to 10.

Fig. 8. Matchstick shapes.

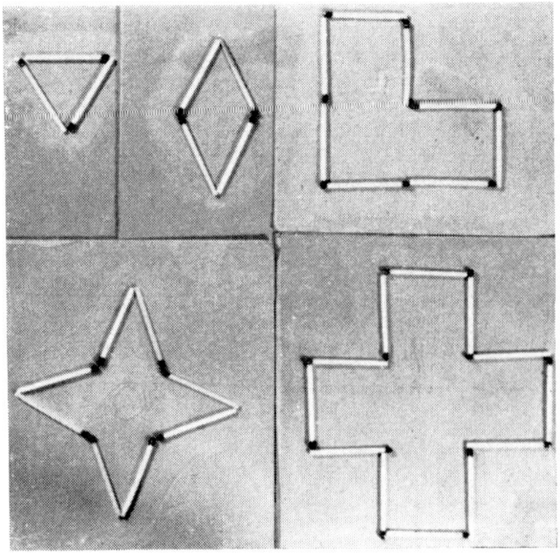

Fig. 9. Child completing shapes.

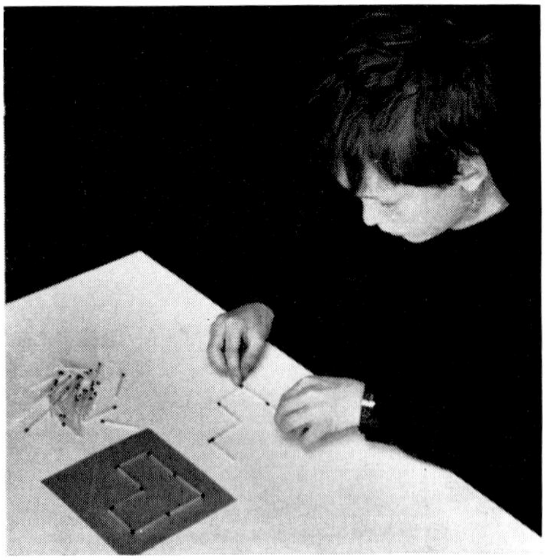

Skull and Limb Asymmetry

Skull symmetry was noted next in the examination. The examiner was asked to note any asymmetry (rated 'slight' or 'marked') of the bony structure of the face or skull vault. As part of this examination he was instructed to stand behind the child and look down at his forehead to see if the frontal prominences were equal in size and shape. Head circumference was not routinely measured, although it should certainly be included as a regular part of the examination of any child with developmental delay or neurological disorder.

Limb symmetry was not assessed until later (immediately after completing that part of the examination in which the child remains seated), but it may be conveniently described here. The hands were placed side by side and then against one another in order to compare for size; the feet were also compared for size. The girth and the muscle bulk of the two arms and then of the two legs were contrasted. The length of the arms was examined by getting the child to stand upright with his arms by his side and then to raise his arms above his head. When any asymmetry was suspected, the upper limbs were measured from the tip of the acromial process to the tip of the radial styloid and the lower limbs from the anterior superior iliac spine to the tip of the medial malleolus (while standing).

Stereognosis

A 'Yale' key was placed in the child's right hand while his eyes were closed. His hands or eyes were then covered by the examiner to ensure that the child could not see the object as he felt it. The child was encouraged to move the object around in his hand but he was not allowed to transfer it to the other hand or to use the other hand in any way. If the child did not recognise the object, it was placed in his left hand; if he still did not identify it, he was allowed to look at it. Astereognosis was rated only if he could then name the object. The exercise was repeated, using a penny in the left hand, then a rubber in the right, followed by an empty matchbox in the left. If the overall judgement of stereognosis was in doubt after using these four objects, the examiner was instructed to use additional ones.

Although these tests were included in the screening examination, in the light of further experience we would now omit them. No child showed astereognosis who did not also show some other neurological abnormality, and it would be preferable to apply the testing of stereognosis only to children known to have some disorder.

Speech and Language

Speech and language involve several distinct functions and, if an accurate appraisal is to be made, it is essential to differentiate them appropriately with separate ratings and descriptions.

Comprehension

Before testing comprehension of speech it is necessary to ensure that the child can hear a conversational voice. This should be observable during the interview with the child, but in all cases it was also systematically examined. The child was asked to stand in a corner of the room facing the wall and told that the examiner wanted to see how good his hearing was. It was explained that he was going to say some numbers which the child had to repeat. The examiner then stood six feet away and said six numbers, including high-tone sounds, in a quiet conversational voice, and a further six numbers in a whisper. If the child could not hear adequately with either ear, fuller testing was carried out.

Comprehension and response to sounds ('hearing behaviour') were observed informally during the whole of the interview but were also tested more systematically by telling the child to carry out a series of eight standard tasks of increasing complexity. ('Stand up; turn around; sit down; go to the door and knock once; bring me the matchbox which is on the table; put both hands on top of your head and stick out your tongue; (put your hands down now); sit down; put one hand on your lap and the other behind your head. Finally, the child was presented with three pieces of paper of clearly different sizes and was told: 'Crumple up the biggest one and throw it on the ground, give the medium sized one to me and put the smallest one in your pocket.') Acuity of hearing and ability to perform the acts had been previously determined and the commands were given without gesture. The last task proved rather unsuitable as young and retarded children often failed it through inability to remember such a lengthy instruction. When in doubt, the examiner used additional tests to evaluate comprehension of spoken language. If verbal commands were poorly understood, comprehension of gesture was tested (but not coded). Comprehension of written language was not assessed.

Vocalisation

Where the child had no speech, the amount, nature and quality of his vocalisations were assessed, but they were not coded in view of the few cases of this kind.

Production of Language

The nature of the child's language usage was observed throughout the interview according to the following categories: mode used (speech, gesture, etc.); syntactical complexity; semantic complexity; amount of language; abnormal types of speech (echolalia, neologisms, etc.); and use of communicative language (to ask questions, to comment, etc.).

As an aid to the assessment of language, the examiner had an aide-memoire in front of him throughout the interview. He had to note the number of words per sentence until the child used a sentence of ten words or more. The aide-memoire listed various parts and aspects of speech which were checked on the first occasion they were used by the child.

Complexity of spoken language was assessed on several scales: the maximum length of sentence used, a score reflecting whether certain parts of spoken language were ever used, and an overall rating for which the examiner took into account how much and how often the child used appropriately complex and correct language. The overall rating proved the most useful in differentiating children with language retardation.

In addition, there was a scale for the adequacy of the child's powers of description. For this it was essential that the child be given an opportunity to describe something which interested him. He was asked to tell the examiner what he did on an outing that he had mentioned, how he got to school, how he played a particular game, or what his favourite television programme was about. In an interview of this length it was almost always possible to get a child to talk adequately for these assessments, provided he was able to talk and did not have a gross psychiatric disorder.

The child was also asked to name fifteen common objects, but this proved to add very little of value for the evaluation. Echolalia was coded separately and provision was made for the coding of any other abnormality.

Word-sound Production

Throughout the interview the examiner was asked to note the child's articulation. No specific test words or sentences were used, although this might have been a valuable addition to the examination. Consonant omissions or substitutions (dyslalia) were coded as 'none', 'slight' or 'severe', and examiners were asked to differentiate articulation problems from local pecularities of speech.

Dysarthria (abnormal word-sound production due to local structural abnormalities or to neurological abnormalities affecting the function of lips, tongue or palate) was separately coded, again according to the degree of severity.

Phonation and Rhythm of Speech

These two additional aspects of speech were noted but were not separately coded.

Tremor

In addition to the observation of tremor during the testing of fine and gross motor co-ordination, the child was asked to stand with his feet together, eyes shut, arms extended and fingers stretched out in front of him. He was reassured that he would not fall and that if he felt unsteady the examiner was there to steady him. The position was maintained for forty seconds. Choreiform movements as well as other forms of tremor or involuntary movement were distinguished, described and coded. Ataxia was carefully noted and its type described in the schedule.

Laterality

Hand, foot and eye laterality were separately assessed by means of three tests in each case. For eye laterality the child was asked to look through a kaleidoscope, through a hole in a card and to sight down a toy rifle. The eye first used for each task was noted to give a score of 0 to 3 for the number of times the left eye was used.

Hand laterality was assessed on the hand used in drawing (see page 29), in throwing a rolled up piece of paper (see test for co-ordination page 36), and to knock on the door (see page 34). Foot laterality was tested by asking the child to kick a crumpled piece of paper on the floor twice and to hop on one leg.

These tests were enjoyed by most children and provided a useful opportunity to aid rapport by interrupting the more formal tasks and examinations. However, in the light of subsequent findings hopping was later dropped from the tests used in the assessment of foot laterality.

Right-left differentiation was assessed separately during the psychological examination (see chapter 5).

Large Muscle or Gross Motor Co-ordination

The child's gait was observed as he came along to the interview room and any movements and actions during the interview were also noted for possible evidence on co-ordination. In addition, a few specific actions were required of the child. He was first asked to remove his shoes and socks (see page 31). A large piece of good quality paper was then crumpled and placed in a free space on the floor a short distance from the child, who was asked to kick it to the door (or some other suitable object), pretending that the door was a goal. The foot used was noted for laterality. The child was then asked to fetch the paper, place it as before and again kick it into the 'goal'. Finally he was asked to throw and catch it. Kicking, throwing and walking/turning were separately coded and the actions also allowed observation of how the child bent down (relevant for assessment of balance). The child was asked also to hop (unsupported) first on one foot and then on the other; this, too, was separately coded.

In addition to the individual codings, the findings were used in making overall ratings of dyspraxia, tremor and ataxia.

Mirror Movements

Because of their possible use as a measure of cerebral immaturity, mirror movements were included in the examination. They were assessed, following the manner of Fog and Fog (1963), by observing movements in the opposite hand when the child was asked to squeeze a clothes peg and then a small bulldog clip between the thumb and index finger of his preferred hand, and again with his non-preferred hand. Associated movements in the opposite hand were rated 'none', 'homologous' (the same movements) to either a slight or marked degree, or 'heterologous' (extension of the fingers of the opposite hand accompanying flexion of the fingers grasping peg or clip).

It became apparent that heterologous movements were rather variable in manifestation and closely comparable to mild homologous movements. A child showing heterologous movements on one test generally showed mild, but less often marked, homologous movements on another test. Accordingly, heterologous movements were combined with slight homologous movements in calculating reliability. Thus, for each test there was a score with a range of 0 to 2, the four tests giving a total score with a range of 0 to 8.

The positioning of the hand to be observed was important; it was placed on the lap midway between pronation and supination and the fingers in a relaxed slightly flexed position (Figs 10 and11).

Muscle Tone

The concept of muscle tone has been the subject of considerable criticism, but the phenomena observable by the conventional tests for 'tone' remain useful indicators of neurologic function. In testing for tone, 'flappability', resistance to passive stretching and range of passive movement were examined.

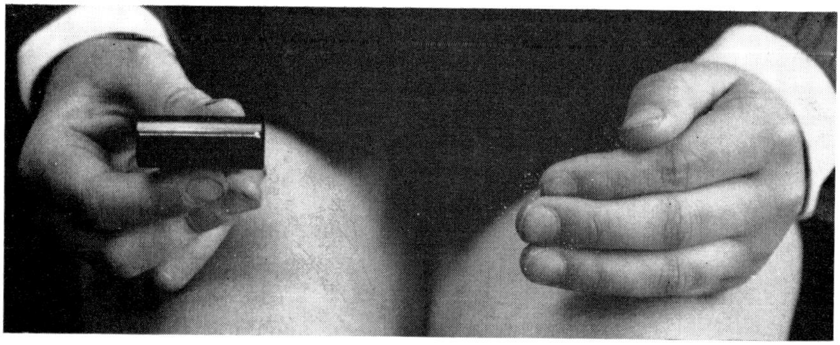

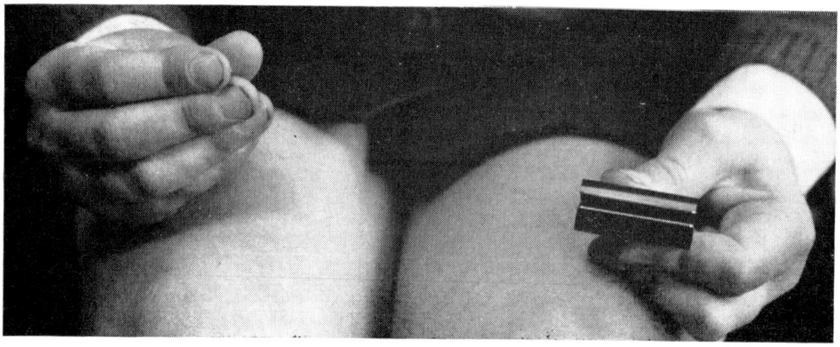

Fig 9 (top). Position of hands for testing mirror movements
Fig. 10 (bottom). Mirror movements - note contraction of fingers of opposite hand.

Tone of the upper limb was tested as follows: (a) the hand was flapped while holding the lower forearm; (b) the wrist was slowly plantarflexed and dorsiflexed; (c) while grasping the child's hand in the manner of a handshake (using the same hand as that of the child) the arm was pronated and supinated and then flapped; (d) the elbow was flexed and extended; and (e) the wrist was dorsiflexed and the fingers bent back as far as they would comfortably go. In carrying out these manoeuvres it was essential for the child to allow his arm to go limp. This was most readily accomplished by talking to the child about something else so that he was not concentrating on the upper limb movements.

Tone of the lower limb was tested by (a) holding the thigh just above the knee with the leg hanging down and flapping the leg; (b) plantarflexing and dorsiflexing the ankle; (c) flexing and extending the knee; and (d) testing the range of movement of the ankle.

Tone was recorded separately for the right and left upper and lower limbs as 'normal', 'slight hypotonia', 'marked hypotonia', 'slight hypertonia' or 'marked hypertonia'. There was an additional coding for the type of abnormality (*e.g.* rigidity, spasticity).

Throughout the examination particular attention was paid to examining for each sign without regard to other findings and to recording each finding before proceeding to the next item in order to avoid 'halo' judgements and hence false associations between signs.

Power

Considerable opportunities for assessing muscle strength were afforded during tests of co-ordination, but a few specific tests were also carried out. Power may be tested either by getting the child to make a movement against the examiner's resistance (kinetic power), or by holding a position and preventing the examiner moving the joint (static power). In general it is easier to get young children to understand and to co-operate in static power testing, so this method was used.

The child was asked to extend his fingers fully and to prevent the examiner flexing them, and then to do the same with dorsiflexion of the wrist. In the same way the child was asked to flex his fingers over the examiner's fingers and prevent their extension. Flexion and extension of the elbow were tested likewise, while similar manoeuvres were used with dorsiflexion of the great toe and then of the ankle, and with flexion and extension of the knee. In all these actions, care, attention and time were necessary to get and maintain the child's full co-operation.

Codings of 'no', 'slight' or 'marked' weakness were made separately for right and left upper and lower limbs.

Deep Tendon Reflexes

Tendon reflexes were obtained in the usual way with a patellar hammer having a rubber-edged metal disc attached to a springy plastic handle. The limbs were arranged so that they were relaxed, supported and free of constriction. The wrist and elbow were in mid-position for testing the upper limb reflexes, the leg hung freely from sitting position for the knee jerk, and the knee was partially flexed with the foot at right angles to the leg for the ankle jerk.

The briskness of the jerk was determined by the weight of the blow required to elicit the jerk and not by the range of movement obtained. The reflex was rated as normal if a brisk (albeit slight) response was obtained with a smart light blow of the tendon hammer, either with or without 'reinforcement'. A minimal but perceptible response was rated 'diminished', and no response as 'absence' of that reflex. A 'slight' or 'doubtful' increase was rated if a brisk response was obtained with only a very light blow and a 'definite marked' or 'very marked' increase if a brisk response was obtained with a minimal tap of the hammer or of a finger. Patellar and ankle clonus were examined for in the usual way and coded as present if found.

Inversion of the supinator was rated only if there was both flexion of the fingers and absence of contraction of the brachioradialis.

Plantar Response

The child was made as relaxed as possible and the lower limb positioned as for testing the ankle jerk. A 'Yale' key was run firmly up the outer border of the foot, starting from the heel and ending by crossing over the distal end of the metatarsals towards the base of the big toe. This movement was repeated if the response was in doubt. A rating of 'flexor' or 'extensor' was made if there was at least one clear flexor or extensor response of the big toe, even if other movements were equivocal, provided that there was not a clear response in the opposite direction. Full extensor responses with fanning of the toes were differentiated from extensor responses without fanning.

Overall Rating

The items already described constituted the minimum requirements for a neurological examination. Scarcely any sensory testing was included as it is quite rare in the age group 5 to 15 years to find a child with sensory abnormalities and no abnormality on any of the listed signs. However, in each case the examiner had to make a final rating on the presence and severity of neurological disorder (none, dubious, slight or marked). Marked abnormality was rated with definite and obviously handicapping disorders (*e.g.* post-polio flail arm or a spastic hemiparesis). Slight abnormality was rated for definite disorders which were either not handicapping at all or only slightly handicapping (*e.g.* a mild but definite hemiparesis or definite gross clumsiness). A rating of dubious abnormality was made for isolated signs which were slight and of uncertain significance (*e.g.* slight clumsiness only, or hypotonia or slight generalised hyperreflexia). Lastly, a diagnosis was made. This often required a fuller examination than that described here, but it was left to the discretion of the examiner to decide what further tests to include.

CHAPTER 3

The Neurological Examination: Reliability

When a new diagnostic procedure is introduced, the first concern of those who use it is that it should be adequately standardised, reliable and valid. In general, techniques like the neurological examination, which were introduced before the importance of a statistical assessment of these attributes was realised, tend to have escaped methodical evaluation. However, unless the examiner knows which parts of a procedure vary most from observer to observer, and is aware of the relationship between individual tests and an overall assessment, and of the way in which individual tests tend to be associated with each other, he suffers from a lack of reference points in assessing the results he obtains. Oldham (1968) has shown, too, that the discovery of unreliability in measurement can be a potential asset in understanding the nature and significance of clinical signs.

A number of studies (reviewed by Witts 1959) have aimed at measuring observer error and variation in such different fields as radiology, respiratory disorder and carcinoma of the breast, but the clinical examination of the central nervous system has been examined in this way only to a very limited degree and has been found as subject to error as other clinical examinations. In a study of old people, McCance *et al.* (1968) found considerable unreliability in the elicitation of plantar responses. Kuzma *et al.* (1965), in developing methods to assess deterioration and evaluate possibly useful methods of treatment in multiple sclerosis, devised a new series of tests to measure muscular power, co-ordination and fatiguability. They also paid attention to the more traditional methods of examination such as the elicitation of reflexes. Four examiners (two neurologists and two physical therapists) gave eight patients a neurological examination once each on eight successive half-days. In 27 of the 60 tests employed, including the supinator, biceps and knee reflexes, there were significantly different observer means, despite a period of training before the study began. Deep tendon reflexes were amongst the procedures most difficult to assess reliably. It is of interest, too, that the two neurologists differed as much, and on occasions, more, from each other, than did the physical therapists from the neurologists.

Methodological evaluation of other aspects of the neurological examination does not seem to have been reported in either children or adults. The Isle of Wight study offered a good opportunity to examine the issues involved, and a study of the reliability of the examination was therefore carried out during the educational part of the survey.

Neurological Examination

Following a series of pilot studies of the neurological examination, a schedule was produced for coding individual signs, for making summary judgements of neurological abnormality and for recording a diagnosis if any abnormality was found. At the same time, a series of examination notes was produced in order to standardise as far as possible the technique of examination and the order in which the signs were to be elicited. The neurological examination is described in chapter 2.

Altogether, 94 items were noted on scales with ranges varying from 2 to 11 points. Ratings were made immediately after the relevant signs had been elicited and were not changed in the light of subsequent findings, so that, for example, if the examiner rated normal tone and power in the legs, but found increased knee and ankle reflexes and extensor plantar responses, he was not allowed to make a re-assessment of tone and power.

Reliability Study

The reliability study was carried out in two stages. Initially, 89 children on the Isle of Wight aged 10 and 11 years, most of whom had been selected because of educational or intellectual retardation (though some formed part of the random control group described in chapter 4) were examined independently by two of the authors (MR and PG) at intervals ranging from one day to one month. Only the name and age of the child was known to the examiner at the time the examination was carried out, and the second examiner was kept in entire ignorance of the findings made by the first.

Preliminary analysis of the results of these examinations showed that there were problems in assessing reliability. As only a minority of the children suffered from any neurological abnormality, the uneven distribution of scores made calculation of reliability difficult. It was also apparent that the reliability of some individual signs was much lower than the overall judgement on neurological disorder. To determine the reasons for this, PG and MR examined a series of children together. It was found that there were minor differences in the method of eliciting certain signs and that one examiner tended to rate more reflexes abnormal than the other.

Further standardisation of the clinical examinations and of the rating procedure was carried out and then, at intervals varying from one day to two weeks, the same two authors independently examined 27 children aged between 7 and 13 years attending a school for the physically handicapped in North London. Again, only the name and age of each child were known to the examiner prior to the examination, and the two examiners carried out their assessment in ignorance of each other's findings. The neurological examination of these children was not preceded by a psychiatric assessment so no attempt was made to assess the neurological aspects of speech and language.

Method of Assessing Reliability

There are many different ways of expressing observer variability and the use of different methods has sometimes led investigators with almost identical findings to come to opposite conclusions regarding the repeatibility of signs (Meade and Gardner 1968). We have attempted to deal with this problem by presenting the findings as fully as space allows and by expressing reliability in several ways in order to demonstrate its different aspects.

The methods may best be illustrated by one detailed example. Tables 1 and 2*a* show the findings in the case of hand laterality. Eighty-eight children were examined by examiner 1 and on another occasion by examiner 2. The diagonal shows that they agreed on '0' for 52 cases, on '1' for 6 cases, on '2' for 2 cases and on '3' for 10 cases, a total of 70 cases. The overall percentage agreement was calculated on the basis of the number of assessments agreed (140: 70 for each examiner) divided by the total number of assessments (176: 88 for each examiner), namely 0·80 or 80 per cent. A similar calculation was done for each point on the scale, using the total number of times that point was assigned by either examiner as the denominator. This enabled a determination of which point on the scale gave rise to the greatest disagreement. In this case (as is usual) agreement was highest at the extremes of the scale (90 per cent for '0' and 83 per cent for '3') and lowest for intermediate points (48 per cent for '1' and 33 per cent for '2').

TABLE 1
Left-handedness in Isle of Wight children: raw data

Number of times left hand used						
		Examiner 1				Total no. cases
		0	**1**	**2**	**3**	
	0	52	5	0	0	57
Examiner 2	**1**	3	6	1	0	10
	2	2	3	2	1	8
	3	1	1	1	10	13
Total no. cases		58	15	4	11	88

To assess the frequency of major disagreements it was necessary to look at the number of times the examiners disagreed by at least 2 points, in this case 4 out of 88 (made up of 3 cases where examiner 1 rated '0' and examiner 2 rated '2' or more, and 1 case where examiner 1 rated '1' and examiner 2 rated '3').

An overall measure of agreement may be obtained by calculating the product-moment correlation between the two ratings, in this case 0·84. However, this figure is influenced by skew (the extent to which ratings occur mainly at one end of the scale), agreement being greater by chance alone when the skew is very marked.

Observer threshold must also be taken into consideration. Disagreements may be due either to the lack of repeatability of the observations ('observer error') or to the fact that the examiners are both making repeatable observations but are doing so on differently calibrated scales, *i.e.* with different thresholds for rating abnormality. This possibility may be checked by calculating the mean rating for each examiner (in this case 0·64 for examiner 1 and 0·59 for examiner 2) and testing for the significance of the difference between the means using a 't' test (which for this item fell well short of statistical significance).

TABLE 2

Inter-rater reliability on hand, foot and eye laterality

	Total no. cases	*Point on scale*	*Times assigned*	*Percentage agreement*	*Overall percentage agreement*	*Product-moment correlation*
(*a*) **Hand laterality** (No. of times left hand used)						
(i) Isle of Wight children	88	0	115	90	80	0·84
		1	25	48		
		2	12	33		
		3	24	83		
No. of disagreements of at least 2 points: 4/88						
(ii) Physically handicapped children	26	0	23	87	73	0·89
		1	7	29		
		2	5	0		
		3	17	94		
No. of disagreements of at least 2 points: 1/26						
(*b*) **Foot laterality** (No. of times left foot used)						
(i) Isle of Wight children	81	0	121	99	98	0·98
		1	4	50		
		2	37	97		
No. of disagreements of at least 2 points: 1/81						
(ii) Physically handicapped children	23	0	29	97	87	0·92
		1	5	40		
		2	12	83		
No. of disagreements of at least 2 points: 0/23						
(*c*) **Eye laterality** (No. of times left eye used)						
(i) Isle of Wight children	85	0	103	91	87	0·87
		1	10	60		
		2	8	50		
		3	49	89		
No. of disagreements of at least 2 points: 5/85						
(ii) Physically handicapped children	26	0	18	89	89	0·83
		1	0	–		
		2	3	67		
		3	31	90		
No. of disagreements of at least 2 points: 2/26						

N.B. No difference in observer threshold on any laterality measures.

Hand, Foot and Eye Laterality

As noted in Tables 1 and 2*a*, there was good reliability on the assessment of hand laterality and the study of physically handicapped children gave rise to a similarly high reliability (r=0·89). Nevertheless, it is important to note that a few children used different hands on the three tests in the two examinations, so a single test of hand laterality would be unsatisfactory.

The findings for foot* and eye laterality were closely similar (Table 2*b* and *c*) and none of them showed any difference in observer threshold between the two examiners. The observation of which hand is used in a task gives little opportunity for differences in judgement and any unreliability in the assessment largely resides in the intrinsic variability of children's hand, foot and eye preferences.

Developmental Abnormalities

The neurological examination contained several items which concerned developmental functions, *i.e.* functions which develop with increasing brain maturation. In any task of this kind the young child encounters difficulties, but his skill gradually increases with age. Abnormalities can only be gauged by assessing the degree of the child's impairment in the developmental task in relation to his age. For this reason, it is often appropriate to use a series of tasks graded in difficulty.

(A) CONSTRUCTIONAL DIFFICULTIES

This approach was followed in the test of constructional difficulties (see page 32). Table 3*a* shows that in the Isle of Wight children this proved to be a highly reliable judgement (r=0·93). There were no 2 point disagreements between grouped scores on the scales (0, 1-3, 4-7, 8-10) and only thirteen 2 point disagreements out of 87 when the full 11 point scale was considered.

Reliability was good (r=0·80), but not quite so good, with regard to the physically handicapped children. Performance on constructional tasks seemed to be more variable in children with overt neurological disorder. In neither group of children was there any difference in observer threshold.

(B) LIMB 'DYSPRAXIA'

Based on the performance of 8 separate motor tasks†, an overall judgement was made on the presence or absence of limb dyspraxia, *i.e.* a central abnormality of motor co-ordination not explicable in terms of weakness, alteration of tone, abnormal movements or tremor. In the Isle of Wight children this was found to be a moderately reliable judgement (r=0·78) and there was only one 2 point disagreement out of 86 cases.

In the physically handicapped children, reliability was somewhat lower (r=0·68) with two 2 point disagreements out of 26 cases. Both examiners found it difficult to assess inco-ordination beyond that which could be attributed to varying degrees of paresis and spasticity. Judgement was much easier when the child had no overt neurological condition. Again, in neither group was there any difference in observer threshold (Table 3*b*).

*Initially, it was intended to assess foot laterality by judging which foot the child first used when asked to hop, but it became clear that the foot a child used for this purpose was very weakly related to the foot used in kicking, which was obviously the stronger and preferred foot. We therefore restricted our assessment of footedness to the foot used in two tests of kicking.

†Threading beads; holding pencil; touching fingers with thumb; finger-nose test; kicking ball of paper; throwing ball of paper; hopping on one foot; walking and turning.

TABLE 3
Inter-rater reliability on developmental abnormalities

		Total no. cases	Point on scale	Times assigned	Percentage agreement	Overall percentage agreement	Product-moment correlation
(*a*)	**Constructional difficulties**						
(i)	Isle of Wight children	87	0	70	80	76	0·93
			1 — 3	72	72		
			4 — 7	17	59		
			8 —10	15	93		
			No. of 2 point disagreements: 0/87 (13/87)				
(ii)	Physically handicapped children	26	0	12	50	58	0·80
			1 — 3	26	62		
			4 — 7	6	33		
			8 —10	8	75		
			No. of 2 point disagreements: 2/26 (8/26)				
(*b*)	**Limb 'dyspraxia'**						
(i)	Isle of Wight children	86	0 (none)	106	88	77	0·78
			1 (possible)	25	24		
			2 (definite)	26	77		
			No. of 2 point disagreements: 1/86				
(ii)	Physically handicapped children	26	0 (none)	32	81	77	0·68
			1 (possible)	8	50		
			2 (definite)	12	83		
			No. of 2 point disagreements: 2/26				
(*c*)	**Articulation defect** Isle of Wight children	89	0 (normal)	122	89	78	0·71
			1 (mild abn.)	33	48		
			2 (marked abn.)	21	67		
			No. of 2 point disagreements: 2/89				
(*d*)	**Speech syntax rating** Isle of Wight children	88	0 (no speech)	8	100	58	0·89
			1 — 6	10	20		
			7	20	20		
			8	41	29		
			9	97	68		
			No. of 2 point disagreements: 8/88				
			Difference in observer threshold significant at 10 *per cent level,* $t = 1{\cdot}76$				

(*Continued overleaf*)

TABLE 3 (*continued*)

	Total no. cases	Point on scale	Times assigned	Percentage agreement	Overall percentage agreement	Product-moment correlation
(*e*) **Overall speech complexity**						
Isle of Wight children	88	Normal	106	89	82	0·87
		Less than normal	53	72		
		Markedly retarded	10	60		
		Little or no useful speech	7	86		
		No. of 2 *point disagreements:* 0/88				
(*f*) **Adequacy of description**						
Isle of Wight children	88	0	118	85	76	0·73
		1	41	49		
		2	17	42		
		No. of 2 *point disagreements:* 0/88				
(*g*) **Mirror movements**						
(i) Isle of Wight children	83	0	33	48	63	0·56
		1 — 3	47	47		
		4+	86	77		
		No. of 2 *point disagreements:* 6/83				
(ii) Physically handicapped children	23	0	9	67	65	0·78
		1 — 3	19	63		
		4+	18	67		
		No. of 2 *point disagreements:* 1/23				

N.B. No difference in observer threshold on developmental abnormalties except where marked.

(C) SPEECH AND LANGUAGE

The child's speech and language was largely assessed on the basis of systematic examination of conversation during the interview which preceded the physical examinations (see page 33). Articulation defects, which were due neither to dysarthria following neurological disorder nor to local abnormalities, were assessed. These defects (sometimes termed 'dyslalia') were generally of the type shown by children when they first begin to talk. The assessment was moderately reliable (r=0·71) but the examiners experienced some difficulty in distinguishing very mild articulation defects from speech peculiarities associated with the local dialect. A further difficulty arose from the inconsistencies in children's word-sound production. There was no difference in observer threshold (Table 3*c*).

The assessment of the child's level of language usage had to be made without the aid of tape-recorders as it formed but a small part of the overall neurological examination, and only relatively crude measures were possible. Rating of the longest sentence used by the child was reliable ($r=0{\cdot}91$), but proved too coarse a discriminator to be of much use except in the detection of the few children with severe language disorders. Rating the complexity of the child's language, too, was reliable ($r=0{\cdot}89$) but there was an almost significant difference in observer threshold ($t=1{\cdot}76$, $p<0{\cdot}10$) and the reliability in the middle of the scale fell well short of that at the extremes (Table 3*d*).

An overall rating of speech complexity, based on average sentence length and syntactical complexity, was a better discriminator of children with mild disorders and was more reliable at all points on the scale. The correlation between the ratings of the two examiners was high ($r=0{\cdot}87$) and there was no difference in observer threshold (Table 3*e*).

As well as observing the child's language in ordinary conversation, note was taken of his ability to give an adequate description of some recent activity. Again, there was no difference in observer threshold, but the overall reliability was not quite as high ($r=0{\cdot}73$) (Table 3*f*).

(D) MIRROR MOVEMENTS

Mirror movements were assessed (see page 36), following the manner of Fog and Fog (1963). There was no difference in observer threshold but the inter-observer reliability was only moderate ($r=0{\cdot}56$ for the Isle of Wight children and 0·78 for the physically handicapped children) (Table 3*g*).

It would seem that the relative unreliability of the test resided as much in the phenomenon itself as in observer error, as there was only occasional difficulty in deciding whether mirror-movements had been present. We found no difference in the mirror movements associated with the preferred and non-preferred hand but the extent of associated movement seemed to be related to the amount of effort the child put into his attempt to squeeze the clothes peg or bulldog clip. This suggestion is supported by Hellebrandt and Waterland's observation (1962) that, in the normal adult, associated movements were only demonstrable with maximal effort kept up to the point of exhaustion. The motivation of a child is sometimes difficult to control and it may be that variation in this factor led to some of the disagreement between the two observers.

Cranial Signs

Only a limited number of cranial signs were examined in the present study. As most of them occurred infrequently and referred to qualitative rather than quantitative differences from normality, product-moment correlations were inappropriate and are not included in the Tables.

(A) NYSTAGMUS, STRABISMUS AND PTOSIS

Nystagmus was rated with quite good reliability in both studies and there was no difference in observer threshold (Table 4*a*). Ptosis occurred too rarely for reliability to be assessed meaningfully, but reliability appeared fairly high from the very small number of cases observed.

Strabismus was rated with reasonable reliability in the physically handicapped children but with only moderate reliability in the Isle of Wight children. This might be partly explicable by the less satisfactory co-operation shown by some children in the latter group who had mild intellectual retardation, but it appeared that minor differences in the method of examining for strabismus were more important. Greater attention was paid to technique in the later study of physically handicapped children and it is likely that the increased reliability was in part due to this (Table 4*b*).

TABLE 4
Inter-rater reliability on cranial signs

		Total no. cases	*Point on scale*	*Times assigned*	*Percentage agreement*	*Overall percentage agreement*
(*a*)	**Nystagmus**					
(i)	Isle of Wight children	88	None	153	90	92
			Slight	9	44	
			Marked	13	71	
		No. of 2 *point disagreements:* 2/88				
(ii)	Physically handicapped children	27	None	44	96	85
			Slight	4	0	
			Marked	6	67	
		No. of 2 *point disagreements:* 0/27				
(*b*)	**Strabismus**					
(i)	Isle of Wight children	88	None	153	95	89
			Latent	5	40	
			Overt	18	56	
		No. of 2 *point disagreements:* 6/88				
(ii)	Physically handicapped children	27	None	39	87	81
			Latent	3	0	
			Overt	12	83	
		No. of 2 *point disagreements:* 2/27				
(*c*)	**Facial power**					
	Physically handicapped children	26	Normal	36	89	81
			Possible weakness			
			Right	1	0	
			Left	0	–	
			Bilateral	3	0	
			Definite weakness			
			Right	8	75	
			Left	2	100	
			Bilateral	2	100	

(*Continued*)

TABLE 4 (*continued*)

		Total no. cases	Point on scale	Times assigned	Percentage agreement	Overall percentage agreement
(*d*)	**Facial asymmetry**					
	Physically handicapped children	27	At rest			
			Nil	38	89	85
			Present	16	75	
			Spontaneous movements			
			Nil	42	76	63
			Present	12	17	
			Movements to command			
			Nil	37	81	74
			Present	17	59	
(*e*)	**Tongue: licking upper lip**					
(i)	Isle of Wight children	87	Normal	138	93	85
			Slight abn.	23	52	
			Definite abn.	13	62	
		No. of 2 point disagreements: 2/87				
(ii)	Physically handicapped children	27	Normal	38	95	81
			Slight abn.	7	57	
			Definite abn.	9	44	
		No. of 2 point disagreements: 2/27				
(*f*)	**Tongue: side to side**					
(i)	Isle of Wight children	87	Normal	152	95	91
			Slight abn.	12	33	
			Definite abn.	10	100	
		No. of 2 point disagreements: 0/87				
(ii)	Physically handicapped children	27	Normal	35	74	59
			Slight abn.	14	29	
			Definite abn.	5	40	
		No. of 2 point disagreements: 0/27				
(*g*)	**Skull asymmetry**					
(i)	Isle of Wight children	89	None	118	86	78
			Slight	41	54	
			Marked	0	-	
		No. of 2 point disagreements: 0/89				
(ii)	Physically handicapped children	26	None	41	83	69
			Slight	10	20	
			Marked	1	0	
		No. of 2 point disagreements: 0/26				

N.B. No difference in observer threshold on any cranial signs.

(B) FACIAL POWER AND ASYMMETRY

Reliability on definite facial weakness was high but the rating of possible weakness proved to be quite unreliable, and varied according to the method of assessment. Asymmetry at rest was assessed with high reliability, asymmetry of facial movements to command with moderate reliability, but asymmetry on spontaneous facial movements showed only poor reliability. There was no difference in observer threshold on any of these items (Table 4*c* and *d*).

(C) TONGUE MOVEMENTS

Children were rated on their ability to lick their upper lip and move their tongue from side to side. An appreciable number of children had great difficulty in doing this. The sign was rated reliably in the Isle of Wight children but much less so in the physically handicapped children, probably because of the greater difficulty in assessing these movements when there was tongue weakness or gross generalised co-ordination difficulties (Table 4*e* and *f*).

(D) SKULL AND LIMB ASYMMETRY

Only one child in either group was thought to have marked skull asymmetry, so it was not possible to assess the reliability of this judgement. Furthermore, the rating of slight skull asymmetry was too unreliable for it to be of much diagnostic value (Table 4*g*).

There were no children with marked limb asymmetry in the Isle of Wight group, and the reliability on slight asymmetry was very poor. In the physically handicapped children there were 7 ratings of marked asymmetry with a percentage agreement of 57, and 3 ratings of slight asymmetry on which there was zero agreement. Even with the aid of measurement, limb asymmetry proved to be a difficult rating in the case of minor limb inequalities. Sometimes there were problems in getting paretic limbs into the same position for measurement on both sides, and always (particularly in the obese) there was appreciable error inherent in the identification of the necessary bony landmarks for measurement.

Receptive Functions

The reliability of peripheral sensory testing was not examined. Comprehension of language was assessed but too few children showed abnormalities for reliability to be measured. Astereognosis was rated 'dubious', 'possible', 'probable' or 'definite'. No children showed definite astereognosis but there was moderately good agreement on the few children who showed possible or probable abnormalities in stereognosis. A larger number of children with perceptual abnormalities must be studied before any conclusion can be drawn on the reliability of such judgements.

Motor Co-ordination

The child's motor co-ordination was judged from his performance on eight different tasks (see pagees 29, 36 and Table 5). Most of these were moderately or highly reliable and only three produced any 2 point disagreements. Curiously, these three tests included the two traditional tests of co-ordination (touching each finger

TABLE 5
Inter-rater reliability on co-ordination (physically handicapped children)

Variable	No.	*Point on scale*	*Times assigned*	*Percentage agreement*	*Overall percentage agreement*	*No. of 2 point disagree-ments*	*Product-moment correlation*
Threading beads	27	Normal	29	90	85	0/27	0·77
		Slight abn.	17	82			
		Def. abn.	8	75			
Holding pencil	27	Normal	41	83	70	0/27	0·58
		Slight abn.	10	20			
		Def. abn.	3	67			
Touching fingers with thumb	26	Normal	21	57	54	1/26	0·71
		Slight abn.	15	27			
		Def. abn.	17	71			
Finger-nose test	27	Normal	37	81	70	3/27	0·57
		Slight abn.	4	0			
		Def. abn.	13	62			
Kicking ball of paper	26	Normal	18	89	81	0/26	0·89
		Slight abn.	11	55			
		Def. abn.	23	87			
Throwing ball of paper	26	Normal	33	73	58	1/26	0·65
		Slight abn.	10	0			
		Def. abn.	9	67			
Hopping on one foot	26	Normal	6	67	85	0/26	0·86
		Slight abn.	8	50			
		Def. abn.	38	95			
Walking and turning	26	Normal	10	100	88	0/26	0·87
		Slight abn.	5	20			
		Def. abn.	37	92			
Overall judgement on cerebellar dysfunction	26	No abn.	37	92	85	0/26	0·88
		Possible/ slight abn.	8	50			
		Marked abn.	7	86			
Tremor	27	None	41	88	78	2/27	0·61
		Slight	6	33			
		Marked	4	50			
		Gross	3	67			

N.B. No difference in observer threshold on any tests of co-ordination.

in turn with the thumb and the finger-nose test) and the finger-nose test was the only one where there was more than one 2 point disagreement. The most likely reason for this finding is that these were the tasks which young children had most difficulty in understanding.

The assessment of tremor was only moderately reliable in the physically handicapped children, reflecting the difficulty of assessment in a paretic or spastic limb. As previously reported (Rutter *et al.* 1966), the reliability of judgements on choreiform movements in a normal population is at about the same level, or slightly better.

The overall judgement on cerebellar dysfunction (which took account of nystagmus as well as limb co-ordination) was highly reliable.

Power and Tone of Limbs

Judgements on muscle power were highly reliable in both the Isle of Wight and the physically handicapped children. In only one out of 432 assessments was there a 2 point disagreement. Nevertheless, it should be noted that there was a nearly

TABLE 6
Inter-rater reliability on power of limbs

	Total no. cases	*Point on scale*	*Times assigned*	*Percentage agreement*	*Overall percentage agreement*	*Product-moment correlation*
(*a*) **Upper limbs**						
(i) Isle of Wight children	81	Normal	298	97	95	0·77
		Slight weakness	22	64		
		Marked weakness	4	100		
		No. of 2 *point disagreements:* 0/162				
		No difference in observer threshold				
(ii) Physically handicapped children	27	Normal	63	79	72	0·82
		Slight weakness	27	44		
		Marked weakness	18	89		
		No. of 2 *point disagreements:* 0/54				
		Difference in observer threshold significant at 10 *per cent level,* t = 1·88				
(*b*) **Lower limbs**						
(i) Isle of Wight children	82	Normal	290	97	94	0·82
		Slight weakness	20	50		
		Marked weakness	10	80		
		No. of 2 *point disagreements:* 0/164				
		No difference in observer threshold				
(ii) Physically handicapped children	26	Normal	46	83	75	0·80
		Slight weakness	24	50		
		Marked weakness	34	82		
		No. of 2 *point disagreements:* 1/52				
		No difference in observer threshold				

significant difference in observer threshold ($t = 1{\cdot}88$, $p < 0{\cdot}10$) on the rating of upper limb power in the physically handicapped children.

The recognition of abnormalities in muscle tone was only slightly less reliable, but disagreements on whether the alteration in tone was 'slight' or 'marked' were fairly frequent. There was no difference in observer threshold (Tables 6 and 7).

TABLE 7
Inter-rater reliability on tone of limbs

	Total no. cases	*Point on scale*	*Times assigned*	*Percentage agreement*	*Overall percentage agreement*	*Product-moment correlation*
(*a*) **Upper limbs**						
(i) Isle of Wight children	87	Marked hypotonia	12	67	86	0·79
		Slight hypotonia	22	36		
		Normal	302	93		
		Slight hypertonia	8	0		
		Marked hypertonia	4	100		
		No. of 2 *point disagreements:* 0/174				
(ii) Physically handicapped children	27	Marked hypotonia	16	38	57	0·85
		Slight hypotonia	18	22		
		Normal	43	74		
		Slight hypertonia	23	70		
		Marked hypertonia	8	50		
		No. of 2 *point disagreements:* 0/54				
(*b*) **Lower limbs**						
(i) Isle of Wight children	87	Marked hypotonia	10	40	86	0·62
		Slight hypotonia	18	44		
		Normal	306	93		
		Slight hypertonia	10	0		
		Marked hypertonia	4	100		
		No. of 2 *point disagreements:* 0/174				
(ii) Physically handicapped children	26	Marked hypotonia	7	29	67	0·75
		Slight hypotonia	11	36		
		Normal	46	83		
		Slight hypertonia	17	47		
		Marked hypertonia	23	78		
		No. of 2 *point disagreements:* 1/52				

N.B. No difference in observer threshold on tone.

Tendon Reflexes and the Plantar Response

Although there were differences in the level of reliability of different reflexes, the general pattern was very similar. In every case agreement was considerably less good in the Isle of Wight study than in the later study of physically handicapped children. This was due in part to the larger proportion of children with marked abnormalities in the latter study. For example, in many cases the agreement on individual points on the scale was fairly similar, but differences in observer threshold were much greater in the Isle of Wight study. For all reflexes except the knee jerk, the threshold difference was highly significant in the Isle of Wight children, and was almost entirely accounted for by differences in the rating of diminished reflexes. In some cases there was also a minor (but non-significant) difference in the rating of slightly increased reflexes (Table 8).

Following the Isle of Wight study, considerable attention was paid to increasing the standardisation of the method of examination and of the coding of reflex responses. The observer difference in rating diminished reflexes was eliminated but a difference in the threshold for rating increased responses remained.

It is important to note that this difference scarcely ever gave rise to major disagreements in rating reflexes. There were no 2 point disagreements in the 257 ratings of deep tendon reflexes in the physically handicapped children and very few even in the Isle of Wight study. In most cases the disagreement was between possible/slight abnormality recorded by one examiner and no abnormality (or less often definite/marked abnormality) recorded by the other.

The situation with regard to the plantar reflex was similar. Equivocal responses were generally unreliable, and in the Isle of Wight study a difference in observer threshold further reduced the level of agreement.

TABLE 8
Inter-rater reliability on reflexes

	Total no. cases	*Point on scale*	*Times assigned*	*Percentage agreement*	*Overall percentage agreement*	*Product-moment correlation*
(*a*) **Supinator**						
(i) Isle of Wight children	88	Absent	7	57	54	0·20
		Diminished	53	0		
		Normal	249	72		
		Increased	34	12		
		Much increased	9	44		
No. of 2 *point disagreements:* 2/176						
Difference in observer threshold significant at 0·1 *per cent level, t* = 6·55						
(ii) Physically handicapped children	26	Absent	12	67	58	0·66
		Diminished	5	0		
		Normal	63	76		
		Increased	11	18		
		Much increased	13	46		
No. of 2 *point disagreements:* 0/52						
Difference in observer threshold significant at 10 *per cent level, t* = 1·88						

(*Continued*)

TABLE 8 (*continued*)

		Total no. cases	Point on scale	Times assigned	Percentage agreement	Overall percentage agreement	Product-moment correlation
(*b*)	**Biceps**						
(i)	Isle of Wight children	88	Absent	8	50	65	0·45
			Diminished	36	0		
			Normal	269	78		
			Increased	30	40		
			Much increased	9	11		
			No. of 2 *point disagreements:* 0/176				
			Difference in observer threshold significant at 0·1 *per cent level,* $t = 3{\cdot}69$				
(ii)	Physically handicapped children	26	Absent	10	40	62	0·72
			Diminished	10	40		
			Normal	61	78		
			Increased	8	0		
			Much increased	15	53		
			No. of 2 *point disagreements:* 0/52				
			Difference in observer threshold significant at 5 *per cent level,* $t = 2{\cdot}25$				
(*c*)	**Triceps**						
(i)	Isle of Wight children	88	Absent	15	40	60	0·28
			Diminished	44	9		
			Normal	252	77		
			Increased	34	24		
			Much increased	7	0		
			No. of 2 *point disagreements:* 3/176				
			Difference in observer threshold significant at 0·1 *per cent level,* $t = 5{\cdot}34$				
(ii)	Physically handicapped children	26	Absent	12	67	56	0·73
			Diminished	4	0		
			Normal	66	76		
			Increased	14	0		
			Much increased	8	0		
			No. of 2 *point disagreements:* 0/52				
			Difference in observer threshold significant at 5 *per cent level,* $t = 2{\cdot}04$				
(*d*)	**Knee**						
(i)	Isle of Wight children	88	Absent	15	53	76	0·56
			Diminished	17	24		
			Normal	223	76		
			Increased	71	43		
			Much increased	24	33		
			No. of 2 *point disagreements:* 1/176				
			No difference in observer threshold.				

(*Continued overleaf*)

TABLE 8 (*continued*)

	Total no. cases	Point on scale	Times assigned	Percentage agreement	Overall percentage agreement	Product-moment correlation
(ii) Physically handicapped children	26	Absent	25	88	65	0·87
		Diminished	6	33		
		Normal	43	70		
		Increased	9	22		
		Much increased	19	53		
No. of 2 *point disagreements:* 0/51 (*one child had one leg only*). *Difference in observer threshold significant at* 10 *per cent level, t* = 1·67						
(*e*) **Ankle**						
(i) Isle of Wight children	88	Absent	14	57	63	0·36
		Diminished	23	0		
		Normal	254	79		
		Increased	51	24		
		Much increased	6	0		
No. of 2 *point disagreements:* 2/176 *Difference in observer threshold significant at* 0·5 *per cent level, t* = 2·95						
(ii) Physically handicapped children	25	Absent	20	90	62	0·80
		Diminished	6	33		
		Normal	43	65		
		Increased	5	0		
		Much increased	26	54		
No. of 2 *point disagreements:* 0/50 *Difference in observer threshold significant at* 10 *per cent level, t* = 1·96						
(*f*) **Plantar reflex**						
(i) Isle of Wight children	84	Flexor	266	84	74	0·47
		Equivocal	53	23		
		Extensor	17	47		
No. of 2 *point disagreements:* 5/168 *Difference in observer threshold significant at* 0·1 *per cent level, t* = 4·01						
(ii) Physically handicapped children	25	Flexor	34	59	55	0·66
		Equivocal	33	36		
		Extensor	31	71		
No. of 2 *point disagreements:* 1/51 *No difference in observer threshold.*						

Overall Neurological Judgement

As found in a parallel study of the reliability of the psychiatric interview with the child (Rutter and Graham 1968), overall assessments of abnormality were found to be more reliable than most individual items. Table 9 shows that the two examiners agreed quite well in their assessment of whether the child had 'no', 'dubious', 'slight' or 'marked' neurological abnormality. Nevertheless, although there was no overall difference in observer threshold as measured by the 't' test, there was a significant difference in the frequency with which the two examiners rated 'dubious' abnormality. As with individual signs, disagreement was at its highest for borderline abnormality.

Agreement on the presence or absence of an upper motor lesion was moderately good (although again there was often disagreement on 'dubious' lesions and differences on whether a definite lesion was rated 'slight' or 'marked'). Agreement on the presence or absence of a lower motor lesion was even better (r=0·92 compared with r=0·75) (Table 10).

Table 11 shows the final diagnosis made by the two examiners in their own terminology for the 27 children at the school for physically handicapped children. Ordinarily a firm diagnosis would only be made on the basis of a history and (if necessary) the results of special examinations. In this case, in order to assess the reliability of the clinical examination itself, no further information was available to the examiners. There was complete agreement (apart from minor differences in terminology) in 18 of the 27 children (67 per cent) and partial agreement in a further 6 cases (22 per cent). In only 3 cases (11 per cent) was there substantial disagreement (cases 22, 23 and 24).

In the preliminary Isle of Wight study, lesion localisation was not coded but a note on diagnosis was made systematically whenever a lesion was thought to be present. In only 2 out of the 24 cases in which either examiner made a diagnosis of definite neurological abnormality was there any disagreement on localisation of the lesion, when one examiner thought a minimal hemiparesis was present and the other did not.

TABLE 9
Inter-rater reliability on overall neurological judgement

	Total no. cases	*Point on scale*	*Times assigned*	*Percentage agreement*	*Overall percentage agreement*	*Product-moment correlation*
(i) Isle of Wight children	89	Normal	92	85	79	0·88
		Dubious abn.	45	62		
		Slight abn.	28	79		
		Marked abn.	13	92		
		No. of 2 point disagreements: 1/89				
Difference in observer threshold on rating of dubious abn. significant at 5 *per cent level, C.R.* = 2·279						
(ii) Physically handicapped children	27	Normal	8	75	70	0·80
		Dubious abn.	3	0		
		Slight abn.	6	33		
		Marked abn.	35	86		
		No. of 2 point disagreements: 2/27				
		No difference in observer threshold				

TABLE 10
Inter-rater reliability on type of lesions in physically handicapped children

		Total no. cases	*Point on scale*	*Times assigned*	*Percentage agreement*	*Overall percentage agreement*	*Product-moment correlation*
(*a*)	**Upper motor neurone lesion**	27	Normal	128	84	67	0·75
			Dubious	17	24		
			Slight	18	0		
			Marked	53	64		
		No. of 2 point disagreements: 12/108					
		No difference in observer threshold					
(*b*)	**Lower motor neurone lesion**	27	Normal	165	93	86	0·92
			Dubious	17	24		
			Slight	2	0		
			Marked	32	88		
		No. of 2 point disagreements: 2/108					
		No difference in observer threshold					

Discussion

These findings suggest that, given adequate standardisation of methods and an adequate period of training, a satisfactory level of agreement between observers can be reached on most items of the neurological examination as used with children. Nevertheless, the agreement was far from perfect even on the most objective and easily measured signs, and there was often considerable disagreement where slight deviations from normality were concerned.

Together with the rather poor reliability of some individual signs, this fact indicates that it is unwise to place too much emphasis on the presence of slight isolated abnormalities when considering the possible presence of an organic brain disorder. Our findings suggest, for example, that isolated findings of slight deviations in reflexes, muscular tone and plantar responses may not be as reliable as is sometimes thought. In particular, comparisons of the rate of these signs from one study to another are likely to be misleading in view of differences in observer threshold. Such differences persisted in our study of physically handicapped children in spite of rigorous attempts to eliminate them.

It is, of course, well known that many factors, including differences in the subject's state of relaxation, the temperature of the room and the technique that is employed, influence reflexes and tone. However, an appreciable degree of unreliability remains even when care has been taken to exclude their effects. The level of competence of the examiners may also be of importance, and it would be of considerable interest if this study were to be repeated by neurologists more practiced than ourselves.

It is notable that the greatest problems in reliability resided in items of the traditional neurological examination rather than in the developmental assessments of higher functions. It might be argued that a greater effort was made to obtain high

TABLE 11
Agreement on neurological diagnosis
(Children at school for the physically handicapped)

EXAMINER A	EXAMINER B
1. Right hemiparesis	Right hemiparesis
2. Choreo-athetosis. Bilateral spasticity	Spastic athetotic quadriplegia
3. Muscular dystrophy	Progressive muscular dystrophy
4. Mixed spastic lesion with gross tremor, probably cerebellar. ? posterior fossa lesion	Mid-line posterior fossa lesion Constructional dyspraxia.
5. Constructional dyspraxia	Constructional dyspraxia
6. Lower motor neuron paralysis of left leg — ? polio	Left leg paralysis — ? old polio
7. Spastic quadriparesis. Hydrocephalus	Hydrocephalus. Spastic diplegia
8. Nil neurological	Nil neurological
9. Lower motor neuron paralysis of left leg — ? polio	Lower motor neuron paralysis left leg — ? polio
10. ? Muscular dystrophy. Unexplained arm deformity	? Muscular dystrophy Athetoid cerebral palsy
11. Spastic quadriparesis. Nystagmus	Nystagmus with bilateral pyramidal lesion
12. Right hemiparesis	Right hemiplegia
13. Muscular dystrophy. ? Dystrophia myotonica	? Benign congenital hypotonia. ?? Dystrophia myotonica
14. Nil neurological	Nasal speech only
15. Left spastic hemiparesis	Spastic athetotic left hemiparesis
16. Progressive muscular dystrophy	Progressive muscular dystrophy
17. Nil neurological	Dubious hypotonia in upper limbs only
18. Spastic and cerebellar lesion. ? Friedreich's ataxia.	?? Friedreich's ataxia ?? Brain-stem lesion
19. Spastic and cerebellar lesion. Friedreich's ataxia	Spastic athetotic quadriplegia
20. Spastic diplegia	Spastic diplegia. Constructional dyspraxia
21. Haemangiomatosis — primarily non-neurological defect	?? Cervical pachymeningitis
22. Nil neurological	Hydrocephalus. ? Spastic monoplegia. Venous anomaly, left leg.
23. Hydrocephalus. ? spastic diplegia. Constructional dyspraxia	? Progressive muscular dystrophy? Atonic C.P. Constructional dyspraxia
24. Minimal left hemiparesis	?? Benign congenital hypotonia. ? Atonic C.P.
25. Spastic quadriplegia	Spastic athetotic quadriplegia
26. Nil neurological	Nil neurological
27. Right hemiparesis	Right hemiplegia

reliability in these less well established signs, though this did not happen as far as we are aware. However, such an objection could not apply to the study of physically handicapped children. Particular attention was paid to improving the reliability of some traditional signs (particularly deep tendon reflexes) and this had only very partial success; reliability was still only moderate and significant differences in observer threshold remained.

This study may be of relevance to a consideration of the value of the so-called 'soft' sign, a term which has been used variously to describe a sign that is difficult to elicit, a sign that occurs in relative isolation and a sign that is a reflection of a function (usually a higher cognitive function) not normally assessed in the routine neurological examination of adults. As far as the last usage is concerned, the present findings are encouraging in showing that language, speech, motor co-ordination and constructional abilities can all be assessed with good reliability; in most cases these assessments proved more reliable than assessments of slight abnormalities in reflexes and tone. These signs are clearly not 'soft' in the sense of being unreliable. Their 'softness' consists of the problems in their interpretation, an issue considered in the next chapter.

On the other hand, slight abnormalities on signs usually regarded as 'hard' have been shown to be 'soft' with regard to reliability. The adjectives 'hard' and 'soft' as used for different neurological signs are open to so much misinterpretation that they had better be dropped. What seems to be important in determining observer variation and error is not so much the level of function involved as the degree of standardisation in technique and the care taken in measurement.

Although the assessment of some slight individual abnormalities was found to be rather unreliable, it is important to note that most marked abnormalities were highly reliable, and furthermore that the disagreement on individual signs only rarely led to disagreements on the final neurological designation and diagnosis. The neurological examination is a highly efficient means of detecting moderate or marked abnormalities and it is also highly efficient in differentiating between different types of abnormalities.

Finally, it should be said that a sign upon which observers reach very high agreement is not necessarily a valuable sign when investigating neurological functions: it is highly likely that two pathologists could agree very well on measuring the weight of the brain, but it would not by any means follow that brain-weight was the best indicator, or even a useful indicator, of brain function. In the following chapter we shall consider the validity of individual neurological signs.

CHAPTER 4

The Neurological Examination: Validity

The standard neurological examination of adults has evolved gradually over the last two hundred years. For the most part, the tests now used have been based on experimentally confirmed structural and functional concepts of the central nervous system (Brain 1955). Because of this, apart from a lively controversy in recent years over the interpretation of the Babinski response (Fulton and Keller 1932, Holt 1961, McCance *et al.* 1968, Madonick 1960, Nathan and Smith 1955, Scholten 1965), there have been relatively few attempts to assess the validity of the neurological examination as used in the clinical situation. However, the fact that a particular type of brain lesion has been shown to give rise to a particular neurological sign does not necessarily indicate the validity of that sign in clinical practice. The validity of any sign is, to some extent, dependent upon the reliability with which the sign can be clinically demonstrated (see chapter 3). Furthermore, the interpretation of a sign must be based not only on the frequency with which a particular brain lesion gives rise to the sign, but also on the frequency with which the sign is found in the *absence* of that brain lesion. It is well known that many signs may be influenced by fatigue, general bodily disturbances, temperature and other 'non-neurological' circumstances in the individual and his environment. As far as children are concerned an additional, and most important, variable is the child's level of development.

Increasingly, during the last few years it has been recognised that the neurological examination of the infant and child must include a variety of developmental assessments which are not usually part of the adult examination (André-Thomas *et al.* 1960, Egan *et al.* 1969, Gesell and Amatruda 1947, Illingworth 1961, Knobloch and Pasamanick 1962, Paine and Oppé 1966, Peiper 1963, Prechtl and Beintema 1964). These modifications owe much to the work of psychologists (Bayley 1968, Griffiths 1954), but the need to relate the findings to the age and developmental level of the child (as recognised in the development of any adequate psychometric instrument) has not always been fully appreciated by clinicians. Perhaps more than anything else this has contributed to the confusion which surrounds the concept of 'minimal cerebral dysfunction' (Bax and Mac Keith 1963) and the interpretation of 'equivocal', 'minor', or 'soft' neurological signs (Bender 1956, Paine 1968, Strauss and Lehtinen 1947).

The increasing use of ancillary investigations such as echoencephalography, radioactive scanning of the brain, pneumoencephalography, and carotid and vertebral angiography could perhaps be taken as an indication that neurologists have become dissatisfied with the validity of the neurological examination. These techniques, however, are largely used to localise lesions, whereas this chapter is principally concerned with the examination as a means of determining the presence rather than the locus of a neurological disorder.

Previous Studies of the Validity of the Neurological Examination of Children

Several different approaches have been followed in previous attempts to assess the validity of various measures of neurologic function. In the infant, the greatest reliance has usually been placed on *predictive* validity, *i.e.* the extent to which neurological examination in infancy predicts neurological disorders evident in later childhood (Holden and Solomons 1962, Knobloch and Pasamanick 1967, Marstrander 1968, Prechtl 1965, Rosenblith 1966, Schulte *et al.* 1965). False negatives and false positives both occur. Assessments of the infantile neurologic examination have been few, but the examination seems to have some degree of limited predictive validity. Multiple asymmetries have a stronger association with subsequent neurological disorder than do syndromes of apathy and hyperexciteability, but the latter abnormalities are also significantly associated with later neurologic dysfunction, particularly if cases where they are due to overt disease outside the nervous system are excluded. This approach is a useful test of the validity of examinations in infancy but is of little use in the age period (5 to 15 years) covered by the present study.

A second approach has been to relate neurological signs to prenatal or perinatal complications on the assumption that such complications are associated with brain damage (Beintema 1968, Knobloch and Pasamanick 1966, Marstrander 1968, Pasamanick and Knobloch 1966, Prechtl 1965, Rodin *et al.* 1963). The results are not entirely consistent but there can be little doubt that most neurological signs are somewhat more common in children with low birth weight or born following certain prenatal complications*. Although intellectual and social differences have not always been well controlled, the results do provide circumstantial evidence that 'minor' as well as 'major' neurological signs may be due to organic brain damage. Equally, however, the finding that such signs also occur quite often in otherwise apparently normal children who experienced no prenatal or perinatal complications suggests that the association between 'brain damage' and 'minor' signs is sometimes weak. 'Minor' signs cannot be taken as a necessary indication of brain abnormality.

A recent popular approach has been to examine the pattern of intercorrelation between different neurologic signs (Beintema 1968, Klonoff *et al.* 1969, Lucas *et al.* 1965, Paine *et al.* 1968, Rodin *et al.* 1963, Schulman *et al.* 1965). The studies have been quite consistent in showing rather low correlations between the various indicators of neurologic dysfunction. Thus, co-ordination and EEG abnormalities, perceptual deficits and abnormal reflexes show little association one with another. These findings tend to negate the idea of a single syndrome of brain dysfunction, a concept with which few neurologists would have concurred. As the pattern of intercorrelations will be strongly influenced by the types of cases included in the analysis, such studies allow no conclusions on the validity of the neurological examination other than that different signs measure different types of neurologic dysfunction—a banal and unsurprising result.

A more satisfactory (but less used) test of validity is the comparison of normal and neurologically abnormal groups in relation to individual signs. Kennard (1960)

*For this purpose it is irrelevant whether a prenatal neurological disorder causes short gestation or low birth weight or whether perinatal disorders lead to neurological damage.

compared the neurologic findings for a group of 123 children who were patients in a mental hospital and 65 children in ordinary schools who were scholastically successful and without behavioural abnormality. She found that extra-ocular weakness, tremor, reflex irregularities, athetoid movements, speech difficulties, hyperactivity, left handedness, auditory dysfunction and nystagmus were all much more common among the patients, whereas dysdiadochokinesia, graphesthesia and whirling were about equally frequent in cases and in controls. In both cases and controls, most minor neurologic signs were also related to low intelligence. Unlike most other signs, visual defects, extra-ocular muscle dysfunction, reflex abnormalities, intention tremor and the Babinski response were not associated with low IQ. Klonoff *et al.* (1969) found that the abnormalities found on many neuro-psychological tests (Reitan and Heineman 1968) were related to the age and, to a lesser extent, the IQ of the children. It was probably for this reason that the tests differentiated children with chronic brain syndromes from normal controls better in the older age groups than in the younger groups. Hertzig *et al.* (1969) found that 'soft' neurologic signs were much more common in children attending a special educational facility for the 'brain injured' than in control children attending normal schools, showing that the educational designation of 'brain injury' had some meaning. However, the authors' conclusion that the signs also provided 'clear evidence of central nervous system abnormality' is dubious in that no account was taken of possible IQ differences between cases and controls. Without further evidence it cannot be assumed that both the low IQ and 'soft' signs are due to structural damage of the brain, although this may be so.

ISLE OF WIGHT STUDY

It was this last approach upon which we laid most emphasis in the present investigation. In a series of studies of educational, intellectual and neurological disorders, (Rutter *et al.* 1970) neurological examinations were carried out in the same standardised manner (see chapter 2). In each case the examiner knew only the name and age of the child (and not the reason for his selection). To avoid the possibility of 'halo' effects, all examiners were instructed to examine for each sign without reference to other findings, and to record each finding before proceeding to the examination for the next sign.

For present purposes, the children were divided into five groups:

(a) *Control group*. Initially this group consisted of 159 nine and ten year old children who had been randomly selected from the children in this age range resident on the Isle of Wight. Full neurological examinations were available for 147 of the children. The other 12 did not differ in any important respects from the 147 children, who can be regarded as representative both of the original 159 and of the total population of Isle of Wight children aged nine to ten years (Rutter *et al.* 1970). One of the 147 children was known to have epilepsy and has been excluded for present purposes. A further 21 children were also excluded because they had intellectual retardation or specific reading retardation (see below). This is, therefore, a 'super-normal' control group of children with no known neurologic or cognitive disorder.

It might have been preferable to have used a truly random control group, in order to provide a valid picture of neurological abnormality in the general population. For this reason the results were initially analysed for the original control group before any exclusions. In all cases the findings were closely similar to those for the 'super-normal' group, the rate of abnormalities never being more than two per cent different. Nevertheless, as our main interest in this context was the frequency of individual signs in children for whom there was no suspicion of neurological abnormality (because of epilepsy or educational failure), results are given in the Tables with respect to the 'super-normal' control group.

(b) *Children with intellectual retardation.* In 1964, all nine and ten year old Isle of Wight children were given a battery of group tests of intelligence and educational attainment (Rutter *et al.* 1970). Children scoring at least 2 standard deviations below the mean on these tests were seen individually and given 4 sub-tests of the Wechsler Intelligence Scale for Children (similarities, vocabulary, block design and object assembly). The intellectually retarded group consisted of all the nine and ten year olds with WISC IQs of 51 to 85 (based on the 4 sub-tests), after exclusion of those children known to have neurological disorder or epilepsy, leaving a total of 71.

(c) *Children with specific reading retardation.* The nine and ten year old children described above, who were seen individually as a result of poor performance on group tests, were also given the Neale Analysis of Reading Ability test. The level at which a child should be expected to read on the basis of his chronological age and intelligence can be determined by the use of a multiple regression formula (Yule 1967). Using this technique, specific reading retardation was defined as an attainment on either reading accuracy or comprehension which was 24 months or more below the level predicted on the basis of each child's age and short WISC IQ. Again, children with any neurological disorder or epilepsy were excluded, leaving a total of 108 children.

(d) *Children with neurological disorder.* These children were identified as a result of multiple screening procedures (see chapter 6) and in all cases the diagnosis was confirmed by a clinical history from the parents (obtained at an interview) and by an individual neurological examination. Nearly all these children had obvious motor disabilities. In the absence of a history indicating neurological disorder, isolated signs were not sufficient for such a diagnosis. This group included children with disorders both above and below the brain stem, but excluded all children with a short WISC IQ of 50 or less. In order to control for age differences the group was split into 2 parts: (i) a 'cohort' group of 22 children aged 9 to 12 years (and thus comparable in age to the other groups, and (ii) a 'non-cohort' group of 20 children aged 5 to 8 years or 13 to 15 years.

(e) *Children with epilepsy.* These children were selected in the same way as those with neurological disorder. The group included all children who had had a fit in the year prior to the study, and also all children who had had a fit since the age of 5 years and who were still taking anticonvulsants regularly although they had not had a fit in the previous year (see chapter 8). There were no children with a short WISC IQ of 50 or less and all children with a neurological disorder apart from their epilepsy were excluded (such children were included in the neurological disorder group). Again the group was subdivided into a 'cohort' group of 32 children aged 9 to 12 years and a 'non-cohort' group of 29 children aged 5 to 8 years or 13 to 15 years.

Although each group was defined in terms of one particular test or examination, all groups received all the same assessments (namely neurological examination, intellectual testing and measurement of reading ability).

The Value of the Individual Sign

For each individual sign, the frequency of its occurrence in each of the above groups was determined. The validity of any sign as an indicator of neurological disorder was judged by the strength of its association with neurological disorder. Thus a 'good' sign should rarely occur in the absence of any neurological condition and should usually occur in its presence.

Put in operational terms this means that for a sign to be a good indicator, it should have a very high frequency in the neurological group (*i.e.*, it should give rise to very few false negatives) and a very low frequency in the control group (*i.e.*, it should give rise to very few false positives). If in addition the sign is frequent among children with intellectual retardation (but with no known neurological disorder) it may be concluded that the clinical significance of the sign can only be judged after the child's developmental level is taken into account.

Laterality of Hand, Eye and Foot

It is generally said that poorly established, inconsistent or mixed laterality of hand and foot is more commonly found in children with almost any variety of organic brain syndrome than in the general population (Paine and Oppé 1966), and that it is particularly associated with developmental dyslexia (Critchley 1964) and developmental disorders of speech and language (Ingram 1959*b*). Furthermore, it has been suggested that incomplete or bilateral cerebral dominance is the cause of various disturbances in the development of motor or intellectual functions in childhood—a suggestion which, however, remains largely conjectural (Benson and Geschwind 1968).

The present findings (see Table 12*a*) show that left handedness and left footedness are significantly more common in children with neurological disorder. Obviously early paralysis or damage to the preferred limb will shift handedness or footedness. However, there was no increase in left eyedness; eye preference has only a weak association with hand and foot preference and it has been said that in most individuals the preferred eye will be the one with the least refractive error (Benson and Geschwind 1968). It is clear, too, that the frequency of left handedness in the general population is too high for it to be a very useful indication of neurological disorder. Of every 1,000 children in the child population about 41 will be left handed, and, assuming a rate of neurological disorder of 5 per 1,000, only just over 1 of these 41 will have neurological disorder.

While left handedness was associated with neurological disorder, inconsistent handedness and footedness were not. This finding, however, is not of much help in deciding whether incomplete cerebral dominance is associated with neurological disorder, as there is at best only a weak association between the preferred hand and the dominant hemisphere for speech in left handed children (Zangwill 1962).

Inconsistent handedness was not particularly associated with specific reading retardation. Although this finding runs counter to much clinical teaching it should be noted that all epidemiologically based studies have been in agreement in failing to find any significant excess of left handedness or mixed handedness in children with reading difficulties (Belmont and Birch 1965, Douglas *et al.* 1967, Malmquist 1958, Rutter *et al.* 1970).

Whether or not left handedness and mixed handedness are more frequent in children with delayed language development remains uncertain. While clinic studies strongly suggest the existence of a meaningful association between inconsistent or poorly established hand preference and language delay, so far there have been no adequate epidemiological studies.

TABLE 12
Comparison between groups on neurological signs

	Control	*Intellectually retarded*	*Reading retarded*	*Neurological*		*Epileptic*	
				Cohort	*Non-cohort*	*Cohort*	*Non-cohort*
	%	%	%	%	%	%	%
(*a*) **Laterality of hand, eye and foot**							
HAND Right	81	72	71	68	70	91	69
Inconsistent	15	21	19	10	5	9	6
Left	4	7	10	23*	25**	0	24**
FOOT Right	88	87	84	70	62	88	76
Inconsistent	2	5	5	10	0	6	3
Left	10	8	11	20	38*	6	21
EYE Right	65	55	59	46	53	69	59
Inconsistent	6	12	14	19	5	0	7
Left	29	32	27	36	42	31	35
HAND-FOOT Inconsistent laterality	19	25	24	30	25	16	10
HAND-EYE Inconsistent laterality	44	59	50	64	54	37	34
Total no. children	125	71	107	22	20	32	29

(*Continued*)

TABLE 12 (*continued*)

	Control	Intellectually retarded	Reading retarded	Neurological		Epileptic	
				Cohort	Non-cohort	Cohort	Non-cohort
	%	%	%	%	%	%	%
(*b*) **Developmental abnormalities**							
Motor impersistence (score of 2 or more)	2	23***	20**	(71)*	—	(29)	—
Oseretsky test (1 S.D. or more below the mean)	19	52***	35**	(100)*	—	(57)	—
Poor right-left differentiation	29	68***	64***	(57)	—	(100)*	—
Constructional difficulties	5	35***	18**	32***	40***	19*	38***
Limb 'dyspraxia'	1	16***	8	55***	35***	6	14**
Articulation defect	5	17*	20*	24	15	9	11
Speech complexity	6	32***	20**	28**	30**	6	7
Adequacy of description	2	20***	12**	32***	25***	9	25***
Mirror movements	14	24*	24*	24	35*	6	16
(*c*) **Cranial signs**							
Nystagmus	3	10*	5	14*	5	0	3
Strabismus	10	7	5	19	15	16	10
Facial power	4	5	7	24**	40***	6	7
Facial asymmetry	8	6	9	19	37**	13	13
Tongue power	0	1	1	5	10*	0	0
Tongue side to side	4	4	3	23**	50***	3	7
Licking top lip	6	5	6	23*	32**	6	14
Skull asymmetry	9	10	14	20	18	7	7
(*d*) **Co-ordination and power**							
Limb asymmetry	1	7*	2	35***	18**	0	0
Threading beads	7	7	8	41***	50***	6	3
Holding pencil	1	1	1	5	20***	0	7
Finger-thumb	4	10	11	79***	65***	12*	17*
Finger-nose	8	5	5	45***	40***	0	14
Kicking	0	3	1	50***	53***	3	0
Throwing	0	1	0	14***	27***	3	0
Hopping	0	4	4	63***	60***	3	3
Walking	0	1	2	62***	70***	3	0
Cerebellar dysfunction	4	10	6	14	10	0	3
Abnormal power arms	2	3	5	50***	50***	3	3
Abnormal power legs	1	3	3	73***	53***	0	3
Tremor	10	8	7	10	15	6	3
Total no. children	125	71	107	22	20	32	29

(*Continued overleaf*)

TABLE 12 (*continued*)

	Control	Intellectually retarded	Reading retarded	Neurological		Epileptic	
				Cohort	Non-cohort	Cohort	Non-cohort
	%	%	%	%	%	%	%
(*e*) **Increased tone**							
Right arm	3	3	5	41***	50***	6	3
Left arm	3	3	5	45***	55***	6	3
Right leg	4	3	5	64***	45***	0	7
Left leg	4	3	5	68***	63***	0	4
(*f*) **Increased reflexes**							
Supinator: Right	8	9	11	18	30*	13	6
Left	7	6	8	27*	30**	6	10
Biceps: Right	6	11	8	27*	40**	6	13
Left	6	9	7	27*	35**	6	10
Triceps: Right	7	6	7	27*	25*	6	7
Left	8	6	6	36**	25	9	3
Knee: Right	11	19	19	28	45**	12	10
Left	13	19	18	37*	43**	12	10
Ankle: Right	6	11	10	28**	30**	15	24*
Left	6	11	11	37***	42***	19	20
Plantar response (equivocal or extensor)	12	22	13	61***	68***	6	12
(*g*) **Decreased reflexes**							
Supinator: Right	33	15*	13*	23	25	25	14*
Left	32	17*	12*	23	35	28	13*
Biceps: Right	33	25	20	14	30	22	7*
Left	32	25	21	19	45	22	7*
Triceps: Right	22	11	7*	19	25	13	10
Left	21	11	7*	19	35	13	14
Knee: Right	11	4	4	23	20	9	7
Left	10	2	2	18	16	6	3
Ankle: Right	13	10	9	19	20	9	7
Left	11	11	9	19	16	9	10
Total no. children	125	71	107	22	20	32	29

Significantly different from control group: * p. < ·05; ** p. < ·01; *** p. < ·001.

( ) = *Numbers lower than column total.*

N.B. In all cases the percentages refer to mild and severe abnormalties pooled.

Developmental Abnormalities

Table 12*b* shows the frequency of various developmental abnormalities in each of the groups. All these signs concern delays in the development of normal functions (Rutter 1967, 1968) rather than the emergence of neurological features which are abnormal in themselves. During infancy the child cannot speak, has poor motor co-ordination, cannot tell his right from left and is unable to reproduce geometric shapes, but all these functions are present in the normal adolescent. The development of these functions follows an orderly pattern and is related to the continuing growth and maturation of the brain. Developmental disorders are all much more common in children with neurological disorders than in the control group children, but they are also nearly as frequent in intellectually retarded children as they are in children with neurological disorder.

In these respects the intellectually retarded child behaves like a much younger normal child and developmental functions are often related as much to a child's 'mental age' as to his chronological age. Developmental delays may be due to damage to the brain but may also be associated with intellectual immaturity. The clinical significance of the delay can only be assessed in relation to the child's chronological and mental age. Where developmental delays occur in an older child in the presence of normal intelligence, the delay is much more likely to indicate neurological disorder.

However, it is important to note that these disorders may occur in isolation in children without apparent cerebral disease and of normal intelligence (Rutter *et al.* 1970), as is indicated by the frequency of the disorders in the control group and in the reading retarded group. The aetiology of these developmental disorders is not known but it has been suggested that they may be related to an incomplete or delayed maturation of the brain (British Medical Journal 1962). Different parts of the brain normally develop at different rates and at different times (Falkner 1966, Marshall 1968, Minkowski 1967) and it is possible that the developmental disorders are due to an unusually delayed development of just one part of the brain in the same way that some otherwise completely normal children are exceptionally slow in cutting their teeth or are unusually late in reaching puberty (Rutter *et al.* 1970). It is evident that these functions cannot be considered as necessarily indicating brain damage, although they may do so.

In assessing the significance of a developmental delay, the degree of impairment in the developmental function must be considered. A three year old will not have a fully adequate command of language, but some language is to be expected and it is therefore necessary to measure how much language he possesses in assessing this function. An attempt was made to do this by the clinical measurement of the child's speech complexity, adequacy of descriptive language, motor co-ordination (limb 'dyspraxia' is used here to describe co-ordination difficulties which are not due to paresis, abnormalities of tone or tremor) and constructional difficulties (see chapters 2 and 5). The clinical assessment took into account the child's age but not his IQ (which was not known to the examiner).

The necessity of quantifying and standardising the assessment of developmental delays mean that the neurological examination takes on some of the features of a psychometric test. Indeed, it is in the developmental field that the psychologist has most to offer. One of the advantages of a psychometric approach is that it is a straightforward matter to determine the degree of impairment which provides the best differentiation of groups: a 1 standard deviation below the mean cut-off point was used in Table 12*b* but it can be seen from Table 13 that a 2 standard deviation below the mean cut-off point provides a better differentiation. Tests of motor co-ordination, motor impersistence and right-left differentiation were used in the study, and other psychometric measures of developmental function are available or could be developed (see chapter 5).

Of all the studies of developmental signs, mirror movements measured in the manner described by Fog and Fog (1963) were the least useful as an indication of neurological disorder, although the pattern of associations was similar to that found with the other developmental signs.

Cranial Signs

Cranial signs followed a different pattern (see Table 12*c*). On all items, abnormalities were more common in the neurological group than in the control group, but there was no marked increase of abnormalities in the intellectually retarded group or reading retarded group. On two items (strabismus and facial asymmetry) there was an increased rate of abnormality in the epileptics but the difference from the control group fell well short of statistical significance.

There were three main problems in the use of cranial signs as indicators of neurological disorder. Some of the signs may be due to non-neurological disease; for example, nystagmus may be due to amblyopia coming on in early life, to labyrinthine disease, to weakness of the ocular muscles, to familial factors or to a variety of other abnormalities. Although the examiners were asked to note in each case the nature of the nystagmus and to take this into account in making their overall neurological diagnosis, the type of nystagmus was not coded. Similarly, in the case of strabismus only a crude judgement of 'absent', 'latent' or 'overt' was coded, although the examiner was always expected to determine the nature of the strabismus, whether paralytic or non-paralytic and, if paralytic, of which muscle or muscles. Thus, the coding system used (because of the relatively small number of cases with nystagmus or strabismus) underestimates the amount of diagnostic information which may be obtained by a careful and skilled neurological assessment.

A second difficulty stems from the pooling of mild and severe abnormalities. As discussed below in relation to Table 13, severe abnormalities are quite rare in the control group but still relatively common in the neurological disorder group. Not much reliance can be placed on the clinical significance of very mild abnormalities, but severe abnormalities are quite good indicators of neurological disorder.

Thirdly, the poor validity of mild abnormalities is probably due, in part, to their poor reliability. It was shown in the last chapter that two examiners agreed much more often on severe abnormalities than they did on mild ones. If two examiners cannot agree on their clinical assessment of whether there is a mild degree of skull asymmetry, it is very unlikely that valid differences between the groups will be found. In fact there were only small and non-significant differences between the control group and the neurological group in the frequency of mild skull asymmetry, but all the children with marked skull asymmetry were found in the neurological group.

Co-ordination and Power

The pattern of findings for tests of co-ordination and power (other than tremor) were closely similar to those for cranial signs, except that many of the abnormalities occurred less frequently in the control group and were thereby better indicators of neurological disorder. As before, severe abnormalities are much better indicators than mild abnormalities (see Tables 12*d* and 13).

Even mild abnormalities differentiated the neurological and control groups quite well. Nevertheless, the presence of a single mild abnormality of co-ordination or power is, in most cases, more likely to be associated with normality than with neurological abnormality. Certain signs which never occurred in the control group (for example, abnormalities of throwing, hopping and walking) are better indicators of neurological disorder.

Limb asymmetry was rarely found in the control group but occurred in one in four of the children with neurological disorder. Inequality in the size or length of limbs, particularly if marked, is a fair indication of possible neurological abnormality, and an assessment of asymmetry forms an essential part of the neurological examination of children. Nevertheless, it is important to bear in mind the difficulties in reliably assessing small differences in the size of limbs; some difference in size is normal if one limb is exercised more than the other (as in a child who plays a lot of tennis).

Tremor was of no value as an indicator of neurological disorder.

Tone

The findings on tone followed a closely similar pattern to those for co-ordination and power (see Table 12*e*).

Reflexes

Increases in any of the tendon reflexes were significantly more common in the neurological group than in the control group. The usefulness of an increased tendon reflex as an indicator of neurological disorder was much less than that of altered tone, power or co-ordination because of the relatively high frequency with which increased reflexes were found in the control group; in all cases, however, the reflexes in control children were only slightly increased and a marked increase was a very strong indicator of neurological disorder (see Table 12*f* and *g*, Table 13).

With diminished reflexes the pattern was different. In the case of upper limb tendon reflexes, diminished reflexes were, in fact, slightly (but not significantly) more common in the controls than in the children with neurological disorder. Furthermore, diminished reflexes were in some cases significantly less frequent in children with intellectual retardation, specific reading retardation or epilepsy than in controls. These groups were ones with some tendency to an increased rate of developmental motor abnormalities (see Table 12*b*, *c* and *d*). The most likely explanation of this phenomenon is that children with intellectual retardation, reading retardation or epilepsy have a tendency to rather brisker reflexes than normal children, but that this tendency was concealed by errors in the examiners' concepts of normality of reflex activity which tended to include as 'normal' reflexes which were unduly easily elicited and to rate as 'diminished' normal reflexes which were rather difficult to elicit.

Equivocal plantar responses occurred too often in the control group for this sign to be of much use as an indicator of neurological disorder.

Marked Neurological Abnormalities

Isolated mild abnormalities found on a single examination are of little clinical significance. However, as shown in Table 13, which includes only a representative selection of signs, marked neurological abnormalities of almost any kind were fairly good indicators of neurological disorder. The rarity of their occurrence in the control group implies that, even in isolation, a single marked abnormality should be taken as a pointer towards probable neurological disorder. This does not apply, however, to signs like strabismus which may be due to non-neurological as well as neurological disease or damage, nor does it apply to developmental abnormalities which must still be assessed in relation to the child's age and intelligence. It also does not apply to absent tendon reflexes, probably because in some cases reflexes were present but could not be elicited because of the child's lack of co-operation or for other extraneous reasons.

In view of controversies over the meaning of the Babinski response it was noteworthy that none of the intellectually retarded children and only two of the controls showed a definite extensor plantar response, confirming earlier views that this is a fairly good (but not pathognomonic) sign of neurological disorder (Holt 1961). Like other signs, however, caution should be expressed in any neurological judgement based on its presence as an isolated phenomenon.

TABLE 13
Marked neurological abnormalities

	Control	*Intellectually retarded*	*Neurological*	
			Cohort	*Non-cohort*
	%	%	%	%
Motor impersistence (score of 5 +)	0	1	(72)	—
Oseretsky (2 S.D. below mean)	5	26	(100)	—
Overt strabismus	2	4	14	15
Definite facial weakness	1	1	10	5
Tongue side to side (marked abn.)	0	0	14	30
Threading beads (marked abn.)	0	0	9	25
Finger-thumb (marked abn.)	0	0	23	15
Marked limb asymmetry	0	0	25	12
Hopping (marked abn.)	0	1	47	45
Marked weakness legs	0	0	41	32
Right supinator jerk (marked increase)	0	0	9	20
Right supinator jerk (absent)	7	0	9	5
Right knee jerk (marked increase)	0	0	14	25
Right knee jerk (absent)	1	2	23	10
Right leg (marked hypertonia)	0	0	5	15
Right leg (marked hypotonia)	0	0	18	10
Definite extensor plantar	1	0	42	36
No. of children	125	71	22	20

( ) = *Numbers lower than column total*

The State of the Child

It was not possible in the present study to examine the effect of the state of the child and the circumstances of the examination on the assessment of neurological abnormalities; Beintema (1968) and others have shown how important the infant's state is in relation to the neonatal neurological examination. Because of the changes necessary in the infant's adjustment to extra-uterine life and because of the physiological instability during this period, neurological examinations carried out in the first two or three days of life give much less valid results than those carried out at one week of age. Such variation is less likely to be important in the older child. Nevertheless, it is probable that, as in the infant, ambiant temperature, the degree of alertness, the amount of fatigue or nervous tension and whether or not there has been recent exercise might influence the assessment of tone and reflexes. Such factors require further study.

The Localisation of the Lesion

The above comparisons were valuable in assessing the utility of different signs as indicators of neurological disorder. They provided no direct information on the associations between signs and brain lesions and they told us nothing of the nature or location of lesions associated with different signs. This can only be provided by experimental ablation studies, by correlating neurological findings in life with post-mortem studies of the brain and spinal cord, or by the use of special techniques (such as cortical stimulation during craniotomy). These studies have been carried out with respect to many of the standard items in the adult neurological examination but there have been virtually no studies of this kind in relation to developmental or other signs peculiar to the neurological examination as adapted for use with infants and children.

The present findings are to some extent dependent upon the types of conditions included in the group of neurological disorders. There were very few children with cerebellar disorders, so that most cerebellar signs were in the 'possible or slight' category which proved to be a poor indicator of neurological disorder. The only child with marked cerebellar signs was in the neurological group by virtue of other neurological abnormalities.

Patterns of Signs

In ordinary clinical practice more emphasis is placed on the presence of meaningful patterns of abnormal signs than on the presence of isolated abnormalities. The present findings allow some estimate of the validity of this approach, at least in relation to the more common syndromes. Using the total group of children with neurological disorder it was possible to determine how often signs were associated one with another and in what pattern or patterns (Table 14). This neurological group included not only children with cerebral palsy (a restriction which might artificially inflate association because of the exclusion—by definition—of patterns which did not fit the concept) but all children (whose IQ was at least 51) with a definite neurological disorder, regardless of the nature of the disorder or whether it matched a recognised syndrome.

TABLE 14
Tone-power-reflex pattern in children with neurological disorder

	(*a*) *LEGS*		(*b*) *ARMS*	
	Observed frequency	*Expected frequency*	*Observed frequency*	*Expected frequency*
Reflex increase alone	4		7	
Reflex decrease alone	3		7	
Hypertonia alone	5		2	
Hypotonia alone	2		3	
Weakness alone	1		1	
Extensor plantar alone	2			
Reflex increase + weakness	1		1	
Reflex decrease + weakness	1		0	
Reflex increase + extensor plantar	0			
Reflex decrease + extensor plantar	0			
Reflex increase + hypertonia	2		1	
Reflex increase + hypotonia	0		0	
Reflex decrease + hypertonia	0		0	
Reflex decrease + hypotonia	0		3	
Weakness + hypertonia	2		2	
Weakness + hypotonia	0		2	
Weakness + extensor plantar	2			
Hypertonia + extensor plantar	3			
Hypotonia + extensor plantar	0			
Hypertonia + extensor plantar + weakness	4			
Hypotonia + extensor plantar + weakness	0			
Reflex increase + hypertonia + extensor plantar	2			
Reflex decrease + hypertonia + extensor plantar	0			
Reflex increase + hypertonia + weakness	1		11*	1·72
Reflex decrease + hypertonia + weakness	0		0	
Reflex increase + hypotonia + weakness	3		3	
Reflex decrease + hypotonia + weakness	12*	2·04	13*	2·58
Reflex increase + hypertonia + weakness + extensor plantar	12*	1·51		
Reflex increase + hypotonia + weakness + extensor plantar	0			
Reflex decrease + hypertonia + weakness + extensor plantar	0			
Reflex decrease + hypotonia + weakness + extensor plantar	2			
None	19		28	
TOTAL	83		84	

Significantly different: * p. < ·01

Table 14*b* shows the observed and expected frequency (calculated from the product of the separate frequencies of individual signs) of different patterns of signs for the upper limb. Whereas it was not uncommon to get some signs (especially increased or decreased reflexes) in isolation, two combinations of signs (reflex increase and hypertonia and weakness, and reflex decrease and hypotonia and weakness) were very common and occurred at many times the frequency expected if the associations between signs were only at the chance level. These two patterns are the well recognised syndromes of upper motor neurone disorder and lower motor neurone disorder. Weakness very rarely occurred as an isolated phenomenon (1 out of 33 instances) and in most cases (24 out of 33) weakness was present in one or other of these two syndromes. Hypertonia was usually associated with hyperreflexia and hypotonia with hyporeflexia but alterations of tone in either direction did occur (in isolation or with weakness) without any reflex change. Furthermore, there were three children in whom reflex increase was associated with a decrease of tone (and weakness). The opposite combination (reflex decrease and tone increase) never occurred.

There were similar findings for tone-power-reflex patterns in the lower limbs, except that (as expected from clinical teaching) the upper motor neurone pattern usually included an extensor plantar response as well as hyperreflexia, hypertonia and weakness. Again both patterns occurred at many times the frequency expected by chance. Although an extensor plantar response was usually associated with hyperreflexia and hypertonia, there were two instances in which it was associated with hyporeflexia and hypotonia (and weakness). Cerebral palsy sometimes occurs in a hypotonic form (Paine and Oppé 1966).

These findings strongly support the validity of these patterns of signs, although they also emphasise that not infrequently the pattern is incomplete and occasionally appears paradoxical. The number of children with nystagmus or intention tremor was too small to examine other possible patterns (*e.g.*, cerebellar dysfunction). Pattern analyses of this kind cannot determine the mechanisms involved in the production of patterns.

Aggregation of Neurological Signs

In clinical neurology, the appraisal of individual signs and of the ways in which they occur together forms the basis for diagnosis. However, particularly in relation to equivocal or 'soft' neurological signs, there has been a tendency to produce an aggregate 'score', the assumption being that although no one equivocal sign is very significant, a child with a lot of signs is more likely to have neurological disorder (Hertzig *et al.* 1969). It was possible to test this assumption from present findings.

A composite neurological score for each child was obtained by calculating the number of signs found to be present, giving a weight of one point to each and then summing the individual weights. In order not to weight any particular aspect of the examination too heavily, certain signs were considered together so that even if biceps, triceps and supinator jerks on one side were all increased, a score of 1 was obtained if this was the only abnormality. The score thereby obtained had a range of 0 to 30.

It can be seen from Table 15 that apart from one child whose total composite neurological score (T.C.N.S.) was 9, all the control children scored 7 points or less, with a mean score of 2·6. It may seem rather surprising that children in the general population without known neurological or cognitive disorder should score so highly. However, as shown in earlier tables, most of these abnormalities were minor variations in reflex or co-ordination or tremor.

By contrast, the mean T.C.N.S. of the cohort neurological children was 11·7, the difference from the control group being highly significant (p. < ·001). Only one of the 22 children had a T.C.N.S. of less than 5 and 15 of the 22 children with neurological disorders had a score of 8 or more (*i.e.*, greater than all but one of the 125 control children). Clearly there is some clinical meaning in the total number of neurological signs present in any one child.

However, the neurological and control groups represent extremes in this context and it would be very surprising if there were not a difference in score between the two groups. More important, perhaps, is the fact that a substantial minority of the children with neurological disorder had low scores. Obviously some signs have more significance than others and this important difference is lost in the use of a composite score (although a score using different weights for each item could be devised).

TABLE 15
Total composite neurological score

T.C.N.S.	*Controls* %	*Intellectually retarded* %	*Reading retarded* %	*Neurological cohort* %	*Epileptic cohort* %
0 — 4	84	80	81	5	75
5 — 7	15	13	18	27	19
8 — 10	1	4	1	10	3
11 or more	0	3	0	59	3
Total no.	125	71	108	22	32
Mean score	2·64	2·97	2·65	11·73*	2·78

Significantly different from control group: * p. < ·001.

If the T.C.N.S. is to be of any use as a screening instrument, it must not only differentiate children with obvious handicapping neurological disorder from normal children, but it must also differentiate those with minimal and less obvious disorders; it does not seem to do this very satisfactorily. There were no significant differences between the intellectually retarded and controls, reading retarded and controls, or epileptics and controls, even though many people would regard these conditions as indicating possible 'minimal cerebral dysfunction'. Although there were a few more children with very high scores in these groups than among the controls, too many children had very low scores for the T.C.N.S. to be of much use as a screening instrument.

A very high number of minor neurological signs makes it likely that the child has some kind of neurological disorder, but a moderate number of minor signs is quite compatible with normality. It is more important to distinguish which signs are abnormal and in this connection neurological judgement based on a knowledge of the significance of each type of abnormality is more important than a single sum of the number of abnormalities.

Special Tests

Special tests such as the electroencephelogram (EEG) or pneumoencephelogram (AEG) were not used in the Isle of Wight study. However questions of their reliability and validity arise in exactly the same way as for the clinical neurological examination itself. Other investigations have shown the considerable problems in drawing clinical implications from EEG findings (Ellingson 1954, Foley 1968, Paine *et al.* 1968, Schulman *et al.* 1965) or from AEG findings (Storey 1966). In spite of this, these problems (with regard to the clinical examination or to special tests) are largely ignored in the standard text books, and neither 'reliability' nor 'validity' is to be found even in the index of *Neurological Examination of Children* by Paine and Oppé (1966).

'Soft' Neurological Signs

The findings discussed in this chapter and the previous chapter may now be brought together in order to arrive at some assessment of the clinical significance and meaning of so-called 'soft' signs.

Such signs seem to fall into three distinct groups, the pooling of which can only lead to confusion.

The first group consists of signs of developmental delay in one or more functions, such as speech, language, motor co-ordination, perception, right-left differentiation, adventitious motor overflow ('mirror movements'), or extinction to double simultaneous tactile stimulation. For the most part these signs can be quite reliably identified and quantified. They are not equivocal signs (in the sense of uncertainty about their presence or absence) nor do they necessarily concern minor abnormalities. A child who is without speech can scarcely be regarded as having a minor sign of abnormality. However, the interpretation of such signs is entirely dependent upon the assessment of the degree of impairment in relation to the child's chronological and mental age. These functions follow a characteristic course of development in the normal child, and this course may be delayed (and sometimes distorted) by intellectual retardation, specific maturational disorders, organic brain disorders or any combination of these. The difficulties are not solely related to mental age in that there may still be gross delays due to organic brain disorders even after mental age has been taken into account (Cohen *et al.* 1967). Delays in some developmental functions have only a weak association with neurological disorder (Rutter *et al.* 1966, Stemmer 1964), whereas others have much stronger associations. The strength of neurological associations with each developmental disorder can only be determined by considering each disorder separately and this has not often been done. Differentiating pure maturational delays from delays due to neurological disorder can be extremely difficult or even impossible in the individual case.

The second group of 'soft' signs consists of those due to both neurological and non-neurological factors. Nystagmus and strabismus both fall into this category. In many cases a careful delineation of the nature of the sign should allow a diagnosis of the likely cause. Thus, the type of nystagmus due to amblyopia is different from that due to labyrinthine disease and both differ from that due to cerebellar dysfunction. With some of these signs most cases are due to neurological disorder, with others (*e.g.* tremor) only a few. The significance of each sign must be determined separately for each case on the basis of the detailed characteristics of the abnormality and its association with other abnormalities.

The third group of signs consists of slight abnormalities which are difficult to detect. These are often minor examples of classical neurological signs such as slight asymmetries of tone or reflexes, just perceptible hemiparesis, minimal athetosis and mild asymmetry of skull or limbs. The 'softness' of these signs resides in the demonstrated unreliability of judgements concerning their presence. If there is doubt as to whether the abnormality is truly present there will be corresponding doubt as to the significance of the supposed abnormality. Little significance can be attached to the presence of isolated minor signs which have been shown to be present on only one occasion. If the signs have been found repeatedly on independent examinations by more than one physician the likelihood that the abnormality, although slight, is truly present is greatly increased. In such cases the sign can probably be interpreted in much the same way as more obvious abnormalities of the same kind, provided that the abnormality falls outside the range of normal variation. A slight difference in strength and muscle bulk between the right and left arm is normal if the preferred arm is the one that is slightly larger and stronger. If, however, the preferred arm is the smaller or weaker one, then the finding probably indicates neurological disorder.

'Minimal Brain Damage' or 'Minimal Cerebral Dysfunction'

Conclusions regarding the validity of concepts of a syndrome of 'minimal brain damage' follow from the above remarks concerning 'soft' signs and from the numerous studies which have shown that there are not one, but many syndromes of brain damage. To put all the different syndromes into the same ragbag is to lose valuable information. As far as possible, more precise diagnoses should be made. The group of developmental disorders may be subdivided according to which function is affected: developmental disorders of speech and language (Ingram 1959*b*, 1968) involving articulation ('dyslalia'), spoken language ('developmental expressive aphasia') and/or language comprehension ('developmental receptive aphasia') constitute one sub-group (which will require further subdivision in the light of further knowledge); developmental disorders of co-ordination constitute another which may be termed 'developmental clumsiness' (Reuben and Bakwin 1968), 'the clumsy child syndrome' (Gubbay *et al.* 1965, Walton *et al.* 1962), or 'congenital maladroitness' (Ford 1960); specific reading retardation (Rutter *et al.* 1970) which includes specific developmental dyslexia (Critchley 1964) is a third. In addition there are a number of other less common or less well-defined disorders. An appreciable overlap exists between the different developmental disorders and there is a need for some such category as 'developmental disorder—mixed type'.

Where there are persisting and reliably demonstrated slight signs of a mild hemiparesis or athetosis it would seem better to classify the disorder as cerebral palsy (or some more precise designation where appropriate). Similarly, where some identifiable aetiology (such as hydrocephalus or craniostenosis) can be shown, the disorder should be so classified.

Inevitably there will remain some cases which show undoubted organic brain dysfunction of a kind not readily classified under any of the previous headings. Some general heading may still be required for this group but it should only be used where a more precise (and, therefore, more informative) term cannot be applied.

The term 'minimal brain damage' should not be used for categories of behaviour thought to be due to brain damage but in which there is no direct evidence of neurological disorder (Rutter 1968). These should be classified according to the type of psychiatric abnormality shown and not according to speculations about possible aetiology.

CHAPTER 5

Psychometric Assessment of Neurological Characteristics

Assessment of Developmental Abnormalities

The clinical significance of delays in the development of normal speech, language, motor or perceptual functions can only be assessed in relation to the child's age. Quantitative rather than qualitative judgements are required, and the need for some means of scoring neurological assessment has led psychologists to devise tests which attempt to measure developmental functions. A few of these 'Psychological Tests' were included in the Isle of Wight study, our choice of tests being determined by their suitability for 9 and 10 year old children (the age-group used in all our surveys except that of neuro-epileptic disorders), their relevance to educational performance, and the need for little apparatus and little time. The last considerations might not be important in a clinical setting, but they were crucial for a large-scale survey involving children in widely scattered locations.

ISLE OF WIGHT STUDY

The reliability of these tests was assessed by re-examining some of the children within a month of the first assessment. The children constituted a sub-sample of those in a randomly chosen control group from the general population and those suspected of intellectual or educational retardation. Because the reliability studies included few children with marked deviance, they provided a harsh measure of reliability for tests primarily designed to pick out deviant children rather than to differentiate within the normal distribution. In each case, the psychologist seeing the child knew only his name and age and the two examinations were always carried out by different psychologists.

Validity was assessed (a) by determining the level of agreement between the psychometric test scores and the clinical assessment of similar or related functions, and (b) by determining if children with different neuro-educational disorders differed in their performance on the tests. The tests do not differ qualitatively from many of the individual items in the neurological examination described in chapter 2. The work of the psychologist, in this context, differs from that of the neurologist more in approach and in method than in content.

The groups used for this purpose were: (a) a randomly selected control group* of 9 and 10 year old children; (b) 9 and 10 year old children with intellectual retardation; (c) 9 and 10 year old children with specific reading retardation; (d) 9 and 10

*In this chapter, unlike the last, the full control group was used in order to provide adequate normative data. The findings for the 'super-normal' group (which excluded children with intellectual or educational retardation) were given in chapter 4.

year old children with neurological disorder; and (e) 9 and 10 year old children with epilepsy. These groups were defined in chapter 4. In the last two groups, only those suspected of possible intellectual or educational retardation were seen and the numbers were too small for some purposes.

In order to examine the utility of quantified measures of developmental functions, the findings for two of the tests used (motor co-ordination and motor impersistence) are described in some detail.

A Short Form of the Oseretsky Test of Motor Proficiency

The Oseretsky Test of Motor Proficiency was primarily intended as an index of motor development (Lassner 1948). Oseretsky (1931) devised an 85 item scale which was intended to give not only a general motor age but also a profile of specific strengths or weaknesses in various areas of motor competency. These areas were not empirically defined and, not surprisingly, factor analytic studies (Vandenberg 1964) have failed to establish their independence, although the scale went some way towards fulfilling the need for measurement of a child's motor development.

A major revision was published by Sloan in 1955, which resulted in 49 of the items being discarded on the grounds of unreliability, poor correlation with age, the possibility of physical injury or the need for costly equipment. The remaining 36 items succeeded in discriminating between the performance of children at different ages. However, as a clinical instrument, Sloan's version presents considerable difficulties:

(a) it takes at least an hour to administer to a *normal* child;
(b) it involves the use of too much equipment when testing cannot be done in a clinic;
(c) a few ambiguities in instructions and scoring criteria remain; and
(d) there are no truly normative data. (Sloan's population was chosen on the basis of availability rather than representativeness.)

What we required was a simple, easily administered, but objectively scorable measure of a child's motor proficiency at the age of 9 to 10 years, to test the hypothesis that motor clumsiness is associated with educational difficulties. With this aim in mind, we studied Sloan's data and eventually chose 12 items which satisfied two criteria: (1) that the item discriminated well in the chosen age range, and (2) that as little equipment as possible was required.

These items were piloted on children on the mainland, and ambiguities in both instructions and scoring systems were removed. For example, Sloan's suggestion that a tennis ball should be used in the test of catching was found to produce misleading results when the child's hand was too small to accommodate a ball of this size. We therefore substituted a squash ball. Again, an insistence that children start with their right hand in some tests (as required in Sloan's version) discriminated against left handers; 'preferred' hand (or foot) was therefore substituted for 'right' throughout. In some cases, too, it was necessary to provide more detailed instructions as to what level of accuracy was required in order to score a pass. Table 16 lists the 12 items which were selected.

TABLE 16

Items used in the shortened form of the Oseretsky test

1. Walking backwards about six paces (Fig. 12)
2. Crouching on tiptoe (Fig. 13)
*3. Standing on one foot (Fig. 14)
4. Touching nose with index finger (eyes closed) (Fig. 15)
*5. Touching fingertips with thumb of same hand
6. Standing heel to toe (eyes closed) (Figs 16 and 17)
7. Closing and opening hands alternately
*8. Catching a squash ball in one hand
*9. Tapping (making dots on paper)
*10. Sorting matchsticks from one box to another (Fig. 18)
*11. Drawing vertical lines between sets of parallel, horizontal lines
*12. Placing 20 coins in a box (Fig. 19)

**Scored separately for each limb.*

Description

The test consisted of items involving both gross motor control such as in balancing on one leg, and fine motor control such as in picking up matchsticks one at a time from one box and placing them in another. The maximum score for passing an item correctly on the first trial was 3 points. Since in 7 of the items each hand or foot was scored separately, the total maximum score was 57 points. The examiners were each provided with a manual (see Appendix C) giving detailed instructions concerning the administration of each item and detailed criteria for failure. The test was demonstrated to them, and all examiners tested children not included in the study before testing of survey children was begun.

Normative Data

Table 17 provides the normative data based on our control group. A two-way analysis of variance, summarised in Table 18, shows that the total score did differentiate between 9 and 10 year old children. However, there was no significant sex difference nor was there a significant interaction between sex and age. In the light of these findings, it seemed justifiable to combine the scores of the sexes within each

TABLE 17

The Oseretsky test: control group data based on 147* cases

Group	*No.*	*Mean score*	*S.D.*	*Mean age*
Younger boys	37	37.41	6.59	9 y 7 m
Younger girls	38	38.97	5.78	9 y 8 m
Total younger group	75	38.20	6.20	9 y 8 m
Older boys	36	41.03	5.58	10 y 7 m
Older girls	36	41.92	5.03	10 y 7 m
Total older group	72	41.47	5.29	10 y 7 m

**Includes one randomly selected child with epilepsy.*

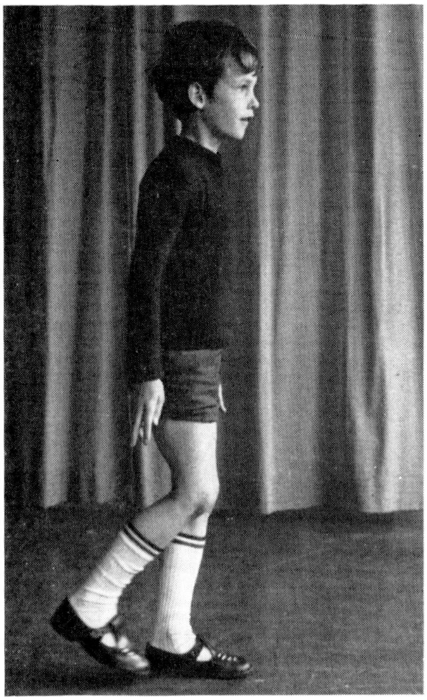
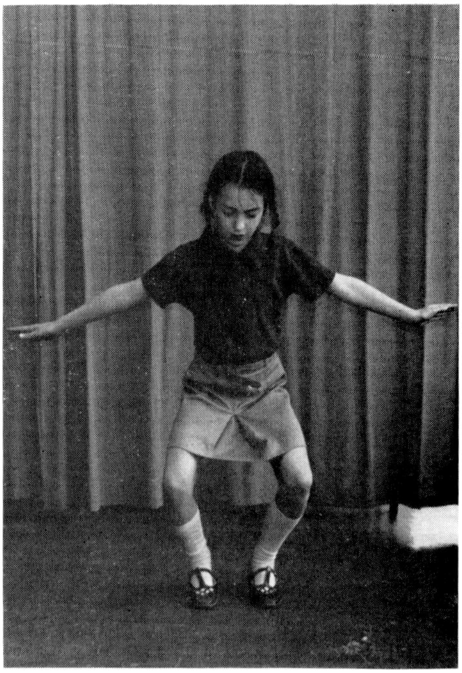
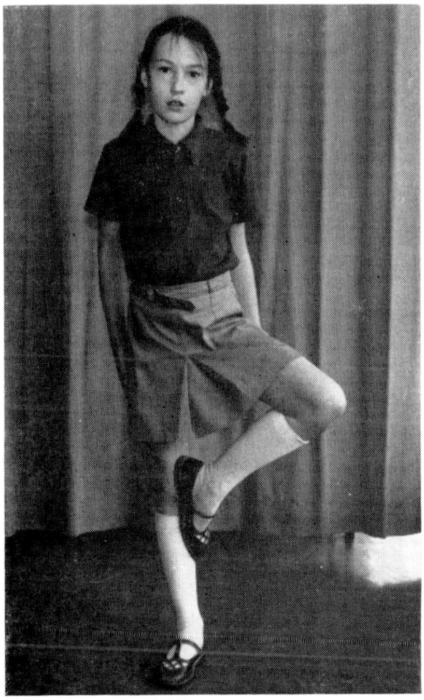
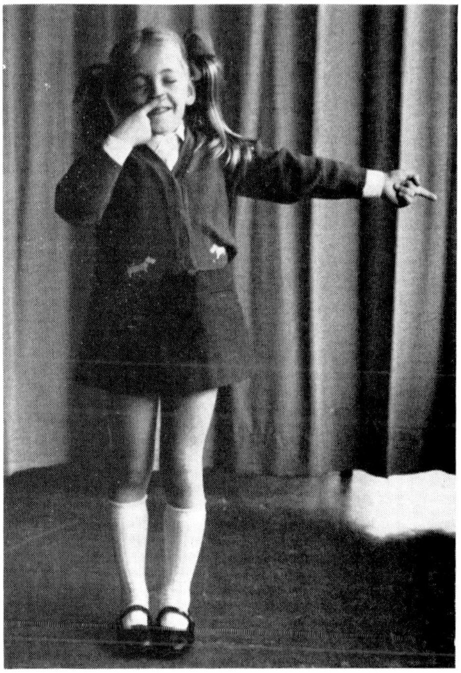

Fig 12 (top left). Walking backwards. **Fig. 13** (top right). Commencement of crouching on tiptoe. **Fig. 14** (bottom left). Standing on one foot. **Fig. 15** (bottom right). Touching nose.

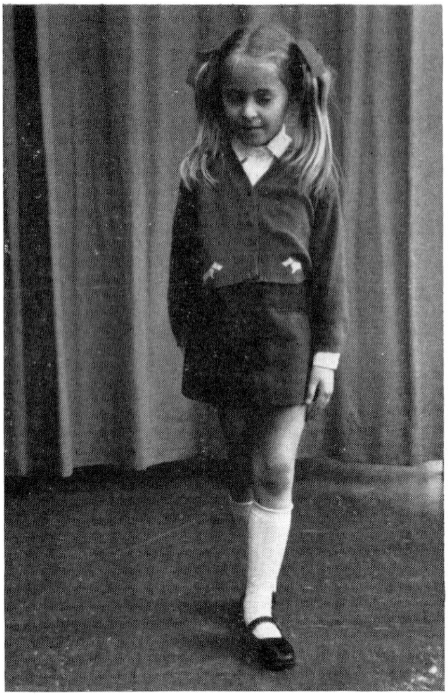
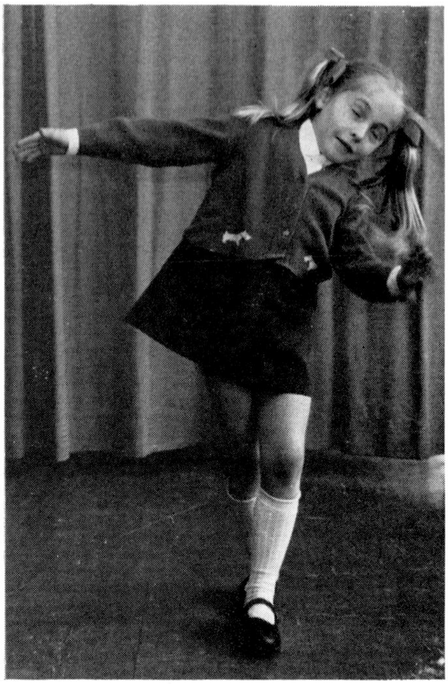
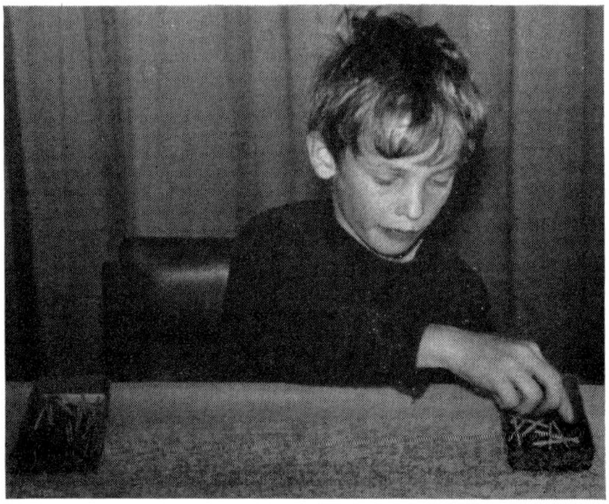
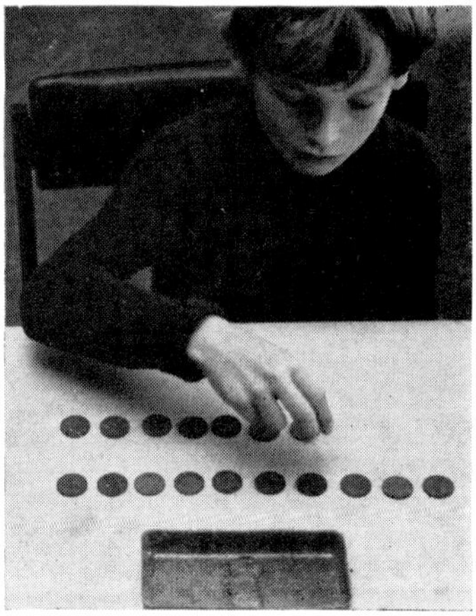

Fig. 16 (top left). Standing heel to toe (passed).
Fig. 17 (top right). Standing heel to toe.
(failed because of gross bodily movements).
Fig. 18 (bottom left). Sorting matchsticks.
Fig. 19 (bottom right). Putting coins in box.

TABLE 18
Two-way analysis of variance of the Oseretsky test control group sample

Sources	*ss*	*df*	*V*	*F*	*P*
Between sexes	54	1	54	1.62	N.S.
Between ages	393	1	393	11.79	0.001
Sex and age	6.4	1	6.4	0.19	N.S.
Within sets	4,765.6	143	33.33		

age group to yield more stable estimates of normal performance at these ages. Thus, in selecting the 12 items from Sloan's version, we appear to have been successful in producing a short list which differentiated between 2 groups of normal children aged, on average, 9½ and 10½ years.

Reliability Study

Table 19 presents the results of a study of reliability: 74 children were retested by a different psychologist 1 to 29 days (mean = 7·8 days) after the original administration. As expected, the group mean scores did increase by nearly 3 points on the second testing, but this increase was not statistically significant.

The test-retest correlation of 0·69 is almost as high as that reported by Sloan (1955) after one year, and is higher than most in the literature (Castell 1962). Since we wanted to identify *abnormally* clumsy children, this test-retest correlation based on a sample of normal children was judged adequate for our purposes.

TABLE 19
Oseretsky test-retest reliability on 74 children

	Mean score	*S.D.*	*r*
1st testing	38.59	5.94	+0.69***
2nd testing	41.34	5.65	

****Significant at the* 0·1 *per cent level.*

Validity

AGREEMENT WITH NEUROLOGICAL ASSESSMENT OF MOTOR CO-ORDINATION

A clinical evaluation of limb 'dyspraxia' was made during the neurological examination of each child. This was defined as a degree of inco-ordination, abnormal in relation to the child's chronological age, which could not be accounted for in terms of lack of proprioception or other sensation, paresis, tremor or alteration of tone. Only 1·4 per cent of the control group showed such 'dyspraxia'. On the other hand, 28·9 per cent of the 45 children found to be clumsy on the Oseretsky test (short form) were 'dyspraxic'. The difference between the groups was highly significant (p. < 0·001). The test was therefore measuring aspects of inco-ordination similar to those thought to be clinically relevant on neurological examination. The test allows no differentiation between different types of inco-ordination (for example that due to paresis, that due to a central defect of motor control and that due to tremor).

INDIVIDUAL TEST ITEM AND TOTAL SCORE

The correlations between each individual test item and the total raw score were all positive, moderately high (0·24 to 0·57) and highly significant (p.<0·001).

CORRELATIONS WITH AGE, IQ, AND EDUCATIONAL ATTAINMENT IN THE CONTROL GROUP

Of all the correlations between the total score and a wide variety of intelligence and attainment measures in the control group, only age correlated significantly at the 1 per cent level (r= +0·31). This confirms the findings of the analysis of variance (see above). The correlation between total score and WISC IQ in this normal group was virtually zero (r= -0·002).

GROUP DIFFERENCES

Using the raw scores on this short form of the Oseretsky test, it was possible to construct an operational definition of clumsiness. Children who scored two standard deviations or more below the mean score for their age were designated 'severely clumsy', and children whose scores lay between one and two standard deviations below the mean were classed as 'moderately clumsy'; all other children were regarded as normal in their motor performance. Of all the children tested, 56 (including 11 with WISC full-scale IQs of 50 or less) were identified as 'severely clumsy'; this group comprised 37 boys and 19 girls. This gives a minimal prevalence rate for the total population of 2·5 per cent.

Table 20 shows the mean score for the control group, the intellectually retarded children, and the reading retarded children. Both the last two groups differed significantly from the control group at the 0·1 per cent level. However, this tells us nothing about the number of individual children with abnormal clumsiness in each group. Table 21 gives a better idea of the utility of the tests in differentiating individuals from each group. The rate of clumsiness was several times higher in the intellectually retarded and reading retarded groups than in the control group (the difference in the first case being significant at the 0·1 per cent level and in the second at the 1 per cent level).

TABLE 20

Group differences on mean 'Oseretsky' score

Group	*No.*	*Mean score*	*S.D.*
Controls	146	39.79	6.00
Intellectually retarded	71	33.54***	8.25
Reading retarded	108	36.23***	7.95

****Significantly different from control group at the* 0.1 *per cent level. Mean difference between intellectually retarded and reading retarded group also significant at the* 0.05 *per cent level.*

The number of neuro-epileptic children in this age group was too small for a very meaningful assessment of the rate of clumsiness. However, it can be seen from Table 21 that the rate was high in both groups, especially in the neurological group.

TABLE 21
Proportion of clumsy children in each group

Group	*Designation on basis of Oseretsky test score*			
	Normal %	*Moderately clumsy* %	*Severely clumsy* %	*No. of children*
Controls	80	15	5	146
Intellectually retarded	49	26	25***	71
Reading retarded	64	24	12**	108
Neurological disorder (age 9-10 years)	0	0	100*	7
Epileptic (age 9-10 years)	43	29	29	7

*Significantly different from control group (pooling moderately and severely clumsy): *at 5 per cent level; **at 1 per cent level; ***at 0·1 per cent level.*

Although there was no association between IQ and clumsiness in the control group, there was an association between *very low* IQ (50 to 85) and clumsiness. This emphasises the fact that associations within the normal range of any variable are no indication of associations at the extremes of the range. However, low IQ is not an adequate explanation of the high rate of clumsiness in the children with specific reading retardation (whose mean IQ of 103 was only slightly below that of the control group), epilepsy or neurological disorder.

It may be concluded that this shortened version of the Oseretsky test agrees well with an independent neurological assessment. It appears to be a valid measure of motor inco-ordination which differentiates between normal children of different ages and which is sufficiently reliable to warrant its use as a research tool. To be of greater diagnostic value it will have to be tested on a larger number of neurologically handicapped children of normal intelligence. If, as seems the case, it measures both gross and fine motor co-ordination and if reliable sub-scores can be developed, it could be of great use in pin-pointing specific areas of motor deficit.

A Test of Motor Impersistence

Inability to carry out purposive movements in the absence of apparent weakness or damage of the muscles involved has been recognised as a sign of neurological disorder for over a century. Since the papers of Jackson (1878) and Lewandowsky (1907), there have been sporadic reports of patients unable to close their eyes on command. In 1924 Pineas extended this concept by reporting a patient who could close his eyes but could not keep them closed. Zutt (1950) and Berlin (1955) reported similar phenomena in relation to mouth opening and tongue protrusion. Fisher (1956) coined the term 'motor impersistence' to describe this symptom. He, like others before him, noted that its presence was more common in patients with non-dominant (usually right-sided) hemispheric lesions.

Up to that time, all the reports had been of a clinical qualitative nature. It remained for Benton and his co-workers to standardise the observations and put them in quantified form. They devised a battery of nine sub-tests to assess motor persistence. Subjects were required to sustain nine different voluntarily initiated motor acts (such as closing eyes, protruding tongue, or keeping mouth open) for specified time periods (Joynt *et al.* 1962). A comparison was made between 101 adult neurological or neurosurgical patients thought to have lesions of one or both cerebral hemispheres and an age-matched group of 74 patients with a variety of physical disorders which did not involve the brain. Only 2 per cent of the control group failed two or more tasks compared with 23 per cent of the brain-damaged patients. Motor impersistence was considerably more frequent where there was mental impairment. There was no significant association with the side of lesion but there was a slight tendency for marked impersistence to be more common with right sided (15 per cent) or bilateral lesions (16 per cent) than with left sided lesions (6 per cent).

Thus, standardised tests confirmed the earlier clinical finding in adults, though no strong association with side of lesion was found. Garfield (1964) was the first person to study the phenomenon systematically in children. He used a sample of 140 children attending a paediatric clinic, with a WISC IQ between 80 and 119 to establish norms for children aged 5 to 11 years on eight of the motor persistence tasks used with adults by Joynt *et al.* From a neurology clinic, he selected 25 children from the same age and IQ range, whose diagnosis of brain damage was substantiated by paralyses of the extremities due to cerebral lesions. Children whose paralyses would directly interfere with their performance on any of the eight tasks were excluded. Since the normal group was of significantly higher IQ and since in adults impersistence had been found to be associated with mental impairment, a sub-group of 25 normal children was matched with the brain-damaged group for age, sex and IQ.

On six of the eight tasks, the brain-damaged children were found to be significantly less persistent than the matched controls.

When pathological impersistence was defined as a deviant score on two or more of the tasks, 4 of the 140 normal children (3 per cent) and 17 of the 25 brain damaged children (68 per cent) were impersistent. That is, 153 of the 165 children studied were correctly classified on the basis of this dichotomous score, giving a total screening efficiency of 93 per cent. However, 32 per cent of brain-damaged children (8 out of 25) would be mis-classified.

Benton *et al.* (1964) then investigated the influence of chronological age and intelligence. First, they compared 21 seven to twelve year old retarded children with 21 normal children matched for sex and chronological age. The mean IQs of the two groups were 44 and 101 respectively. On all eight tests of motor impersistence, the normal children performed at a markedly superior level. The second comparison was between 55 normal children and 55 retardates matched for mental age (mean = 7·5 years) and sex. On two of the eight tasks the normal children did significantly better, and there were no differences between the groups on the other six tasks. Both chronological and mental age, but particularly the latter, were important determinants of motor impersistence in children.

Some retarded children showed marked impersistence which did not seem to be accounted for in terms of either low mental age or chronological age. An investigation of the effect of cerebral dysfunction was made on 22 'cultural familial retardates' (*i.e.* children whose WISC IQ fell in the range 55 to 84, who showed no evidence of cerebral pathology and who had at least one sib or parent retarded in intellectual functioning) and 22 'brain-damaged' retardates matched for chronological age and IQ (Garfield *et al.* 1966). On six of the eight tests the cultural-familial retardates showed superior performance, on one task (head-turning during sensory testing) there was no difference, and on the other (saying 'ahh' for as long as possible) the difference was reversed ($p. < 0{\cdot}01$). On this occasion, using a cut-off point of 4 or more deviant scores as indicating pathological impersistence, eleven of the brain-damaged retardates and only two of the cultural-familial retardates were identified as impersistent, giving a total screening efficiency of approximately 70 per cent.

Thus, even at younger age levels, there is evidence that severity of motor impersistence is associated with cerebral lesions. Since the phenomenon is undoubtedly related to the level of intellectual functioning, it would appear that a more severe criterion of impersistence is required at lower IQ levels before 'brain-damaged' children can be identified.

The psychological processes which underly this phenomenon have remained uncertain. Fisher (1956) opted for the direct explanation that motor impersistence is due to impaired cortical motor control. Garfield considers that the tests may be a measure of distractibility or short attention span, a developmentally acquired capacity, increasing with age (Garfield 1964, Garfield *et al.* 1966).

Our Adaptation

As with the Oseretsky Test of Motor Proficiency, the first step in developing this test further was the examination of the published findings of previous workers. One of the eight sub-tests used by Garfield (head-turning during sensory testing) appeared to have little discriminative value, and consequently we decided to use the remaining seven items. These are described in detail in Appendix D, together with scoring criteria.

Garfield did not lay down explicit scoring criteria, but defined an impersistent response on any single sub-test in terms of a score characterising 5 per cent or less of the normal population. Children who, on this definition, failed two or more tasks were regarded as 'pathologically impersistent.' We established cut-off points in an exactly similar fashion using norms derived from results obtained in our randomly selected control group.

In each of the sub-tests, with one exception, 9 year old children did not differ in their capacity for persistence from the 10 year old group. However, on the test involving saying 'ahh' there was a difference between the 9 and 10 year old children, and scoring criteria were modified accordingly.

TABLE 22
Reliability of motor impersistence score

		Second test score			
		0	**1**	**2** *or more*	*Total*
	0	44	7	3	54
First test score	**1**	5	2	5	12
	2 or more	3	2	3	8
	Total	52	11	11	74

Reliability

The reliability of the motor persistence score was tested in the same way as the short form of the Oseretsky test; 74 children were seen twice by different psychologists, the second test being within 29 days (mean = 7·8 days) of the first test (Table 22).

As it happened, the population contained too few impersistent children for an adequate assessment, but within this largely normal group there was evidently considerable unreliability. The good discrimination between groups (see below) suggests that reliability may be much higher for deviant children. This is also suggested by an examination of the seven sub-tests. On the first sub-test *all* children received perfect scores and it was only on items 4, 6 and 7 that more than two or three children were impersistent. Numbers 4 and 7 (fixation of gaze in lateral visual fields and saying 'aah') were found to be highly reliable, whereas number 6 (fixation on examiner's nose during confrontation testing of visual fields) was not.

Validity

AGREEMENT WITH RATINGS OF COGNITIVE IMPERSISTENCE AND MOTOR RESTLESSNESS

No direct test of the validity of the test of motor impersistence is possible in that it is not known what basic function is being tapped. However, Table 23 shows the ratings of hyperkinesis, fidgetiness, and cognitive impersistence in normal children and those found to have motor impersistence on the test. There was no association between motor impersistence and general overactivity, but there was an association with fidgetiness and squirminess as rated by both parents and teachers. Fidgetiness might be taken as a more global assessment of motor impersistence. There was also some association between motor impersistence and cognitive impersistence, as assessed by ratings of short attention span and distractibility. High associations would not be expected in view of the only moderate reliability of the cognitive assessment.

GROUP DIFFERENCES

Children who scored 2 or more on the motor impersistence test were defined as 'impersistent'. When the different groups studied were compared (Table 24) it was found that there was a much higher rate of impersistence in the groups of children

TABLE 23

Associations between motor impersistence and cognitive impersistence/motor restlessness

	Impersistent *% with characteristics*	*Persistent* *% with characteristics*
Parental scale		
Overactivity	50	50
Fidgetiness	55*	33
Poor concentration	65	53
Total no.	(20)	(83)
Teachers' scale		
Overactivity	43	34
Fidgetiness	62*	34
Very poor concentration	57	31
Total no.	(21)	(87)
Psychiatric interview		
Fidgetiness	67	56
Short attention span	19	11
Distractibility	19	11
Total no.	(21)	(87)

Significantly different: *$p. < \cdot 05$.

TABLE 24

Motor impersistence in children with neurological or educational disorder

Group	*Score of 2 or more on Motor Impersistence Test* %	*Total no. of children*
Controls	5	146
Intellectually retarded	23***	71
Reading retarded	20**	108
Neurological disorder (age 9-10 years)	71*	7
Epileptic (age 9-10 years)	29	7

Significantly different from control group: **at* 5 *per cent level:* ***at* 1 *per cent level;* ****at* 0·1 *per cent level.*

with intellectual or reading retardation than in the control group. The neurological group was too small for an adequate evaluation, but it was notable that impersistence was most frequent in these children, the difference from the control group being significant at the 5 per cent level.

As with clumsiness, there was an association between motor impersistence and very low IQ, but there were also associations with specific reading retardation and neurological disorder which could not be accounted for in terms of IQ differences.

To a considerable extent, motor impersistence and clumsiness tended to occur together (Table 25). Nearly half the clumsy children (defined on the basis of a score on the short Oseretsky test 2 standard deviations below the mean) showed abnormal impersistence compared with only one in 20 of the controls. Conversely, over a quarter of the impersistent children were severely clumsy on the short Oseretsky test compared with one in 20 of the controls and 14 per cent were rated as 'dyspraxic' on the neurological examination compared with 1·4 per cent of the controls.

TABLE 25
Associations between motor impersistence and clumsiness

	Impersistent %	*Severely clumsy on short Oseretsky* %	*'Dyspraxic'* %	*No. of children tested*
Controls	5.4	4.8	1.4	146
Severely clumsy children (2 S.D. below mean on short Oseretsky)	42.2***	–	–	45
Impersistent children	–	28.8***	14.1***	64

****Significantly different from control group at* 0·1 *per cent level.*

In general, then, our findings in a total population support those of Garfield and Benton based on clinic samples. Motor persistence is a developmental phenomenon which improves with age and which can be measured through the use of standardised tests. Persistence is impaired in children of very low IQ and even more so in children with cerebral disorders. It remains uncertain exactly what physiological function is being assessed by tests of motor persistence. The finding that it is closely associated with motor co-ordination and somewhat less so with cognitive persistence suggests that it may be due to impaired cortical motor control, as Fisher (1956) suggested, but the matter requires further consideration.

Other Psychometric Tests of Neurological Characteristics

Several other items in the neurological and psychological examinations also involved quantification of neurological characteristics as described, *e.g.* constructional abilities and language impairment.

In addition, in the psychological examination the children's ability to differentiate right and left was tested using five tests described by Williams and Jambor (1964). The measure was only moderately reliable (r=0·39) in the mostly normal group of 74 children used in the test-retest reliability study, but the large inter-group differences suggested (as with motor impersistence) that it was probably more reliable in picking out deviant children.

However, as a clinical test to assess function in an individual child, rather than as a research procedure to differentiate groups, five questions are probably insufficient, bearing in mind the opportunity for the child to get the answer right by a lucky guess (unlike the impersistence and clumsiness tests). The five questions include three on right-left differentiation on the child and two on the examiner, and as the latter discriminate better, at least twice the number of questions on this is desirable.

Like motor co-ordination and motor persistence (with both of which it was significantly associated), right-left differentiation is a phenomenon which is poorly developed in the young child and in which performance improves with increasing age. By 9 and 10 years most children get perfect scores and although there was a very slight age difference in scores in this study, it fell well short of statistical significance. The age difference was more marked (although still not significant) in the educationally retarded children who differentiated right and left less well. There was no significant sex difference though boys tended to be poorer than girls in right-left differentiation. Children with intellectual retardation, specific reading retardation, or a neuro-epileptic disorder all did very poorly on the test compared with normals (see Table 2, page 43).

Discussion

Psychometric Assessment of Neurological Characteristics

These tests cover a wide range of cognitive, motor, perceptual and language functions, but they share certain common characteristics.

(a) They measure developmental features, *i.e.*, skills acquired by children as they grow older and as their brain structure and function approach maturity.

(b) Whether or not a child's performance is abnormal depends on quantitative assessment of his degree of impairment in relation to the age-norms, rather than on qualitative considerations.

(c) Performance on the test is generally more closely related to mental age than to chronological age; the functions measured by the test develop together with other more general intellectual capacities.

(d) Children with cerebral disorders perform particularly poorly on the tests, even after IQ is taken into account.

(e) In most cases the tests show a high degree of reliability and validity.

These characteristics apply to many features of the neurological assessment of children, apart from the few for which we used specific tests. Numerous other tests of developmental functions have been devised, *e.g.* the measurement of 'mirror-movements' (Fog and Fog 1963) or other aspects of motor 'overflow' (Cohen *et al.* 1967) which require a similar psychometric approach. Techniques for assessing inter-sensory development and audio-visual integration have been developed (Birch and Belmont 1964, 1965 *a* and *b*; Birch and Lefford 1963; Blank and Bridger 1964, 1967). Double simultaneous touch perception (Bender *et al.* 1951) has been used in the neuropsychological evaluation of children for some time. Frostig *et al.* (1961, 1964) devised tests of visual perception thought to be related to reading skills. Stott (1966) provided another modification of the Oseretsky test and Wepman (1958) produced a test of auditory discrimination. Until recently, there has been a dearth of adequate tests of speech and language but now several have become available. Language comprehension can be assessed by a picture vocabulary test (Dunn 1965) and McCarthy and Kirk (1961) pioneered analyses of different aspects of language ability with their

Illinois Test of Psycholinguistic Abilities. Perhaps most useful of all in the area of speech and language are Reynell's test of language comprehension and expression (1970), Renfrew's articulation test (1966) and Ingram's test of phonetic maturation (1970).

The above tests vary greatly in sophistication and standardisation but they all represent attempts to introduce precision into the assessment of developmental characteristics. Accurate measurement of developmental characteristics is likely to require properly standardised tests, and the psychologist has a crucial role to play in their development and administration.

Tests of 'Brain-damage'

An enormous amount of time and energy has been expended by psychologists in devising tests of 'brain-damage' for use with adults (Meyer 1957) and with children (Herbert 1964). Psychiatrists, in particular, have often been concerned to determine whether a child's emotional or behavioural problems are due to organic brain dysfunction and this concern has provided the chief impetus to the development of tests of 'brain-damage'.

Several reviews have clearly demonstrated that attempts to devise such tests have been singularly unsuccessful (Graham and Berman 1961, Herbert 1964, Meyer 1957, Yates 1954) and it may be worthwhile to consider why this has been so.

In the first place, tests of brain damage have usually been validated on their differentiation between normal children (often of average intelligence) and children with cerebral palsy (usually of below average intelligence), but they have been used clinically to determine the presence of brain damage in psychiatrically abnormal children without overt neurological abnormalities. It is hardly surprising, therefore, that where the neurological examination is ambiguous, psychological tests tend also to give ambiguous results; and where neurological abnormalities are clearly present, a psychological test of 'brain-damage' is unnecessary.

At one time it was thought that cerebral damage usually caused psychological deficits which were different from normal in kind rather than in degree (Goldstein 1940). It is now clear that this is not the case (Reitan 1968). Supposedly pathognomonic signs of brain damage occur in many individuals without cerebral injury, while most of the psychological deficits associated with cerebral disorder are quantitatively but not qualitatively different from those found in normal people.

The concept of a test of 'brain-damage' also implies that damage to the brain leads to a uniform psychological picture. This is manifestly not so. The nature, locus and extent of the lesion and the age of the child at the time the lesion developed all profoundly affect psychological consequences (Birch 1964). There is no one type of 'brain-damaged' child (Wortis 1956). The symptoms of brain-damage are extremely varied. Consequently, the designation of 'brain-damage' is very uninformative.

As a consequence of these and other considerations, there has been a tendency in recent years to move away from global assessments of 'brain damage' to a more precise description of a child's neuro-psychological difficulties. The tests described in this chapter serve this purpose. They make no pretence of diagnosing the cause of a child's problems, but they do define the character and extent of impaired functions.

Some might consider that this is not sufficient and that a psychological test should be able to say not only how much a child is impaired in his language development, for example, but also whether this is due to 'organic' or other factors. This view lies behind Reitan's attempt to devise a battery of tests aiming to diagnose specific neurological deficits and to differentiate these from similar handicaps of psychogenic origin (Reitan 1968, Reitan and Heineman 1968). These promise to provide a useful delineation of a child's difficulties which should offer valuable guides to treatment. However, whether they can diagnose the cause of the deficits is more doubtful. Knights and Tymchuk (1968) found that children's performances on the tests were significantly correlated with IQ and that the tests appeared to be sensitive to impairment regardless of whether the impairment was due to a brain lesion or some other factor.

It seems highly improbable that psychological tests can be devised to diagnose the aetiology of a handicap unless the nature of the handicap differs according to its cause. This sometimes happens, but more frequently the end-results of different processes are similar. In any case, one must beware of implying a mental dualism in which 'organic' disorders are associated with abnormalities of the brain and 'psychogenic' disorders with something vaguely outside the head. Both involve defects in brain function although only the first involves structural abnormalities. Even this distinction is not absolute. Experiential factors can lead to structural change. For example, it seems that early visual deprivation can lead to irreversible cellular changes in the retina (Riesen 1965). There is also some suggestion that environmental differences may, in some circumstances, lead to changes in brain anatomy and brain chemistry (Rosenzweig *et al.* 1967). Psychological impairment may sometimes prove to be irreversible, and conversely it is apparent that structural lesions may lead to purely transitory impairment (see chapters 1 and 7).

This is not to suggest that a differentiation between structural brain disorders, psychogenic disorders and social disorders is unimportant. On the contrary, this differentiation has most important consequences for treatment and for prognosis. However, the diagnosis is not an either/or decision which can be made on some test. Rather, the relative contribution of different factors to the development of a disorder must be decided on the basis of a determination of the nature of the impairment and the history of its development. Psychological tests have an important role to play in this decision, but the findings have to be considered in relation to all the other findings, anamnestic, clinical, laboratory and experimental.

The Role of the Psychologist in the Neurological Clinic

The role of the psychologist in neurological practice may now be summarised in terms of description, diagnosis and treatment.

Perhaps the most important contribution of the psychologist lies in the accurate description of a patient's handicaps. This has already been discussed in terms of the use of specific tests of developmental features of a neurological kind. These tests are of value not only in defining a child's handicap, but also in measuring his progress during and after treatment. As well as devising and using standardised tests, the psychologist should be able to aid the neurologist in adapting his clinical examination to take advantage of psychometric techniques, where this is appropriate.

As shown in chapter 9, many children with neurological disorder have intellectual or educational retardation. The use of cognitive and attainment tests allows an accurate evaluation of these difficulties. Psychiatric disorder is also relatively common in association with cerebral palsy and epilepsy (see chapter 12). The psychologist may be able to devise appropriate tests to measure behaviour or emotions and his training should enable him to make systematic observations. However, psychological tests are of very little use in psychiatric diagnosis. Although claims have been made for the value of projective tests, studies have consistently shown them to be of little practical value (Cronbach 1949, Jensen 1964, Payne 1955, Zubin *et al.* 1965). The uselessness of tests of brain damage has already been discussed.

Although psychological tests are not of much use in providing an overall diagnosis, they may be of considerable value in testing alternative hypotheses about the nature of a child's difficulties, for example, whether his difficulties in learning to read are due to failure to learn or failure to retain what he has learned (Shapiro 1957). This type of diagnostic testing involves the application of research principles to the study of a single case, not by the application of standard tests but rather by the design of experiments to investigate a specific problem in an individual (Shapiro 1951, 1961).

To what extent psychologists should be involved in psychological methods of treatment is controversial (Committee on Training in Clinical Psychology 1947, Eysenck 1968). Conditioning techniques may be useful in treating the behavioural abnormalities sometimes associated with neurological disorder (Becker *et al.* 1967, Bijou 1968, Gelfand and Hartmann 1968, Leff 1968) and, of course, psychologists have an important contribution to make in advising upon specific techniques in remedial teaching, and sometimes in providing such teaching. To what extent conditioning procedures may be useful in treating neurological abnormalities as such is not known, but operant techniques can be used to control muscle action (Connolly 1968, Hefferline 1958, Sasmor 1966) and it is conceivable that they might be of some value in treating motor handicaps in children with cerebral palsy.

PART III

Epidemiology of Neuro-epileptic Disorders

CHAPTER 6

Selection of Children with Neuro-epileptic Disorder

The aim of the study was to investigate all school-age children with any neuro-epileptic disorder. We directed our attention to disorders which (a) were of a type which in childhood usually lasted at least one year (*i.e.* were chronic), (b) were associated with persisting or recurrent handicap of some kind, and (c) were known to have been present during the 12 months preceding the survey (*i.e.* were currently present). This was in line with the definitions used in our surveys of other conditions in Isle of Wight school children (Rutter *et al.* 1970). We were not concerned with acute head injuries without subsequent handicap, nor with disorders in earlier childhood which had left no neurological abnormalities identifiable by clinical examination at the time of the survey. Furthermore, owing to problems of definition and measurement and the need to confine the study to what could be managed with our limited resources, we decided to restrict neuro-epileptic disorders to those in which there was an undoubted abnormality of the brain of a type not due to maturational factors. Thus, we did not deal with developmental disorders except incidentally, although 'developmental dyslexia' was considered in the context of specific reading retardation in a parallel educational study (Rutter *et al.* 1970). Finally, we excluded cases in which abnormal brain function was shown only in behavioural or cognitive abnormalities and those in which the diagnosis of neuro-epileptic disorder had to be made on minor signs of uncertain significance. In practice this meant that we were largely concerned with cerebral palsy and epilepsy.

Age Group

In order to obtain an adequate number of children with these conditions it was necessary to study a wide age group. However, we did not have suitable screening methods for preschool children and after the end of compulsory schooling total population coverage becomes very difficult. In fact a 10 year cohort provided a suitable sized population (11,865) so that the group studied comprised all Isle of Wight children who were in the age group for whom schooling was compulsory at the start of the September term in 1965, *i.e.* children born between 1st March 1950 and 31st August 1960.

Isle of Wight children were defined as those whose homes were on the Isle of Wight, regardless of where they went to school. Because the school medical register which constituted our most comprehensive screening of the population (see below) was not available for children in private schools, it was decided to restrict the survey to children whose schooling was paid for by the local authority (this was over 90 per cent of the population).

Selection of Children

It was not possible to examine every child on the Island, so a two stage procedure was used. First, screening procedures were used to identify all those children who might have a neuro-epileptic disorder; these children were then studied individually to enable a final decision to be made on the presence or absence of disorder and on its diagnosis. The individual study was also used to obtain information on the social, psychological and educational functioning of the children.

Screening Methods

The most appropriate survey methods to identify chronic physical disorders have been discussed in the literature on several occasions (Banas and Dawis 1962, Napier 1962, Yankauer *et al.* 1962). In relation to cerebral palsy, Ingram (1955) has clearly shown the importance of using multiple screening techniques.

The first principle is to use methods which survey *all* the children in the population to be studied, and the second is to use techniques which are appropriate for the identification of the conditions to be investigated. Thirdly, as Ingram showed, it is valuable to have a special check on populations which have a particularly high rate of the disorders in question.

School Medical Register

The school medical examination fulfils the first condition. On the Island at the time of the survey all children received medical examinations shortly after school entry at about the age of five years and again at about the age of eight years. A third examination was held some time after entry to secondary school at the age of 12 years.

The second condition requires more consideration. As usually carried out, the routine medical examination seems to be an inefficient and uneconomical method of identifying children with most physical disorders (Lee 1958, Yankauer and Lawrence 1955). First, the reliability of the examination leaves a lot to be desired (Rutter *et al.* 1970), although it is unlikely that cases of cerebral palsy would be missed. Secondly, episodic disorders such as epilepsy can only be identified on the basis of a medical history (rather than examination). Fortunately, the Island authorities routinely made particular efforts to contact parents by letter and invite them to attend each examination. The letter of invitation also contained a form which the parents were asked to complete and either send back or bring along to the examination. The form listed a number of physical complaints (including fits) and the parent was asked to circle any conditions from which the child suffered. It is an index of the good relationship between schools and parents on the Island that over 90 per cent of the parents of the 159 ten and eleven year old children selected at random from the general population had either completed this form or had attended the school medical examination on at least one occasion.

There is some evidence from other studies that mothers can give an accurate account of their children's state of health, provided that well-phrased questionnaires are used. Ashley-Miller (1965) in a study of eight-year-old Isle of Wight children showed that only an insignificant number of defects is likely to be missed if school medical examinations are restricted to children selected on the basis of questionnaires completed by mothers. Furthermore, in relation to a study of 6 to 13 year old children, Leeson (1965) found that when the judgement of school doctors on whether a child needed an examination is compared with a mechanical judgement based on questionnaires completed by parents, there is agreement in 70 per cent of cases.

Of course, a small number of parents will either forget or deny the presence of health problems in their children, both in answer to questionnaires and in direct interview with a doctor. However, most handicapping physical disorders in these children are likely to be manifest in the school situation or will be detectable on a physical examination, so that very few children with a disorder fulfilling our criteria were likely to be missed. It is also probable that, by concentrating attention on disabilities present during the previous year, a failure to remember a disorder was a less important factor in producing omissions than it would have been if a longer time-period had been taken.

The task of searching school medical records was made very much simpler by the fact that a Register of physically handicapped school children, based on these records, had been established some years ago by Dr. Michael Ashley-Miller who was Deputy Principal School Medical Officer at the time we planned the study. The Register contained cards classified according to the type of physical disorder. It was, therefore, an easy matter to discover how many children at any one time were under surveillance by the school health service for any sort of disorder. It also made it easier to ensure that children who needed more frequent medical examinations were not overlooked.

A check on a sample of school medical records nine months before the survey began showed that chronic physical disorders which were noted on the records were regularly recorded on the Register. We could thus rely on the Register without going back to the original records.

From this Register we selected all children recorded as having had a fit or anti-convulsants since starting school, any sort of neurological disorder, talipes or 'club-foot', shortening of any limb, or any sort of disorder which might have a neurological component. For example, children who had had a severe spinal deformity or disease or encephalitis were included. In addition to the current Register we also searched the records of children who had been on the Register previously (but whose names had been removed because they were no longer thought to need medical supervision).

Other Local Authority Medical Records

Although an effective screening procedure (see below), it was not desirable to use the Register as our only source of cases, both because certain groups of children were not included on the Register (for example, those in units for the mentally subnormal), and because some of the children would not have had a medical examination for several years so that the information would be out of date.

The first difficulty was readily overcome by going directly to sources not included on the Register. Thus, the records of all children at hospitals for the mentally subnormal, at the junior training centre (for mentally subnormal children), not attending school (either because of mental subnormality or because home tuition was being provided), at the Spastics Day Unit or at day or residential special schools were individually studied. All mentally subnormal children not attending school were scheduled to be examined regardless of what the records showed, because they constituted a 'high risk' group. Similarly, all children attending the Spastics Day Unit and all who had been seen in the past at the Unit with a view to their possible admission were examined individually, as were all children receiving special schooling (either day or residential) for total or partial blindness.

Hospital Records

The second disadvantage of the Register, namely, that some children would not have had a medical examination for some years, was overcome by using as many other sources of cases as possible. The most important of these was the hospital record services. Paediatric services on the Island are centered at the Royal County Hospital, Ryde, and we attempted to examine the records of all children who had been seen for the first time by a consultant paediatrician during the three years 1963-65 before the survey began. In the event we were able to examine 378 (84.6 per cent) of the 447 case records for these three years.

The same criteria were used as for the school Register; any child with a condition which might constitute a neurological disorder was selected. All those referred for attacks of any kind involving loss of consciousness were included, regardless of diagnosis. Also all children with limb shortening or with any abnormality of gait or of co-ordination were included.

Speech Therapy and Audiology Lists

Two further 'high-risk' groups were specially checked. To select children with deafness, lists of all children who had been fitted with hearing aids or who had been thought to be deaf were obtained from the audiologist. To screen children with speech and language difficulties, the speech therapist provided lists of all children she had seen, together with details of the speech or language abnormality and the nature of any accompanying disorder. On the basis of this information, all children with a retardation of language and all those where there was any suggestion of an accompanying neurological disorder (such as clumsiness, weakness, tremor or involuntary movements) were selected for further investigation. Children with an articulation defect alone were not selected unless this appeared to be part of a dysarthria due to neurological abnormality.

Head Teachers

The second phase of the screening consisted of asking parents and teachers to complete questionnaires on the physical health of all children selected on any of the procedures mentioned above. As a final check, head teachers were asked to provide the names of any children not on the list of those for whom questionnaires were sent, who suffered from any chronic handicap.

Possible Sources of Selection which were not Used

Although multiple sources of selection were employed, there were still others which could have been used and it is as well to consider why the more important of these were rejected. Under the National Health Service, all children (and adults) are eligible to be on the list of a general practitioner for medical care, and in practice nearly all take advantage of this opportunity. For each person on the doctor's list a medical record has to be completed and obviously this could constitute an invaluable source of information. Unfortunately, doctors vary greatly in the amount and quality of the information they record so that there is a lack of uniformity, and in many cases the information is inadequate for any research purposes. Equally important is the fact that unless the medical cards are coded in some way (and only some doctors do this) it is impossible, without going through every card of every doctor in the area, even to sort out which cards belong to children, let alone children with physical handicaps. As previous epidemiological studies of a comparable nature have not found reporting of cases from general practitioners to be particularly useful (Ingram 1955, 1964) it was decided that the likely benefit would not be sufficiently great to justify the amount of additional work which would be required.

A further possible source of information was the school's record of absenteeism. However, the experience of other workers has shown that this is not a fruitful case-finding method (Yankauer *et al.* 1962) in that the cause of absenteeism is not systematically recorded. Nearly all children have periods of absenteeism each year, so that in effect it means checking on the health of a large proportion of the children.

Screening Questionnaires

For all children discovered on any of the screening procedures to have a possible neuro-epileptic disorder, questionnaires were sent to parents and school teachers.

The parental form consisted of 23 questions*; the first 19 dealt with the child's health and the last four concerned family employment and housing (see Appendix E). For each question answered positively the parent was asked a series of additional questions. For example, if the parent wrote 'Yes' to the question 'Has he/she had a fit at any time in his/her life (*i.e.*, a blank spell, convulsion or any other attack that a doctor has called a fit)?' then the parent was asked to state when the last attack occurred and to give a description.

Similarly, the teachers were asked to reply 'Yes' or 'No' to 20 questions on the child's physical health (see Appendix F) with additional questions about any disorder said to be present. They were also asked to provide information about the number of times the child did not attend school during the previous two terms (Autumn 1964 and Spring 1965).

Individual Study of the Selected Children

On the basis of all available information from the selection sources and from both questionnaires, a decision was made as to whether to include each child in the intensive phase of the investigation. If there was a possibility that any child had a disorder which met our criteria, he was included. In general, where there was conflicting information or where there was any doubt about the presence of the condition, the child was included, so that a personal interview with the parent could help to

*Because the form was also designed to select children with other types of physical disorder as part of a wider survey of handicap (Rutter *et al.* 1970) several of the questions refer to non-neurological conditions.

settle the issue. If the parent and teacher *both* denied the presence of a condition for which the child had been selected, this was usually taken as sufficient evidence that the child was not currently handicapped and further investigation was not pursued. However, precedence was always given to information recorded by a doctor at the time the child was suffering from his disability. If, for example, a paediatrician had recorded at the time the presence of an epileptic fit during the year beginning September 1st, 1964, the child would have been selected for further investigation even if both parent and teacher later denied that such an event had occurred. In addition, if the parental questionnaire was not returned or was inadequately completed, a personal interview with the parent was always sought. All blind, deaf or mentally subnormal children not attending school and children seen at the Spastics Day Unit were individually examined regardless of what the questionnaires or records showed.

The intensive investigation served two purposes: (a) to obtain sufficient information about the possible neuro-epileptic disorder to decide whether it fulfilled our criteria and (b) to obtain information on the child, his family and his schooling in terms of the issues examined for children finally identified as having a neuro-epileptic disorder. The studies undertaken for the second purpose are described in the chapters appropriate to each issue. The parents of all children were visited and interviewed by a member of the research team who was a doctor (or in some cases a graduate in one of the social sciences).

Interview with the Parents

The parents were asked to describe the nature of the child's physical condition and how it had affected the child during the previous 12 months. As there was a wide variety of disorders, it was impossible to completely standardise the questioning in this section of the interview (except for epilepsy), but the interviewers were instructed to obtain as complete a picture as possible of the development of the condition and to determine precisely how the child was handicapped by it. The non-medical interviewers were briefed on what aspects were likely to be important and as to what sort of questions should be asked. Details of contacts with hospitals and general practitioner services were routinely obtained. Medication, special treatments such as physiotherapy and the child's requirements for physical help were all asked about systematically.

Specific questions about fits of any kind were provided in the interview proforma. Parents were asked to provide a detailed description of each variety of attack, together with information on frequency, duration, the presence of an aura or warning before the fit, and whether the child lost consciousness, wet or soiled or injured himself during the fit. Details of any sequelae of the fit were obtained. The age of the child when general practitioner and hospital services were first contacted was also noted.

Neurological Examination of the Child

All the children had a standardised neurological examination (described in chapter 2) which was carried out by physicians who had had post-graduate neurological training. In all cases where the examiner thought the child had a neurological disorder (other than uncomplicated epilepsy) the findings were checked by either PG or MR.

Hospital Records

In all cases where the child had attended hospital (either on the Isle of Wight or elsewhere) for a neuro-epileptic disorder, the records were perused by PG or MR to obtain details of clinical findings and the results of relevant investigations.

On the basis of all available information from records, from an interview with the parents and from a neurological examination of the child a final diagnosis was made by PG and MR jointly.

Number of Children Seen

Altogether, 262 children were scheduled to be included in the intensive phase of the investigation because of suspected neuro-epileptic disorder. When all the information was available and the final diagnosis made, there were 19 children with a lesion below the brain stem, 2 who had a spinal deficit but only a dubious neurological defect, 35 with cerebral palsy, 20 with some other brain disorder, 40 with severe intellectual retardation, 15 who were blind, 14 who were deaf, 9 with a developmental language disorder and 64 with uncomplicated epilepsy; a total of 186 children when overlap between the groups is taken into account.

The children with a suspected neuro-epileptic disorder who were not finally diagnosed as having such a condition were a fairly heterogeneous mixture. The largest group of exclusions consisted of children who had had epileptic fits previously but who had not had a fit or taken regular anticonvulsants during the 12 months preceding the survey. There were also some children suspected of fits who were diagnosed as having faints, vertiginous attacks or some other form of non-epileptic disorder.

Several children had been diagnosed when younger (on apparently good evidence) as having cerebral palsy or some other brain disorder but showed no evidence of this at the time we saw them. It is well recognised that some children with a mild cerebral palsy in infancy can lose all signs of the disorder by middle or late childhood. Similarly, some of the disorders following encephalitis or tuberculous meningitis seemed to have cleared up completely. Presumably in all these cases there was some residual brain damage, but as the children now had no detectable neurological disorder they were excluded.

There were a number of severely clumsy children who showed no other abnormalities on neurological examination. These, too, were excluded as we did not consider that our screening methods were adequate to detect all children with disorders of this kind. There were also children included because of a condition which might have led to neurological complications (*e.g.*, a child with collapsed vertebrae following a spinal abscess) but which, in the event, turned out not to have done so. Finally, some children included because of conditions which might have been confused with cerebral palsy (*e.g.*, talipes) were found to have been correctly diagnosed and to have no signs of neurological disorder.

Nevertheless, the value of casting our net rather wide was shown by the fact that there were a few children previously diagnosed as having some other condition who were found to have a neuro-epileptic disorder. For example, a child noted on the Register as having a '? club foot' was found to have a spinal palsy and a boy with a 'congenital short leg' was shown to have a mild hemiplegia as was also another boy shown on the Register to have a 'congenital weak and short leg'.

Sources of Selection

The sources of selection for the children in each group of those finally diagnosed as having a neuro-epileptic disorder are illustrated in Table 26, and Table 27 shows the number of sources of selection per child in each group. As the main sources of selection were rather different for different conditions, these will be considered separately.

The Register based on the school medical examination was the most useful single source of cases of cerebral palsy, but even so it only selected half the cases (see Table 26). With the addition of the Spastics Day Unit cases (which overlapped with the Register list) a quarter was still left unaccounted for. These were mainly mentally subnormal children who were known through the records of the mental subnormality hospital or junior training centre, but there was one child known only through the authority records of mentally subnormal children at home, another of normal intelligence who received home tuition, one only selected because of personal perusal of the records of the special day school for educationally subnormal children and another only known because the head teacher supplied her name.

TABLE 26
Sources of selection

Sources	*Cerebral palsy*		*Other brain disorders*		*Lesions below the brain stem*		*Epilepsy*		*Blind children*	
	A	B	A	B	A	B	A	B	A	B
Register based on school medical examination	8	16	0	6	6	13	34	56	0	3
Hospital records	0	5	1	6	1	7	8	28	0	2
Special day school (E.S.N.)	1	6	0	4	0	0	0	2	0	1
Speech therapy lists	0	7	1	4	0	1	–	–	0	1
Spastics Day Unit	1	12	0	1	1	3	–	–	0	1
Children at home	2	2	–	–	–	–	–	–	1	1
Mental subnormality hospital	2	4	5	5	1	1	–	–	4	4
Junior Training Centre	2	5	5	5	0	1	–	–	2	2
Special residential schooling	0	1	–	–	–	–	–	–	5	7
Head teacher addition	1	1	1	1	1	1	–	–	–	–
Inclusion in other part of survey	–	–	–	–	1	1	–	–	–	–
Total	17	59	13	32	11	28	42	86	12	22

A = *Number of cases for which it was the only source.*
B = *Number of cases from this source as well as any other source or sources.*

TABLE 27
Number of sources of selection per child

No. of sources	*Cerebral palsy*	*Other brain disorders*	*Lesions below the brain stem*	*Epilepsy*	*Blind children*
One only	17	13	11	42	12
Two	13	3	7	22	–
Three	4	3	1	–	2
Four	1	1	–	–	1
Total no. of children	35	20	19	64	15

The hospital records were of very limited use in selecting cerebral palsied children. This was largely because of the way the records were organised, as a majority of the children had in fact attended hospital at some time in the past. The filing of records was not based on age or diagnosis so that the only way to find children's records (short of going through the records of all people of all ages who had ever attended hospital) was to use the lists of new cases seen by the paediatrician. As we were only able to examine the records for the last three years, all children who had first attended for any reason before that time were missed. Another difficulty stemmed from the fact that some children were seen in other clinics (particularly the orthopaedic and surgical clinics) without ever seeing a paediatrician. In addition a substantial minority of children had been referred directly to hospitals in London rather than on the Isle of Wight (this rarely happened with epileptic children).

The sources useful in the selection of children with other brain disorders were fairly similar except that a smaller proportion were noted on the Register and a larger proportion were found only through the records of one or other of the facilities for mentally subnormal children. One child was found only through the availability of a list of children seen by the speech therapist, one only through the hospital and one only because she was named by the head teacher of the school she attended.

The situation was also fairly similar for children with lesions below the brain stem. However, one child was identified only because she happened to have been included in another survey and too late to be included in the intensive phase of the investigation.

For epileptic children, only the Register and hospital records were of much use as means of selection. Most epileptic children (56 out of 64) were known to the school health authority but one in eight was identified only through the use of hospital records.

Blind children were generally identified either through their placement at a special school or through one of the facilities for the mentally subnormal. It should be appreciated that no attempt was made to detect children with visual defects which did not give rise to the need for special schooling or special placement of some other kind.

Obviously, the mental subnormality units and hospitals were the main source of cases of severe intellectual retardation. In fact, very few children were identified from any other source: four from the Spastics Day Unit (where they were seen with a view to attendance), one from hospital records, one from the list of children wearing a hearing aid, and three because they were being cared for at home. All were known to the authorities as mentally subnormal.

The deaf children were all selected from the audiology clinic list but two had also seen the speech therapist, one had attended the paediatric clinic and one went to the junior training centre.

Finally, all the children with language retardation were notified by the speech therapist. Two of these were also selected from the special school records.

It should be said that the figures indicating source of selection cannot be used to identify the placement of the children at the time of the survey (for this information chapter 9 should be consulted). Some of the information was out of date by the time we received it so that, for example, a child whose name appeared on the Spastics Day Unit roll might, by the time of the survey, have transferred to a residential school.

Checks on Identification of Cases

A number of independent checks were made to cover the possibility that physically handicapped children had been missed by the screening procedure. During an educational survey in the previous year about 450 children (that is nearly a quarter of the total population of 9 and 10 year old children) received neurological examinations. It was therefore possible to look at the results of these individual examinations to determine what children with neurological conditions had escaped our net of screening procedures. Only one child with a possible neurological disorder was discovered; she was included in the intensive phase of the study and on the basis of this fuller information was found *not* to have a handicapping condition which fulfilled our criteria.

During the same educational survey, as part of a general medical study of the children, parents had been asked to complete a comprehensive questionnaire about their child's health. When these forms were scrutinised, no children whose names were not otherwise known to us had been selected by the health questionnaire responses as having even a *possible* neuro-epileptic handicap.

The third check was provided by the psychiatric survey which involved the personal interviewing of the parents of 268 children selected because of possible emotional or behavioural problems. The parents were routinely asked about their child's physical health as well as their behaviour. No additional child with neuro-epileptic disorder was discoverd in this way. Few children with neuro-epileptic conditions could have escaped the net of screening procedures.

CHAPTER 7

Prevalence and Characteristics of Neurological Disorders

There are no obvious or clear-cut boundaries to the concept of 'neurological disorder'. Some unequivocal injuries to the brain do not give rise to any signs on neurological examination. This is illustrated, for example, by ablation studies in animals (see chapter 1) and by studies of individuals who have been subjected to a prefrontal leucotomy or temporal lobectomy. Children who have neurological abnormalities in infancy may appear normal when examined some years later (Solomons *et al.* 1963); similarly, the neurological sequelae of encephalitis may clear up completely as the children grow older (Meyer and Byers 1952). On the other hand, cortical lesions associated with little deficit in infancy may be associated with the later development of spasticity or athetosis (Kennard 1942, Perlstein and Barnett 1952). There are also various motor 'abnormalities' on neurological examination which occur in the absence of any evidence of brain disease or damage and which may be due to maturational delays rather than to a structural brain lesion (Brenner *et al.* 1967, Gubbay *et al.* 1965, Ingram, 1963*b*, Walton *et al.* 1962). As a consequence of these and other considerations it is not possible to arrive at any accurate estimate of the total prevalence of overall 'neurological disorder'.

However, the prevalence of various defined neurological conditions may be determined and some estimate of the overall rate obtained by summation of the individual rates. Even this approach is subject to very considerable difficulties due to the fact that, for the most part, neurological disorders in childhood do not constitute discrete disease entities.

Definition of Cerebral Palsy

This problem is clearly illustrated by considering the definition of 'cerebral palsy' (Ingram 1964, Mitchell 1961, Mac Keith *et al.* 1959). This widely used diagnosis is an artificially derived category, not a disease entity. Nevertheless, it has some administrative usefulness and facilitates comparisons between different studies; for these reasons it was retained in the present investigation and defined as an unequivocally pathological motor disorder in which there was evidence of a non-progressive lesion above the brain stem. As the study was confined to children under the age of 15 years, it was implicit that the lesion occurred in an immature brain. This definition is equivalent to that used by Ingram (1964) and Mitchell (1961) in their epidemiological studies of cerebral palsy.

Motor disorders due to progressive disease (*e.g.* cerebral lipoidosis) were excluded, as were disorders due to lesions at or below the brain stem. Obviously, the decision on these points involved inference based on the clinical examination, history and, in some cases, special examinations, but as far as possible, cases were classified as cerebral palsy only when there was no reasonable doubt as to the diagnosis.

The chief difficulty arose in relation to cases where there was gross motor incoordination or hypotonia but no paresis or spasticity. Some of these children showed severe mental subnormality but others were of normal intelligence. In either case they were excluded on the grounds that the abnormality involved a delay in a developmental function rather than an unequivocally pathological disorder.

No upper age limit was set for the onset of the disorder, since the development of the brain is not complete until adolescence. However, only four cases of postnatal cerebral palsy were diagnosed, the child who was oldest at the time of onset of the disorder being six years of age.

Prevalence of Cerebral Palsy

Thirty-five cases of cerebral palsy were found in a child population of 11,865, making a prevalence rate of 2·9 per 1,000, or 2·6 per 1,000 if only congenital cases are included. There were four cases of postnatal cerebral palsy, one due to a head injury, two to encephalitis and one to a head injury received during an attack of encephalitis. All four children had a hemiplegia, but one also had some minor involvement of the other side.

There are now a large number of prevalence studies of cerebral palsy in the literature. The rates which have been reported vary from 1·0 per 1,000 to 5·9 per 1,000, but this variation is somewhat misleading in view of the differences in methods used to identify cases. Table 28*a* summarises the studies which have used multiple screening methods. The Scottish surveys of Ingram (1955, 1964) and Henderson (1961) are those most closely comparable to the Isle of Wight study. Ingram used the school medical service and public health department, the files of the Scottish Council for the Care of Spastics, general practitioners, hospitals, institutions for the mentally defective and cases seen in personal research projects as his source of cases; Henderson and his colleagues used local authority records, hospital records and enquiries to general practitioners and to longstay hospitals and institutions for the physically and mentally handicapped for case finding. Both studies produced rates of between 2·0 and 2·5 per 1,000. Gudmundsson (1967), Tuuteri *et al.* (1967), Andersen (1954) and Herlitz and Redin (1955) used comparable methods and also produced rates of the same order.

The Schenectady County study has produced the highest rate so far reported (5·9 per 1,000). Case reporting by doctors and by a variety of medical and other clinics and agencies was followed up with a house to house survey of 16 per cent of the population. Undoubtedly, this was one of the most thorough studies there has been. It remains uncertain, however, whether the definition of cerebral palsy used in the Schenectady County study was the same as that used in other investigations.

McGreal (1966) found a city rate of 2·4, which is closely similar to that reported from the other studies using multiple screening methods, but his county rate (1·1) was considerably lower. The reason for the discrepancy between these two rates was not determined, but in many respects this study was less thorough than the others already noted. Children in long-stay institutions for the mentally and physically

TABLE 28
Previous studies of the prevalence of cerebral palsy

Country	*Author*	*Date*	*Rate per* 1,000 (*school age children*)
(a) Studies using multiple screening methods			
Norway	Andersen	1954	1·9
England	Brewis	1966	1·4
Iceland	Gudmundsson	1967	2·3
Denmark	Hansen	1960	1·4
Scotland	Henderson	1961	2·0
Sweden	Herlitz and Redin	1955	2·1
Scotland	Ingram	1955	2·2
Canada	McGreal	1966	2·4 (city)
			1·1 (country)
Finland	Tuuteri *et al.*	1967	2·2 (approx.)
U.S.A.	Schenectady County Study	1949	5·9
(b) Studies where details of methodology are not known or not satisfactory			
New Zealand	Barclay	1956	2·6
England	British Council for the Welfare of Spastics	1948	2·0
			2·0
			2·4
England	Cohen	1953	2·2
England	Cohen	1954	1·9
U.S.A.	Phelps	1941	4·0
England	Smallwood	1953	2·0
England	Woods	1963	1·6—2·5
(c) Largely administrative or clinic studies			
England	Asher and Schonell	1950	1·0 (estimate)
,,	Dunsdon	1952	1·3
,,	Floyer	1955	1·3
,,	Griffiths and Barrett	1967	1·7
			1·5
,,	Holoran	1952	1·6
,,	MacGregor *et al.*	1957	1·2
,,	Woods	1957	1·9
,,	Wright *et al.*	1966	0·9

handicapped were not examined for cerebral palsy and doctors were relied upon to report cases, there being no personal search of records.

The study of Brewis *et al.* (1966) was thorough, systematic and involved several independent sources of cases, but it was not primarily concerned with children or with cerebral palsy. The somewhat lower prevalence of cerebral palsy reported (1·4) is probably explicable in terms of the sampling error inherent in the small size of population studied.

Hansen's study in Denmark (1960) has produced the lowest rate of all the studies using multiple screening methods, namely 1·4 per 1,000. He relied on hospitals, institutions and physicians informing him of all their cases when asked to do so, rather than personally searching their records. This may have resulted in some cases being missed. He excluded cases with an onset after three years and also cases of mental subnormality and retarded motor development with neurological abnormalities (unspecified). Although Hansen was more explicit than other writers in describing excluded cases it is possible that some of these cases might have been included by other investigators.

Thus, with the exception of the last two studies and the American study with a much higher rate, the most thorough investigations are agreed in finding a rate of cerebral palsy of about 2·0 to 2·5 per 1,000 among school age children.

Table 28*b* summarises the findings of another group of studies which appear generally similar to those already discussed but where the methods have been less fully reported. The Phelps study (1941), with a rate of 4·0 per 1,000, probably used methods similar to those used in the Schenectady County study. Otherwise, the findings of this second group of studies are closely similar to the first group.

Table 28*c* shows the findings of studies which have largely used clinic populations or administrative statistics. The rates of cerebral palsy reported are all considerably lower than the average for the first two groups of (more thorough) studies. Holoran (1952) used cases known to the local authority and found a rate of 1·6 per 1,000 for children aged 5 to 15 years; Griffiths and Barrett (1967) used records held by the Midland Spastics Association and found rates of 1·5 to 1·7 per 1,000; Asher and Schonell (1950) in a much quoted study found a rate of 1·0 per 1,000. Although they used multiple screening methods, the methods were unsystematic compared with those of Ingram, Henderson and others in the first group. Woods (1957) used cases referred to a cerebral palsy assessment clinic but, as there was no screening of the general population, her result probably underestimated the prevalence. On the other hand, this was counterbalanced by the inclusion of cases which would certainly have been excluded by most other investigators.

As one might expect, the less thorough studies have produced lower prevalence rates for cerebral palsy. Ingram has shown in his comprehensive survey (1955) that if the school medical service, public health authorities and general practitioners only had been contacted, a rate of approximately 1·0 per 1,000 would have been obtained. The addition of hospital cases raised the figure to about 1·6 per 1,000 and it was only with the addition of other miscellaneous sources that the figure was over 2·0 per 1,000.

Many cases of cerebral palsy are not known to the authorities, and administrative or clinic surveys produce rates of only 1 to 2 per 1,000. It is unfortunate that most studies of this kind have been English so that English reviews of the subject (Illingworth 1958) have concluded (we think wrongly) that these lower figures give the true prevalence of cerebral palsy.

No exact comparisons can be made between many of the studies owing to differences in method and in definition of cerebral palsy. Furthermore, some differences may be accounted for by random error, particularly in the smaller studies. However, it seems reasonable to conclude that the true prevalence of cerebral palsy in school age children is somewhere between 2 per 1,000 and 3 per 1,000.

The Isle of Wight rate is at the top of this range but it does not differ significantly from either the Henderson (1961) or Ingram (1955) surveys (the difference from the Henderson survey falls just short of the 5 per cent level of significance). The region of error in estimates of prevalence rates, even when based on large populations, is often not appreciated. Thus the 95 per cent confidence limits for the Isle of Wight figures are from 2·05 to 4·10 per 1,000. Similarly the limits for Ingram's figures, based on a larger population, are 1·8 to 2·5 per 1,000. The somewhat higher rate of cerebral palsy found in the present study may be explained in part by merely chance variation.

Nevertheless, it is still necessary to consider whether there are reasons why the rate might be truly higher on the Isle of Wight. There is as yet no satisfactory evidence for regional differences in rates. The higher American figures might be taken to indicate higher rates in the U.S.A., but the differences in methods between American and other studies make it unwise to come to this conclusion. In this context, however, it may be relevant that the perinatal mortality rate in the U.S.A. compares unfavourably with the United Kingdom and Scandinavia (Chase 1967). It is also possible that there is a similar explanation for the higher rate on the Isle of Wight, in that the perinatal mortality rate for the Island prior to the survey was above the national average (County Medical Officer of Health 1963, Registrar-General 1964)*. In 1962 the Island rate was 37·2 compared with 28·6 in the country as a whole. However, it is uncertain whether this is a large enough difference to account for the findings.

Another possible factor is the presence of an excellent day unit for children with cerebral palsy on the Isle of Wight. However, the figures do not suggest that this has influenced the rates by causing people to migrate to the Island to obtain good care for their children. In the control group 31 per cent of the children had been born off the Island; among the children with cerebral palsy the rate was closely similar (25 per cent).

Differences in the definition of cerebral palsy are unlikely to have given rise to differences in rates with respect to the two other British studies (Henderson 1961, Ingram 1955) as closely similar criteria were employed. It is unlikely, too, that any cases included here would have been excluded by other investigators (see case histories in Appendix A).

In summary, then, most of the best previous studies found rates of cerebral palsy between 2 and 2·5 per 1,000. The Isle of Wight rate was slightly higher (2·9 per 1,000) but is probably partly explicable by chance variation. The importance of multiple screening methods in any prevalence study has been shown repeatedly. The low rates reported from administrative studies are explicable, therefore, in terms of the inadequacy of their case-finding methods. There is no satisfactory evidence for marked regional variation and the true rate of cerebral palsy, at least in Great Britain, is probably somewhere between 2 and 3 per 1,000. It is highly unlikely that it is below

*The rate has fallen recently and it now approximates the national average (County Medical Officer of Health 1969, Edwards 1968).

2 per 1,000 and, as the present figures are at least as high as those of comparable surveys carried out a decade ago (Ingram 1955, Henderson 1961), it seems unlikely that there has been a decline in the rate of cerebral palsy, as suggested by some (Brandt *et al.* 1964, Woods 1963).

Prevalence of Other Disorders with a Lesion above the Brain Stem

There are a large number of mostly ill-defined conditions, which are not included under the term cerebral palsy as defined above, but which nevertheless are associated with a lesion above the brain stem. In our study there were 20 cases of this kind, giving a prevalence rate of 1·7 per 1,000. In 5 cases there was a well-defined condition (one case of craniostenosis, galactosaemia and cerebral lipoidosis, and two cases of hydrocephalus) but in 15 cases no definite diagnostic label could be attached. Many of these non-specific disorders appeared to be a consequence of perinatal damage and the neuropathology was probably often similar to that found in cases of cerebral palsy. To be included there had to be good evidence for some definite lesion above the brain stem; a developmental disorder of motor co-ordination or language was not enough. Many of these children had been diagnosed as having cerebral palsy at some time in the past and in many respects the similarities with cerebral palsy outweigh the dissimilarities (see chapter 8). Nevertheless, the cases did not fulfil the criteria for cerebral palsy and some had a quite different pathology.

This group of disorders is difficult to define clearly and most previous studies have not dealt with cases not classified as cerebral palsy, so it is not possible to compare the present findings with previous investigations. However, it is noteworthy that Hansen (1960) in his survey of cerebral palsy in Denmark, excluded one case which would fulfil the above criteria for every four cases of cerebral palsy included. Evidently the problem of children with brain disorders other than cerebral palsy is substantial.

Severe Intellectual Retardation

Quite how large this group is obviously depends on the criteria for inclusion. If a complete tally of children with brain disorders is wanted, those with severe intellectual retardation must be added. Post-mortem studies have shown that all or nearly all children with an IQ below 50 have demonstrable pathology of the brain (Crome 1960). The great majority of these children are known to the authorities, so that there is a very good agreement between administrative prevalence and true prevalence. A good estimate of severe intellectual retardation may be obtained in this country by a count of the number of children in mental subnormality hospitals, junior training centres and at home not attending school by reason of a severe degree of mental subnormality (Kushlick 1961, Tizard 1964).

Out of the total population of 11,865 there were 37 children not attending school by reason of mental subnormality, giving a prevalence rate of 3·1 per 1,000 or 3·4 per 1,000 if the 3 mongol children attending school are also included. This rate is closely similar to (but slightly below) the rates found in much earlier studies of children in England and Wales (Lewis 1929), as well as in more recent studies in this country (Goodman and Tizard 1962; Kushlick 1961, 1964, 1965) and elsewhere (Tizard 1966).

The largest single group consisted of the children with Down's syndrome, who accounted for about a third of all cases of severe intellectual retardation, as found in most previous studies (Tizard 1966). There is good agreement between studies that the rate of Down's syndrome in school age children is about 1 per 1,000 (Carter 1958, Penrose and Smith 1966).

The rates for children whose severe intellectual retardation was associated with cerebral palsy (0·8 per 1,000) or with some similar brain condition (0·8 per 1,000) were similar to those for Down's syndrome. There were two children who had an associated lesion below the brain stem (one case of peroneal muscular atrophy and one of muscular dystrophy). It now seems from other investigations that there is a real link between muscular dystrophy and severe mental subnormality (Cohen *et al.* 1968). Finally, there were five children in whom the neurological examination revealed no unequivocal abnormality.

Some of these intellectually retarded children were already counted because of the conditions (such as cerebral palsy) with which the retardation was associated. A further 20 remained, making a rate of 1·7 per 1,000 which must be added to the cerebral palsy rate of 3·0 per 1,000 and the other brain disorder rate of 1·7 per 1,000. The total prevalence of children with pathological disorders of the brain was 6·4 per 1,000.

Total Prevalence of Structural Brain Disorders

This is still a minimal figure as it does not include children with developmental language disorders (a rate of 0·8 per 1,000 in the present study of school age children) some of whom may have had structural brain pathology; nor does it include severely clumsy children or children with very poor visuomotor ability. Severe clumsiness is probably as common as any of the neurological groups so far considered (Brenner and Gillman 1966, Brenner *et al.* 1967) and in some cases it may be due to brain damage of perinatal origin (Gubbay *et al.* 1965, Walton *et al.* 1962). Because we did not screen the total population for clumsiness, our only assessment of prevalence comes from the control group of 147 children. This is too small a number to provide reliable figures but, in keeping with other studies, the neurological examination showed 1·4 per cent to be 'dyspraxic' and the modification of the Oseretsky test defined 5 per cent as severely clumsy. The figure for total prevalence of structural brain disorders also does not account for many other conditions sometimes included under the term 'minimal cerebral dysfunction' (Bax and Mac Keith 1963), nor does it include children with uncomplicated epilepsy (another 5·3 per 1,000, see chapter 8), or, of course, those with lesions below the brain stem (1·6 per 1,000, see page 116).

For children with conditions such as severe language delay, severe clumsiness or epilepsy, there are no satisfactory means of determining what proportion have structural brain pathology. The same applies to children who suffered severe insult to the brain in early life (such as by injury or encephalitis) or who gave evidence of cerebral palsy in early childhood but later showed no abnormality on neurological examination. Clearly, many of these disorders are due to brain disease or brain damage and their inclusion would undoubtedly multiply the minimal figure of 6·4 per 1,000 already obtained for children with a pathological disorder of the brain.

Lesion at or below the Brain Stem

Altogether there were 19 children with disorders involving a lesion at or below the brain stem, including muscle disorders, giving a rate of 1·6 per 1,000 (Table 29). None of the sub-groups was large enough to warrant the calculation of individual prevalence rates. Paralyses following poliomyelitis and muscular dystrophy were the two most common disorders but both were quite uncommon in comparison with cerebral palsy, as found by other investigators (Brewis *et al.* 1966, Forrester 1967).

The very low rate of spinal palsy needs comment in view of the fact that the incidence of spina bifida cystica at birth is somewhere between 2 and 4 per 1,000 in Britain (Laurence *et al.* 1967). In the present study there was only one case of spinal palsy among 11,865 children. Even if two further children with spina bifida, but only a dubious neurological disorder at the time of the survey, are included, this is still a rate of less than 0·3 per 1,000. There are major regional variations in the incidence of spina bifida, partly due to the rates being higher in urban than in rural areas (Edwards 1958, Laurence *et al.* 1967), but the variation is insufficient to explain the very low rate of children with spinal palsy. More important is the fact that in the past very few children with spinal palsy have survived (Jaeger 1953). At the time the survey children were born (1950 to 1959), very few children with spina bifida cystica were being operated on, so that it was too early to see the improved survival rate which has followed modern surgical intervention (Eckstein 1968).

TABLE 29
Prevalence of disorder with lesions at or below the brain stem

Condition	*No. of cases*
Paralyses following poliomyelitis	7
Muscular dystrophy	5
Peripheral nerve palsy	2
Amyotonia congenita	1
Spinal palsy	1
Syringomyelia	1
Freidreich's ataxia	1
Peroneal muscular atrophy	1
Total cases	19
Rate per 1,000	1·6
(Plus 2 cases of spinal lesions with dubious neurological defect)	

Prevalence of Miscellaneous Other Disorders

Developmental Language Disorders

There were 9 children with a developmental disorder of language, a prevalence rate of 0·8 per 1,000. As found by others (Ingram 1959*b*) there was a marked preponderance of boys (8:1). This group includes only those children with substantially impaired language usage at the time of the survey; it does not include those who had been delayed in their language development but who were talking normally at the time of the survey, nor does it include children with a disorder only of articulation or of speech rhythm. Furthermore, it refers only to children with a specific developmental disorder; those in whom the language retardation was associated with severe intellectual retardation, cerebral palsy or other neurological disorder, deafness or psychosis were excluded. Severe language impairment was more frequent in association with these conditions than it was as an isolated, specific developmental disorder. Of the 16 children with virtually no useful speech, none had a specific developmental disorder, although 4 of the 9 children with a developmental language disorder were very severely impaired in their language usage. Thus, the total prevalence of impaired language usage is much greater than the rate for specific disorders.

The rate for specific developmental language disorder in the present study cannot be treated with the same confidence as the rates for other neurological disorders, in that the screening techniques were not particularly designed to pick out children with an isolated language problem. The list of children seen by the speech therapists was the main source of cases and included all the 9 children. Although it is perhaps unlikely in a well served community like the Isle of Wight that many children with a serious persisting language disorder would not be referred for diagnosis or treatment, the number of children with such a disorder who were never seen by the paediatrician or speech therapist is quite unknown.

There are several surveys of speech disorders in children (Grady and Daniels 1964, Morley 1965), but less attention has been paid to serious disorders of language development. The best estimate of the rate of severe language retardation is provided by Ingram's surveys in Edinburgh and Aberdeen (Ingram 1963*c*). Speech therapists, educational psychologists, child psychiatrists and audiologists were asked to report children thought to be of average intelligence who had only a few single words at the age of 3 years and only very limited connected speech by the age of 5 years. The estimated prevalence of severe specific language retardation was 0·71 per 1,000 for Edinburgh and 0·75 per 1,000 for Aberdeen. These figures are close to the present rates (which included children of below average intelligence, provided that their language delay was too severe to be accounted for in terms of intellectual impairment). The true rate for developmental language disorders can only be determined by a large scale survey designed for the purpose, but the present best estimate seems to be that the rate of severe disorders is probably slightly less than 1 per 1,000 among school age children. The rate for mild disorders is, of course, very much greater.

Blindness and Deafness

Blindness and deafness were included in the survey for comparative purposes in connection with the study of association between psychiatric disorder and organic brain dysfunction (see Part IV). It is convenient, therefore, to consider their prevalence here. In both cases only minimal estimates were obtained as heavy reliance was placed on administrative statistics. Blindness was defined as sight so poor as to require special schooling, or in the case of children not at school, so severe as to seriously impair their daily life. Defined in this way there were 15 blind children, a rate of 1·3 per 1,000. Nine of the 15 children also had some neurological disorder and 7 of these 9 had severe intellectual retardation.

Deafness was defined simply in terms of children for whom hearing aids were currently prescribed. There were 14 deaf children, a rate of 1·2 per 1,000. They were very much less handicapped than the blind children and 12 attended ordinary school compared with none of the 15 blind children. Only one deaf child had severe intellectual retardation and no other deaf child had a neurological disorder.

Classification of Cerebral Palsy

The classification of cerebral palsy has been discussed several times (Balf and Ingram 1955; Hansen 1960; Ingram 1964; Mitchell 1961; Perlstein 1952; Phelps 1941, 1949) without any entirely satisfactory resolution of the difficulties which result from the wide variety of manifestations of cerebral palsy, from the lack of clear differentiation between them and from the fact that in any individual child the manifestations tend to change as he grows older. The last difficulty was less important in the present study because attention was confined to children of at least five years of age, by which time most major changes have already taken place.

The number of cases in the present study did not warrant the use of a fine breakdown into numerous sub-categories and so cases were classified according to the part of the body involved, using a scheme based on that of Ingram (1964). The chief difficulty arose where there was both a spastic paresis and athetosis. In these cases, the classification was based on the distribution of the spastic paresis, the category of dyskinesia being retained for cases where athetosis or other involuntary movements constituted the major disability, and where there was little or no accompanying paresis. The classification was based on the limbs where there was impaired function, so that limbs with some abnormality detectable only on detailed neurological examination but no impairment of function were classed as normal limbs.

Categories were defined as follows:

Hemiplegia referred to a unilateral paresis involving either the upper or lower limbs or both. Cases of monoplegia were included.

Diplegia was defined as a more or less symmetrical paresis which was worse in the lower limbs than in the upper limbs.

Bilateral hemiplegia was used for cases where there was a paresis of all four limbs which was most marked in the upper limbs or of equal severity in upper and lower limbs.

Dyskinesia was confined to cases where involuntary movements of the limbs produced the major disability, there being little or no paresis.

Ataxia was the category used when inco-ordination and impaired balance were the main manifestations and where there was little paresis.

The relative frequency of the various types of cerebral palsy is shown in Table 30, where comparisons are also made with the Dundee survey (Mitchell 1961) and the Edinburgh survey (Ingram 1955). Similar findings emerge from comparisons with the numerous other studies in the literature. There is good agreement that about a third of the cases have hemiplegia, about half are diplegic or quadriplegic and that both dyskinesia and ataxia are uncommon varieties. The most marked difference between the Isle of Wight and the Dundee and Edinburgh surveys is the much higher proportion of cases of bilateral hemiplegia in the present study, as well as the lower rate of diplegia. It seems likely that the difference is due, in part, to the ways in which diplegia and bilateral hemiplegia have been differentiated. It may also be that the personal examination of all mentally subnormal children on the Isle of Wight (including those living at home and not attending any school or institution) brought to light more cases of bilateral hemiplegia, a variety of cerebral palsy associated with an exceptionally high rate of severe intellectual retardation.

The number of cases in this survey was too small for a separate examination of the medical, educational and psychiatric aspects of each type of cerebral palsy, so that, with a few exceptions, hereafter the subdivisions have not been maintained.

TABLE 30
Various types of cerebral palsy in the Isle of Wight, Dundee and Edinburgh surveys

Neurological syndrome	*Isle of Wight survey* %	*Dundee survey* %	*Edinburgh survey* %
Hemiplegia	37·1	37·5	36·1
Diplegia	34·3	41·2	43·7
Bilateral hemiplegia	22·9	1·3	3·9
Dyskinesia	2·9	8·4	8·2
Ataxia	2·9	1·7	7·2
Other	0·0	10·0	1·0

Sex Distribution

Twenty (57 per cent) of the 35 children with cerebral palsy were boys. There was a similar sex ratio (12 boys to 8 girls) in the group with other brain disorders. These findings are in keeping with those of other studies; Ingram (1964) found that 61 per cent of children with cerebral palsy were boys, Mitchell (1961) found 54 per cent, Herlitz and Redin (1955) found 55 per cent and Gudmundsson (1967) found 60 per cent.

The sex ratio in cerebral palsy closely parallels that found with perinatal mortality (Butler and Bonham 1963). This probably reflects the fact that a high proportion of cases of cerebral palsy are due to perinatal abnormalities and complications (Drillien *et al.* 1962, Illingworth 1958, Ingram 1964, Mitchell 1961). Several explanations have been offered as to why the male should be more vulnerable to perinatal damage (Gruenberg 1966). Whereas there may be factors specific to the birth process, it is important to note that the young male is more susceptible than the young female to a wide variety of biological hazards. He is more vulnerable to all manner of infections in childhood (Schlegel and Bellanti 1969, Washburn *et al.* 1965) and more commonly has specific delays in development (Rutter *et al.* 1970).

In relation to perinatal mortality and morbidity (including cerebral palsy of perinatal origin) it is likely that the greater physiological immaturity of the male plays an important part. In general, the immature organism is more vulnerable than the mature one and at birth boys are considerably retarded in their development compared with girls (Flory 1935). If immaturity is a relevant variable, it might be expected that the sex difference in morbidity and mortality should be maximal late in pregnancy or after birth and minimal early in gestation. There is some evidence that this may be the case. On the whole, the sex ratio in mortality is more marked for mature births than for premature births (though this might be due to the different causes of death at different stages of maturity; Butler and Bonham 1963), and the sex difference in cerebral palsy is greater for infants born after longer periods of gestation than for those born prematurely (McDonald 1963). Similarly, whereas irradiation after birth affects the skeletal growth of boys more than girls (Greulich *et al.* 1953), there is no sex difference in the effects on growth of foetal irradiation (Wood *et al.* 1967).

Degree of Handicap

Handicap was assessed on the extent to which the child's disability interfered with his daily life. In the case of a multiple handicap it was rarely possible to assess exactly which handicap led to which disability. Attention was accordingly confined to the actual restriction of activities, regardless of whether this seemed to be due to mental, physical or motivational factors. As far as could be judged, motivational factors played only a very minor part in the handicap but intellectual factors were more important. However, in most cases where there was a severe mental defect, there was also a severe physical defect.

The criteria for rating were as follows:

None: No handicap.

Slight: Inability to perform strenuous or stressful activities such as sport, long hikes or physical education; restriction of such activities or difficulty or discomfort in their performance. This rating was used where there was a slight limp, or where surgical shoes were worn.

Moderate: Inability to perform ordinary activities, restriction of such activities or difficulty or discomfort in their performance (but to an extent less marked than that covered by the severe rating). This rating was used where there was a marked limp, where crutches were used or where there was only a limited ability to walk distances. It was also used where the child was slow in his self-care but was independent or, at most, needed minor help with daily activities such as washing his back or brushing his hair.

Severe: Substantial help needed with daily activities such as dressing, undressing, washing, bathing and feeding. The rating was also applicable where the child required special transport or was unable to go out unaccompanied.

Total or almost total incapacity: The child needed help with all or nearly all daily activities.

The degree of handicap is shown in Table 31. There was a slight tendency for the children with other brain disorders to be less handicapped than those with cerebral palsy but the difference fell short of the 5 per cent level of statistical significance.

Much more striking was the large difference between those attending school and those who had been excluded from school by reason of mental subnormality. All the cerebral palsied children who had been excluded from school had a severe handicap compared with only 1 in 8 (12 per cent) of those attending school (p. < ·01). Similarly, of the children with other brain disorders excluded from school, 60 per cent had a severe handicap compared with none of those attending school (p. < ·01).

It is difficult to compare these findings with other surveys owing to uncertainty regarding the comparability of assessments. The proportion of cerebral palsied children with severe handicap in the present series (37 per cent) is similar to that reported by Ingram (37 per cent) but rather higher than that found by Mitchell (23 per cent).

TABLE 31
Degree of handicap

Handicap	*Cerebral palsy*				*Other brain disorders*			
	Excluded from school		*In school*		*Excluded from school*		*In school*	
	No.	*%*	*No.*	*%*	*No.*	*%*	*No.*	*%*
None	0	–	0	–	0	–	1	10
Slight	0	–	10	40	2	20	6	60
Moderate	0	–	12	48	2	20	3	30
Severe	4	40	2	8	3	30	0	–
Total or almost total incapacity	6	60	1	4	3	30	0	–
Total cases	10		25		10		10	

Epilepsy

In the present study, 40 per cent of the children with cerebral palsy had had epileptic fits (not counting those cases where convulsions were confined to the first two weeks of life). The rate of epilepsy was higher (70 per cent) in the children excluded from school than in those attending school (28 per cent). Epilepsy was slightly (but not significantly) more common among the children with other brain disorders (50 per cent) than among the cerebral palsied and, curiously, in the other brain disorder group fits had occurred in more of the children attending school than in those excluded by reason of mental subnormality.

A similar rate of epilepsy has generally been found among cerebral palsied children in other investigations, although the rate in this study was slightly higher than most. Ingram (1964) reported that 32 per cent had fits, Mitchell (1961) found that 25 per cent were epileptic, Andersen (1954) found 35 per cent, Gudmundsson (1967) 24 per cent, Woods (1957) 38 per cent, Tuuteri *et al.* (1967) 30 per cent and Barclay (1956) 29 per cent. The characteristics of the fits are considered in more detail in the next chapter.

Abnormalities of Speech and Language

Very few of the cerebral palsied children attending school were severely retarded in language but, in contrast, 80 per cent of those not at school had little or no useful language. As with every other handicap, language problems were much more common in children with severe intellectual retardation than in those with normal or only mildly subnormal intelligence. The situation among the children with other brain disorders was closely similar (Table 32).

Just over half the cerebral palsied children attending school (52 per cent) had an articulation defect in their speech (the number excluded from school who had speech was too small to warrant analysis). Among the children with other brain disorders attending school, 70 per cent had articulation defects.

Other workers have noted the very high rate of speech and language problems in children with cerebral palsy. Cockburn (1961) found that 19 per cent of the children in the Dundee study had no intelligible speech, compared with 23 per cent in this study. In most studies, too, half or more of the children have been found to have articulation defects (Andersen 1954, Dunsdon 1952, Floyer 1955, Ingram 1955). Illingworth (1958) and Ingram (1964) have discussed the possible causes of speech and language difficulties in cerebral palsy. Obviously, intellectual retardation is an important factor as severe language impairment is much more common in children of low IQ. Hearing difficulties are also a factor in some children, but it seems that deafness is only rarely the main cause of language difficulties except in children with athetosis (Ingram 1964, Ingram and Barn 1960). Aphasic problems due to cortical damage are sometimes important. Paresis or inco-ordination of the articulatory organs may cause dysarthria and dyskinesia may also affect speech through involvement of the respiratory muscles. However, many speech defects are developmental in type, the articulation problems being of the same pattern as those seen in children just learning to speak rather than those due to local abnormalities.

TABLE 32
Spoken language in children with cerebral palsy and other brain disorders

Spoken language	*Cerebral palsy*				*Other brain disorders*			
	Excluded from school		*In school*		*Excluded from school*		*In school*	
	No.	*%*	*No.*	*% of known*	*No.*	*% of known*	*No.*	*%*
Normal	1	10	14	61	0	–	4	40
Less complex than normal	1	10	8	35	1	11	4	40
Markedly retarded	0	–	1	4	2	22	2	20
Little or no useful language	8	80	0	–	6	67	0	–
Not known	–	–	2	–	1	–	–	–
Total cases	10		25		10		10	

Visual Defects

Four of the children with cerebral palsy were blind or nearly blind (two from retrolental fibroplasia, one from optic atrophy and one probably from cortical damage). Three of these children had been excluded from school by reason of mental subnormality. Strabismus was present in about a third of the cerebral palsied children (40 per cent in those excluded from school and 26 per cent in those at school). Altogether 29 per cent of the children with cerebral palsy had some type of visual defect (40 per cent in those excluded from school and 26 per cent in those at school). Visual problems were equally common among children with other types of brain disorder (10 per cent in those excluded from school and 60 per cent in those at school).

No examination was made for visual field defects. It has been found that hemianopia occurs in 10 to 25 per cent of hemiplegics, but very good compensation is usual so that this is rarely a cause of disability (Douglas 1961, Ingram 1964, Tizard *et al.* 1954). Degenerative myopia is also more common in the cerebral palsied, especially in premature children of low birth weight, than in the general population.

It is evident that visual defects—especially strabismus—are very common in children with cerebral palsy. Blindness is present in a substantial minority of those with severe intellectual retardation but really serious and handicapping visual defects are much less frequent among those of normal or near normal intelligence. The causation, nature and treatment of visual defects in cerebral palsied children is very well discussed by Douglas in relation to the findings of the Dundee study.

Other Disabilities

The present study was not intended as a full investigation of the medical aspects of cerebral palsy, so that the defects discussed above are only the most obvious of the medical disabilities found in association with cerebral palsy. In addition, most surveys have shown deafness to be present in 5 to 8 per cent of cerebral palsied children (Ingram 1964, MacGregor *et al.* 1957, Woods 1957), while more intensive studies (of adfflittedly rather selected groups) suggest that serious hearing impairment may, in fact, be as much as twice as common (Fisch 1957, Mowat 1961); high frequency hearing loss is especially common in association with athetosis. Dwarfing of the paralysed limb is also commonly found (Ingram 1964) and this is often associated with sensory and vasomotor disturbances. Contractures are liable to develop in limbs which are not used (as was found in several children in long-stay institutions in this study). Gingival abnormalities, malocclusion and retarded dental development are also all very common (Munro 1961), as are generalised intellectual impairment and specific learning difficulties (see chapter 9) and psychiatric disorder (see chapter 12). Often there are considerable problems in management for the family (see chapter 10).

The frequency and range of medical problems associated with cerebral palsy clearly indicate that the children's handicaps extend far beyond the paralysed limb. The need for a full and expert assessment of each child's disabilities, together with continuing supervision and treatment which takes account of the associated handicaps, has already been discussed by other writers (Henderson 1961). The implications for treatment will be considered again when the psychological, social and psychiatric findings have been discussed.

CHAPTER 8

Epileptic Disorders

Definition

There is no shortage of definitions of epilepsy but they are mostly of a kind which rely on reference to presumed brain dysfunction, such as 'paroxysmal cerebral dysrhythmia' (Gibbs *et al.* 1937). For epidemiological purposes, operational definitions in terms of observable behaviour are always to be preferred, particularly where there is disagreement about what conditions should be included in a category. For example, opinions differ as to whether some types of recurrent abdominal pain or migraine or disturbances of behaviour should be classed as epileptic equivalents. It is not clear from the definition used by the College of General Practitioners (1960) in their survey of epilepsy ('attacks primarily cerebral in origin in which there is a disturbance of movement, feeling, behaviour or consciousness') to what extent such conditions would be included.

Unfortunately the manifestations of epilepsy are so legion that it is extremely difficult to devise an entirely behavioural definition. As we did not wish to include so-called epileptic equivalents and in an attempt to provide criteria involving the minimum of inference, we defined epilepsy as a condition in which there had been at least one overt fit since the age of 5 years and in which the child had had an overt fit during the 12 months preceding the day of interview or had been on regular anti-convulsants during this same 12 months. An overt fit meant an attack involving paroxysmal motor abnormalities and/or total or partial loss of consciousness which was thought to be due to altered brain function and not produced by failure of the cerebral circulation or emotional causes.

Such a definition excludes the rarer types of sensory epilepsy but it was felt that with the methods at our disposal it would be very difficult to differentiate these varieties of epilepsy from other disorders. In order to ensure that the group of children with epilepsy included no-one in whom the diagnosis was in serious doubt, it seemed preferable to exclude all cases in which sensory disturbances were the only manifestation of epilepsy. Cases diagnosed by others as epilepsy were also excluded if they did not meet our criteria. As it happened, the excluded cases did not include any cases of local sensory fits.

Prevalence

Using these criteria there were 86 epileptic children in the 5 to 14 year old child population of 11,865, a rate of 7·2 per 1,000 (the 95 per cent probability limits are 5·7 to 8·9 per 1,000). In 64 of the children, the fits were not associated with any other known brain disease, disorder or injury; these are therefore classed as having 'uncomplicated epilepsy' (a rate of 5·4 per 1,000). In the remaining 22 children (1·8 per 1,000) the fits were associated with cerebral palsy or some other structural brain disorder.

The distinction between 'uncomplicated epilepsy' and epilepsy associated with structural brain disorder is retained throughout this chapter.

Fifty-two of the 86 epileptic children (4·3 per 1,000) had had a fit during the 12 months previous to the date of interview. The remaining 34 children (2·9 per 1,000) had had a fit since the age of 5 years and were on regular anticonvulsants during the previous 12 months.

The study most closely comparable to this one is that by Pond *et al.* (1960). They studied the patients in 14 general practices and defined an epileptic as someone who had had a fit during the 2 years prior to the time of the survey, or who had been on regular anticonvulsants during this period. They found a rate of 7·9 per 1,000 for children aged 5 to 14 years. The findings of the British national survey (Cooper 1965) were similar: 8·2 per 1,000 at 6 years, 4·3 per 1,000 at 7 years, 7·1 per 1,000 at 11 years and 8·2 per 1,000 at 15 years. These figures are based on the occurrence of a fit during the previous year as judged by a school medical officer on information from the mother. The College of General Practitioners' survey produced rather lower figures, the rate for children aged 5 to 14 years being 4·0 per 1,000. Gudmundsson's figures (1966) for Iceland were also rather lower than the Isle of Wight rate. He studied hospital and EEG records and enquired of G.Ps. to pick out epileptics, finding a rate of 4·3 per 1000 for children aged 10 to 19 years. Kurland (1959), in an American study based on Mayo Clinic and private physicians' records, found a rate of 5·8 per 1,000 for children aged 0 to 9 years and 3·5 per 1,000 for those aged 10 to 19 years. Not surprisingly, the figures based on administrative studies are much lower (Ministry of Education 1962, Henderson 1953), a tendency already noted when considering the prevalence of cerebral palsy. It may be concluded that the Isle of Wight findings are in agreement with the most thorough previous surveys and that the rate of epilepsy in school children is somewhere in the region of 5 to 9 per 1,000*.

Sex Distribution

There was only a very slight and non-significant excess of boys among the epileptic children; 12:10 in those with an associated structrual brain disorder and 34:30 in those with uncomplicated epilepsy. The findings of other studies are contradictory. Cooper (1965) and Pond *et al.* (1960), in studies of rather small numbers, found an excess of girls among epileptic children of school age, whereas the College of General Practitioners (1960), Kurland (1958, 1959) and Gudmundsson (1966) found a slight excess of males. Altogether it seems that there is no marked sex difference in the prevalence of epilepsy among school age children, although studies based on larger numbers suggest that epilepsy may be very slightly more common in boys.

Types of Fit

Half the epileptic children (both those with uncomplicated epilepsy and those with an associated structural brain disorder) had only had major attacks (Table 33),

*The rate of fits in preschool children is much higher but most cases of 'febrile convulsions' do not persist after the age of 5 years and so would not be included in these prevalence figures for children aged 5 to 14 years.

i.e. fits in which there was loss of consciousness and convulsions. None of the children with structural brain disease and only 5 per cent of those with uncomplicated epilepsy had pure petit mal. Petit mal was defined as a disorder with episodes of loss of consciousness which began and finished suddenly, lasted only a few seconds, occurred without warning and without after-effects and which were unaccompanied by loss of posture, falling, tongue-biting or incontinence (Gibberd 1966*a*, Holowach *et al.* 1962, Lees and Liversedge 1962). Characteristically the attack consisted of a brief lapse of conversation or action, often with staring, head nodding and/or pallor of the face. Other types of minor epilepsy were put in a separate category (see below). Although petit mal usually begins in childhood and often stops by early adult life (Gibberd 1966*b*, Gordon 1965), as a pure disorder it is nevertheless a quite uncommon type of epilepsy even in childhood. It is somewhat more frequent in association with other types of fit—this was the case in 16 per cent of the children with uncomplicated epilepsy and 5 per cent of those with a structural brain disorder. Of all the varieties of epilepsy, petit mal was least often associated with structural brain disorder.

TABLE 33
Type of epilepsy

Type of fit	*Uncomplicated epilepsy*		*Structural brain disorder*	
	No.	%	*No.*	%
Major only	32	50	11	50
Petit mal only	3	5	0	–
Minor only	12	19	4	18
All 3 types	2	3	0	–
Major and petit mal only	7	11	1	5
Minor and petit mal only	1	2	0	–
Major and minor only	7	11	6	27
Total cases	64		22	

Minor Fits

About a fifth of the children had only minor attacks* (see Table 34). These included all types of fit other than major fits or petit mal, *i.e.* psychomotor fits, focal motor fits and attacks in which there was loss of consciousness with falling but no convulsions.

Psychomotor fits were defined as fits in which there was total or partial loss of consciousness without convulsions and in which the chief manifestations included sensory phenomena (such as peculiar visceral sensations, strange smells or tastes or visual or auditory hallucinations), emotional phenomena (especially fear but also *déja vu* sensations or feelings of strangeness and detachment), and/or behavioural phenomena (such as licking or smacking of the lips, confused or odd movements or

*As this was the group in which there were the most difficulties in diagnosis, case histories are given in Appendix B.

TABLE 34
Minor fits

Type of fits	*Uncomplicated epilepsy*		*Structural brain disorder*	
	No.	*%*	*No.*	*%*
Psychomotor fits	8	13	3	14
Myoclonic fits	3	5	2	9
'Salaam' attacks	1	2	0	–
'Infantile Spasms'	0	–	1	5
Focal motor fits	4*	6	0	–
Other minor fits	8	13	4	18
Total cases with minor fits	24		10	
Total cases	64		22	

**Includes one child who also had psychomotor fits.*

disturbance of speech). There were 11 children with psychomotor fits: 8 with uncomplicated epilepsy and 3 with structural brain disorder (a similar proportion in both groups). Six of the 11 children had only psychomotor fits and the other 5 had major fits also.

In all, 17 per cent of the epileptic children had had psychomotor fits. Apart from Kurland (1959) and Pond (Pond and Bidwell 1960, Pond *et al.* 1960), previous general population surveys have not considered the prevalence of different types of fit so that few comparisons are possible. Pond found a rate of temporal lobe epilepsy similar to ours in children over 10 years but no cases in younger children. Kurland found that 6 per cent of his epileptic children had temporal lobe fits. In the present study, as in Pond's, psychomotor fits were more common in the older children. However, it should be emphasised that psychomotor fits and temporal lobe epilepsy are not synonymous (Glaser and Golub 1955). Many children with a temporal lobe focus do not have psychomotor fits and psychomotor fits are not always associated with a focus in that region. If the character of the aura preceding other types of fit is taken into account in making a clinical diagnosis of temporal lobe epilepsy, as is usually done (Hill *et al.* 1953, Margerison and Corsellis 1966), then the rate of temporal lobe epilepsy would be higher than the 17 per cent for psychomotor fits. This type of epilepsy is probably a good deal more common than suggested by earlier writers (Bridge 1949).

Four children (6 per cent) had myoclonic fits, defined as attacks consisting of a sudden, severe and momentary muscular contraction resulting in a sudden jerk forwards or backwards of head and body with or without an associated jerk of the arm. This rate is comparable with the 4 per cent found by Harper in his clinic series (1968). The rates for myoclonic epilepsy were not given in the previous general population surveys. A fifth child, who had cerebral lipoidosis, was in almost continuous status with very frequent myoclonic jerks. These, perhaps, did not amount to a true myoclonic fit, but if he is included the rate of myoclonic epilepsy is 8 per cent altogether.

One child had 'salaam' attacks, another had 'infantile spasms' and four children had focal motor fits. The remainder had attacks of a less differentiated kind, usually involving falling and some loss of consciousness but no convulsions.

Fits with a Focal Motor Component

Altogether 12 (19 per cent) of the children with uncomplicated epilepsy and 2 (9 per cent) of those with a structural brain disorder had fits with a focal motor component. There was also one child with psychomotor fits which began with a focal sensation confined to one arm. Only 3 children had fits which were solely Jacksonian (*i.e.* fits characterised by the onset of either tonic or clonic spasm in one region of the body and followed by a progressive march from this area to adjacent muscle groups) and did not end in unconsciousness.

In most cases the fits began focally but then spread to the other side and ended in unconsciousness and generalised convulsions. It was notable that attacks with a focal motor component were as common in the 'uncomplicated' group as in the structural brain disorder group. As far as could be ascertained, the focal attacks in the children with uncomplicated epilepsy were not due to any organic intracranial disease and they do not appear to have the same significance as in adults (Gordon 1958).

The same applies to localised after-effects of fits. In 8 children fits were sometimes followed by temporary weakness in one or more limbs (Todd's paralysis). In adults this frequently indicates the presence of a localised brain lesion. However, 7 of these 8 children had uncomplicated epilepsy, there being no detectable evidence of structural brain disease.

The rate of fits in this study with a definite focal component (16 per cent not including psychomotor fits) is similar to that found by Kurland (1959) in the Mayo Clinic study (12 per cent).

TABLE 35
Fits with a focal motor component

Focal component	*Uncomplicated epilepsy*		*Structural brain disorder*	
	No.	*%*	*No.*	*%*
Left sided focal motor	4	6	1	5
Right sided focal motor	4	6	1	5
Both right and left	3	5	0	–
Focal motor—side not known	1	2	0	–
Total cases with focal fits	12		2	
Total cases known	63		21	

Frequency of Fits

In the great majority of epileptic children, the fits were well controlled and over a third had not had a fit for at least a year. Of the 28 children who had major fits in the previous 12 months, only 7 had had 10 or more attacks and nearly half had only had one (Table 36). Minor fits were rather more difficult to control but, even so, of the 21 children with minor fits in the past year only 9 had had 10 or more attacks (Table 37). There was no appreciable difference between the children with uncomplicated epilepsy and those with a structural brain disorder in the frequency of fits.

TABLE 36
Frequency of major attacks in past year

Frequency of major fits	*Uncomplicated epilepsy*		*Structural brain disorder*	
	No.	*% of known*	*No.*	*% of known*
None	42	66	14	67
One attack only	9	14	2	10
2-5 attacks	7	11	1	5
6-9 attacks	0	–	2	10
10 or more attacks	5	8	2	10
Total cases known	63		21	

TABLE 37
Frequency of minor attacks in past year

Frequency of minor fits	*Uncomplicated epilepsy*		*Structural brain disorder*	
	No.	*%*	*No.*	*%*
None	50	79	14	67
One attack only	2	3	1	5
2-5 attacks	3	5	1	5
6-9 attacks	3	5	1	5
10 or more attacks	5	8	4	19
Total cases known	63		21	

TABLE 38
Anticonvulsant medication in past year

Medication	*Uncomplicated epilepsy*		*Structural brain disorder*	
	No.	*%*	*No.*	*%*
None	7	11	2	10
Phenobarbitone only	38	60	8	40
Other only	6	9	1	5
Phenobarbitone and other	12	19	9	45
Type of drug not known	1	2	0	–
Total cases known	64		20	

Anticonvulsant Medication

One in ten of the children was not having any regular anticonvulsant medication. In a few cases this was because none had been prescribed, but more often it seemed to be because the parents had decided to give drugs 'only when the child needed them'. Phenobarbitone was much the most common drug used, usually on its own but sometimes in combination with phenytoin sodium which was the only other drug used at all often (Table 38). Primidone, troxidone and ethosuximide were each being used with a few children.

Age of Onset of Epilepsy

The age of onset of fits was one of the few variables to differentiate significantly the children with uncomplicated epilepsy from those with a structural brain disorder. The modal age of onset for uncomplicated epilepsy was 5 to 8 years but for the children with a structural brain disorder fits most often began in the first 2 years of life (Table 39). This difference was even more marked when the 3 epileptic children with clear-cut post-natal disorders (2 cases of encephalitis and 1 of cerebral lipoidosis) were excluded. Of 16 epileptic children with a structural brain disorder, in 9 (56 per cent) the fits began in the first 2 years compared with only 15 (24 per cent) of 63 children with uncomplicated epilepsy ($p. < \cdot 05$).

These findings are in agreement with those of other studies (Peterman 1946). Although many children have convulsions in the infantile period, very few continue to have fits after the age of 5 years (Cooper 1965, Costeff 1965, Schulte 1966). Of those that do, a disproportionate number have some structural brain disorder. Of the cerebral palsied children who develop fits, a high proportion do so in the first 2 years of life (Mitchell 1961). In contrast, uncomplicated epilepsy more often begins during middle or later childhood (Pond *et al.* 1960).

TABLE 39
Age of onset of epilepsy

Age of onset	*Uncomplicated epilepsy*		*Structural brain disorder*	
	No.	%	*No.*	%
Less than 2 years	15	24	9	47*
2 years to less than 5 years	15	24	3	16
5 years to less than 8 years	24	38	2	11
8 years to less than 11 years	5	8	4	21
11 years or older	4	6	1	5
Total cases known	63		19	

**Significantly different at the 5 per cent level.*

Features of Fits

In most children the period of unconsciousness in major fits usually lasted between 1 and 5 minutes and in only 3 children (all with uncomplicated epilepsy) did unconsciousness usually last over half an hour. Of the 64 children with uncomplicated epilepsy, 9 (14 per cent) were sometimes incontinent in the fit and another 11 (17 per cent) were usually incontinent. Among the children with a structural brain disorder, the proportion with incontinence was somewhat (but not significantly) higher. A fifth of the epileptic children had sometimes suffered a trivial injury as a direct result of a fit, but only 5 per cent of those with uncomplicated epilepsy and 13 per cent of those with a structural brain disorder had ever suffered an injury of any importance. Of the children with uncomplicated epilepsy, 20 per cent sometimes experienced a warning or aura preceding the attack and another 16 per cent usually did so. More of the children with a structural brain disorder were severely intellectually retarded so that it was less easy to determine whether they experienced an aura, but it appeared that about the same proportion did so.

Medical Care

Nearly all of the children had been seen by their family doctor with regard to their epilepsy and three-quarters of them had been seen within two months of their first fit. Most of the children, too, had been referred to hospital at some time, and only 16 per cent of those with uncomplicated epilepsy and 19 per cent of the others had never seen a paediatrician for advice or treatment with regard to fits. This is a rather lower proportion than that found in previous British studies (Pond *et al.*

TABLE 40
Delay before seeing G.P. following first fit

Delay	*Uncomplicated epilepsy*		*Structural brain disorder*	
	No.	%	*No.*	%
Never seen G.P.	1	2	3	14
Less than 2 months	50	78	15	71
2 to 12 months	8	13	2	10
More than 12 months	5	8	1	5
Total cases known	64		21	

TABLE 41
Delay before hospital appointment following first fit

Delay	*Uncomplicated epilepsy*		*Structural brain disorder*	
	No.	%	*No.*	%
Never attended hospital (for epilepsy)	10	16	4	19
Less than 2 months	20	31	7	33
2-12 months	17	27	3	14
More than 12 months	17	27	7	33
Total cases known	64		21	

1960). However, whereas most children saw their family doctor very soon after their first fits, referral to hospital was more often delayed or only initiated when fits recurred (Tables 40 and 41).

Electroencephalographic Abnormalities

About half the children had had an EEG (Table 42). As it was not possible for us to examine the records ourselves, we had to rely on the reports made at the time. These have some comparability in that nearly all the records were taken and reported on at the same hospital. Nevertheless, neither the exact criteria used in deciding upon the presence of abnormalities nor the reliability of judgements on the EEG is known.

A third of the children with uncomplicated epilepsy, but three-quarters of those with a structural brain disorder, were said to have definite generalised abnormalities on the EEG. Focal abnormalities (usually a spike focus) were less common and, unlike general abnormalities, appeared equally in the two groups. Six children (five of whom had uncomplicated epilepsy) had a temporal lobe focus; three of these had psychomotor fits. In addition, two children with uncomplicated epilepsy had an occipital focus and one had both a temporal and occipital focus.

TABLE 42
General abnormalities in electroencephalography

General abnormalities	*Uncomplicated epilepsy*		*Structural brain disorder*	
	No.	%	*No.*	%
No abnormalities	15	45	1	13
Doubtful abnormalities	7	21	1	13
Definite abnormalities	11	33	6	75
No EEG taken	29		11	
Total cases known	62		19	

Fits in School

Only a minority of the children (23 per cent of those with uncomplicated epilepsy and 15 per cent of those with a structural brain disorder who were attending school) had had fits at school during the past year, and very few had had more than one or two fits. Disruption of schooling was an uncommon problem.

CHAPTER 9

Intellectual and Educational Aspects of Neuro-epileptic Disorders

The size and age-spread of the neuro-epileptic group posed many problems for any assessment of the children's psychological and educational characteristics. Because of these considerations we decided to restrict our enquiry to two main areas, those of general intellectual functioning and reading attainment, since indices of these have well documented implications for education.

The Psychological Examination

Apart from a very few whose parents refused permission for them to be seen, all children with neuro-epileptic disorders were examined individually by qualified clinical psychologists using a shortened version of Wechsler's Intelligence Scale for Children (Wechsler 1949) and the Neale Analysis of Reading Ability (Neale 1958).

Wechsler's Intelligence Scale for Children

The WISC is probably the most satisfactory test of general intelligence available for use with school-age children. A great deal is known about it, it is well standardised, and it allows separate measures of different aspects of intelligence (a particularly important point when the children have specific handicaps which interfere with the testing of some types of intellectual function but not others).

The complete test takes about one hour to administer which was more time than was available; we accordingly decided to use a shortened version. Maxwell's factor analysis of Wechsler's original data (1959, 1962) showed, in common with other factor analytic studies (Cohen 1959), that the test measures two major factors which may be called 'verbal' and 'visual-spatial' intelligence. These are closely similar to, but not identical with, Wechsler's postulated groupings of the sub-tests into a verbal scale and performance scale. Each factor is best measured by two sub-tests: similarities and vocabulary for the verbal factor IQ and block design and object assembly for the visuo-spatial or performance factor IQ. The sum of all four sub-tests provides a reliable estimate of full scale IQ.

It has been found that the sum of the four sub-tests gives a good approximation to the results obtained using all ten sub-tests. The correlation between the short form and the full WISC was 0·87 in a study of 9 year old Scottish school-children (Belmont 1968). The test-retest reliability of this short form was found to be 0·86 in a somewhat atypical sample of 140 children retested after an interval of one year (Yule 1967). The time saved in using these four sub-tests rather than the full scale was at least 30 minutes.

Except where otherwise stated, all estimates of intelligence given in this chapter are reported in terms of the sum of the scaled scores for the individual sub-tests. These are directly comparable across age groups, since the raw scores obtained in each sub-test are converted into scaled scores (having a mean of 10 and a standard deviation of 3) separately for each age group. Thus, the verbal scale IQ is the sum of two scaled scores as is the performance scale IQ, whilst the full scale IQ is the sum of all four scaled scores. Likewise, differences between verbal and performance IQs are reported in terms of scaled scores. The reason for this somewhat unorthodox presentation of results is to avoid erroneous inflation of errors of measurement involved in extrapolating the scores to standard IQ units, particularly since the estimates at the extremes vary widely depending upon the method of extrapolating. As Silverstein (1967) has shown, straight prorations from short forms of the WISC (*i.e.* multiplying the sum of the four scaled scores by 10/4 before converting) yield higher estimates above the mean than the scores based on multiple regression. There is also the problem of choosing suitable norms for conversion. Wechsler's original data are now twenty years old and there is evidence that British children score higher than his standardisation sample (Jones 1962, Rutter *et al.* 1970). On balance, we decided to stick as closely as possible to the raw data.

Although it provides the best available IQ test the WISC has some disadvantages, not the least being that it is too difficult for children below the age of six years (Scottish Council for Research in Education 1967) and that there are very few items which differentiate at lower levels of intelligence. Because the difference between failing all items and passing one or two makes for large apparent differences in measured IQ at the 50 to 60 level, to all intents and purposes children with IQs below 50 are untestable. While this is not crucial for most purposes (since less than 1 per cent of the population score at such a low level), it is more important when the proportion of children with low intelligence is higher, as it is in children with neuro-epileptic disorders. In our study, 45 out of 185 children were found to be untestable on the WISC. Of these 45 children, 2 were at ordinary infant schools, 7 attended the day school for educationally subnormal children, 19 attended the junior training centre, 15 were resident in hospitals for the mentally subnormal and 2 were at home not receiving formal education. The high proportion of these children makes it difficult to estimate the average IQ of some groups. However, as differentiation of IQ below 50 is of very limited educational relevance, it was decided to confine the testing of intelligence to the WISC.

Neale Analysis of Reading Ability

The Neale test is a prose reading test in which children have to read aloud a few carefully written short stories, attractively presented with illustrations, and then answer a few questions about what they have read. It is standardised for British children aged 6 to 12 years. Below the age of 6, reading skills are very rudimentary and there is little agreement among experts as to what differentiates a good reader from a better one. As for the upper limit of the test, if a child can achieve a reading age of 11 years on a conventional test he should be able to cope with as much reading matter as will be met in any popular tabloid newspaper. The Neale test was designed specifically as a diagnostic test, and much useful *qualitative* information can be gathered at the same time as the three separate *quantitative* measures of reading ability (rate, accuracy and comprehension). Many of the other widely used tests such as Schonell's Graded Word Reading test (Schonell and Schonell 1950), which take rather less time to administer, seem to measure primarily the accuracy of reading single words out of context. The wider scope of the Neale test, therefore, provides advantages which outweigh the slightly longer time taken to administer it. The reliability of the scale is high in that the retest correlation after an interval of one year is 0·95 for accuracy and 0·93 for comprehension (Yule 1967). Furthermore, as Netley *et al.* (1965) have shown, a score on the Neale test is not affected by previous testing (as opposed to coaching) and it is, therefore, admirably suited for retesting reading to assess progress.

The Children's School Placement

Table 43 shows the school placement of children with neuro-epileptic disorders. Nearly all the children with uncomplicated epilepsy and most of the children with lesions below the brain stem attended ordinary schools. In contrast, only a third of those with cerebral palsy and a quarter of those with some other brain disorder did so.

The school placement of the epileptic children reflects the modern view that the vast majority can be taught without difficulty in ordinary schools (Ministry of Education 1962). With the range of well tested anticonvulsants which are available today, it should usually be possible in the case of uncomplicated epilepsy to control fits sufficiently for them not to disrupt a child's schooling unduly. In fact, many epileptic children never have fits at school (Henderson 1953).

The major difference in school placement between the children with cerebral palsy and those with lesions below the brain stem is the more striking because the physical handicap of both groups was fairly similar. However, the cerebral palsied children had a much higher rate of associated handicaps (such as intellectual retardation and psychiatric disorder). A special school placement is rarely necessary purely on account of a physical disability, even if severe. Usually the presence of multiple handicaps gives rise to the need for special provision.

It is difficult to compare the present figures for school placement with those of other studies in that different countries have different school policies. Table 44 shows the figures for the two other comparable British studies of cerebral palsy. There is good agreement that between a quarter and a third are catered for by one of the

TABLE 43
School placement of children with neuro-epileptic disorder

	Cerebral palsy	*Other brain disorder*	*Uncomplicated epilepsy*	*Lesion below the brain stem*
Ordinary school	11	5	62	14
School for Spastics	7	1	–	3
E.S.N. school	6	4	2	–
Mental subnormality service	10	10	–	2
Other	1	–	–	–
Total	35	20	64	19

TABLE 44
School placement of children with cerebral palsy—comparison with other studies

	This survey %	*Ingram* %	*Cockburn* %
Ordinary school	31	26	50
P.H. school	23	28	15
E.S.N. school	17	25	6
Mental subnormality service	29	21	29

mental subnormality services. This has also been so in studies from other countries (*e.g.* Andersen 1954). There is more variability in the proportion attending ordinary schools but again it is generally about a third.

Table 45 shows the school placement according to the type of cerebral palsy. Half the hemiplegic children attended ordinary school and none of them came under the mental subnormality services. In sharp contrast, no child with bilateral hemiplegia was at ordinary school and all but one were under the care of one of the services for mentally subnormal children. Diplegic children were intermediate with respect to placement; a quarter were in ordinary schools, one in six were outside the educational system and most were in some form of special school. In other studies, too, there has been a similar association between type of cerebral palsy and school placement (Floyer 1955; Ingram 1955, 1964; Woods 1957).

TABLE 45
School placement according to type of cerebral palsy

	Hemiplegia	*Diplegia*	*Bilateral hemiplegia*	*Dyskinesia*	*Ataxia*
Ordinary school	7	3	–	1	–
School for spastics	1	5	1	–	–
E.S.N. school	4	2	–	–	–
Mental subnormality service	–	2	7	–	1
Home tuition	1	–	–	–	–
Total	13	12	8	1	1

The placement of children with developmental or sensory disorders is shown in Table 46. In most of the deaf children, the hearing defect was only partial. When the hearing loss was compensated for by the use of a hearing aid there was no difficulty in their placement in ordinary day schools. The blind children were much more severely handicapped and many had multiple handicaps (including intellectual retardation) which necessitated special provisions of some kind. Just over half the children with developmental language retardation were in ordinary schools, the remainder being at the local day school for educationally subnormal children. Whether these were the right placements is not known. What is certain, however, is that there were very few alternatives. Apart from two small residential schools there is scarcely any provision for children with severe language disorders in Britain.

TABLE 46
School placement of children with developmental or sensory disorder

	Developmental language disorder	*Deafness*	*Blindness*
Ordinary school	5	11	–
Special school (for blind or deaf)	–	2	7
E.S.N. school	4	–	1
Mental subnormality service	–	1	7
Total	9	14	15

IQ Distribution

As shown in Table 47, the distribution of IQ in epileptic children was roughly normal (the prorated mean IQ was 102). In children with lesions below the brain stem, the IQ distribution was also normal (a mean of 107). In marked contrast, there was a heavy preponderance of children of low intelligence in both the cerebral palsy and other brain disorder groups (mean IQs were 78 and 74 respectively after exclusion of children who were untestable on the WISC). However, the variability in IQ was much greater than normal and it should be noted that there were several children with above average or even superior intelligence.

In all tables in this section, the IQ has been assessed on the basis of the child's score on the short form of the WISC except where there was some specific handicap, in which case the score (verbal or performance) least affected by the handicap was

TABLE 47
IQ distribution in neurological groups

IQ	*Cerebral palsy*		*Other brain disorder*		*Uncomplicated epilepsy*		*Lesion below brain stem*	
	No.	*%*	*No.*	*%*	*No.*	*%*	*No.*	*%*
131 or more	0	–	1	5	1	2	0	–
116-130	3	9	1	5	17	29	6	35
101-115	5	15	1	5	9	16	4	24
86-100	3	9	2	10	21	36	4	24
71-85	4	12	1	5	8	14	1	6
51-70	6	18	3	15	2	3	0	–
50 or below	12	36	11	55	0	–	2	12
Total	33		20		58		17	
Not known	2		–		5		2	

used instead of the total score. Thus, where the child was deaf or had a pronounced language defect, the performance score was used; where the child was blind or could not do the performance tests adequately because of motor difficulties, the verbal score was used.

The findings from other studies of cerebral palsy are closely similar (Table 48). About a third of children with cerebral palsy have an IQ below 50 or 55, about a fifth have mild intellectual retardation (IQ 50/55-69) and about a fifth have an IQ of 100 or more.

However, the IQ distribution is very different for different types of cerebral palsy (Table 49). Children with hemiplegia have only a slight excess with low intelligence, diplegic children are more often intellectually retarded and all or nearly all children with bilateral hemiplegia have a very low IQ, results again closely similar to those from other studies (Asher and Schonell 1950; Dunsdon 1952; Floyer 1955; Ingram 1955, 1964).

When only the performance scale was used, deaf children were found to have a normal level of intelligence (mean IQ 109). Blind children, on the other hand, included a high proportion with severe intellectual retardation (due to associated brain

TABLE 48

IQ distribution of children with cerebral palsy—comparison with other studies

IQ	*This study* %	*Ingram* %	*Cockburn* %	*Dunsdon* %	*Floyer* %	*Asher and Schonell* %	*Holoran* %	*Herlitz and Redin* %
100 or more	24	18	26	9	10	25	25	43
85-99	9	14		15	14			
70-84	12	24	25	17	29	28	36	
50/55-69	18	22	21	24	17	24	21	19
Below 50/55	36	22	27	35	29	23	18	38

TABLE 49

IQ according to type of cerebral palsy

IQ	*Hemiplegia*	*Diplegia*	*Bilateral hemiplegia*	*Dyskinesia*	*Ataxia*
116-130	3	0	–	–	–
101-115	2	2	–	1	–
86-100	1	2	–	–	–
71-85	1	3	–	–	–
51-70	4	2	–	–	–
50 or below	1	2	8	–	1
Total	12	11	8	1	1
Not known	1	1	–	–	–

TABLE 50
IQ distribution in children with developmental or sensory disorders

IQ	*Developmental language disorder*	*Deafness*	*Blindness*
131 or more	0	2	0
116-130	0	4	0
101-115	2	3	0
86-100	3	2	5
71-85	0	1	1
51-70	3	1	1
50 or below	0	1	8
Total	8	14	15
Not known	1	0	0

damage) and no children of superior intelligence, though the group was much too small to allow any conclusions about the distribution of intelligence in blind children. By definition, there were no children with more than mild intellectual retardation among those with a developmental language disorder, but the mean IQ was somewhat below average (Table 50).

Pattern of Cognitive Abilities

The WISC measures 'verbal' and 'performance' abilities separately; these are shown in Table 51 for the neuro-epileptic children and in Table 52 for the children with developmental sensory disorder. Table 53 shows the statistical significance of verbal performance (V-P) discrepancies (the numbers in this table are slightly smaller as only children who scored on both subscales are included).

In the cerebral palsied children there was a slight tendency, just significant at the 5 per cent level, for the mean verbal IQ to exceed the mean performance IQ. There was a lesser tendency of the same kind in epileptic children, which fell short of significance. The V-P discrepancies were very much more striking in the deaf children

TABLE 51
Intelligence of children with neuro-epileptic disorder

Group	*Verbal scale*		*Performance scale*		*Total*		*No. of children*
	Mean	*S.D.*	*Mean*	*S.D.*	*Mean*	*S.D.*	
Conrtol	23·3	5·0	22·7	5·3	46·0	8·7	147
Cerebral palsy	14·8	7·7	13·0	7·4	27·6	14·1	24
Other brain disorder	12·6	9·7	13·2	7·9	26·6	16·9	11
Epilepsy	21·4	5·9	19·8	6·7	41·3	10·6	59
Lesion below brain stem	22·8	4·9	21·6	4·1	44·4	7·1	15

TABLE 52
Intelligence of children with developmental or sensory disorder

Group	*Verbal scale*		*Performance scale*		*Total*		*No. of*
	Mean	*S.D.*	*Mean*	*S.D.*	*Mean*	*S.D.*	*children*
Developmental language disorder	8·9	5·6	14·9	6·4	23·8	10·0	8
Deaf	15·5	6·4	22·5	6·5	38·9	11·5	13
Blind	15·0	5·9	13·6	4·7	29·1	11·1	8
Control	23·3	5·0	22·7	5·3	46·0	8·7	147

TABLE 53
Verbal-performance differences

Group	*Mean V-P difference*	*No. of children*
Cerebral palsy	+2·18*	22
Other brain disorder	+0·78	9
Epilepsy	+1·63	59
Lesion below brain stem	+1·20	15
Blind	+3·8	5
Deaf	−6·75**	12
Developmental language disorder	−6·00*	8

Significantly different: *p. < ·05; **p. < ·01.
N.B. *Only children who scored on both subscales are included in this Table.*

and the children with developmental language disorders. In both cases the mean performance score greatly and significantly exceeded the verbal score. This difference has been found consistently in previous studies of deaf or language retarded children (Davies-Eysenck 1966, Luszki 1965, Pickles 1966, Myklebust 1960) and reflects the fact that language abilities as well as general intelligence are required in order to do well on the verbal sub-tests of the Wechsler Scales.

These findings, of course, apply to groups of children. Of much greater interest clinically is the proportion of individual children in each group displaying the 'characteristic' pattern. To look at this, it is necessary first to decide on what is a significant discrepancy between the two scales. Obviously, because of test unreliability and errors of measurement, differences of only one or two IQ points are not worthy of note since they occur in many cases and may well disappear on retesting. The frequency with which discrepancies of any given size on the full WISC may be expected in the general population have been calculated by Field (1960). Maxwell (1959) has made similar calculations for the present short WISC.

Using this short WISC, a difference of 9 between the sum of the two scaled scores on the verbal scale and the sum of the two scaled scores on the performance scale is considered to be statistically abnormal (this is equivalent to 25 IQ points difference between the completed verbal and performance scales). Discrepancies as large as

9 scaled points are expected in only 10 per cent of any population, 5 per cent having higher verbal IQs and 5 per cent having higher performance IQs. Table 54 expresses the verbal-performance differences in these terms. Looking only at statistically abnormal discrepancies, it can be seen that the neuro-epileptic group (not including children with lesions below the brain stem) contains nearly twice the proportion in the control group of discrepancies where the verbal score exceeds the performance score (13/84 compared with 11/147) and about the same proportion in the opposite direction. This difference falls just short of the 5 per cent level of statistical significance. In contrast, nearly all the children with deafness or a developmental language disorder had discrepancies in the opposite direction.

TABLE 54
WISC verbal-performance discrepancy

Group	*Verbal exceeds performance*		*No difference*	*Performance exceeds verbal*		*No. of children*
	Diff. 9+	*Any diff.*		*Any diff.*	*Diff.* 9+	
Controls	11	73	12	62	7	147
Total neuro-epileptic	13	52	6	27	4	85
Total cerebral palsy	3	13	2	4	0	19
Total other brain disorder	0	4	0	3	0	7
Total epilepsy	10	35	4	20	4	59
Deaf and language disorder	0	2	2	15	7	19

Reading Test Results

In considering the reading attainment of these children, certain difficulties must be faced before the data can be interpreted. Whereas the scores on the WISC are corrected for chronological age so that a given quotient (*i.e.* standardised score) carries the same meaning irrespective of the child's age, the reading test results are presented in terms of reading ages and these only within the range of 6 to 13 years, the scores at the upper end being extrapolated from the standardisation data. Thus, whilst it is of some value to know that a child is reading at, say, the 10 year level, this information will be interpreted very differently if the child is 14 years old than if he is 9 years old. Again, there is a strong correlation between intelligence and reading attainment so that one generally expects a bright child to be reading at a more advanced level than a dull child of the same age and school experience. In interpreting any child's reading scores, it is advisable to consider both his chronological age and his intelligence before deciding whether he has a problem with reading.

It has become customary to distinguish between backwardness and specific retardation in reading (Department of Education and Science 1964, Jackson 1966, Miles 1967, Rutter *et al.* 1967*b*, 1970). Reading retardation is a term used to describe a specific disability in reading—specific in that the reading difficulties are not explicable in terms of the child's general intelligence. Reading backwardness is a term used to describe reading which is backward in relation to the average attainment for that age, regardless of intelligence. This group might well include children with a specific disability but it would also include children whose reading problems were associated with a general impairment of intellectual functioning.

Thus a 10 year old child with a reading age of 7 years 6 months would be considered 2½ years backward. However, if the same child was of subnormal intelligence he would not have a *specific retardation* in reading. Conversely, if a 10 year old child of IQ 140 was reading up to his chronological age he might still have some degree of specific retardation because, other things being equal, one expects a bright child to do better scholastically than a dull one.

Many ways of estimating such retardation have been explored. Disparity between mental age and reading age has been used by many authors, and great controversy has raged around the use and abuse of reading and other attainment quotients (Burt 1959, Crane 1959, Levy 1962). All approaches of this kind are subject to statistical criticisms and a more satisfactory technique is provided by the use of a multiple regression formula (Fransella and Gerver 1965, Ravenette 1961, Yule 1967). Knowing the means, standard deviations and inter-correlations among three variables (in this case, age, intelligence and reading), an equation can be derived which allows the prediction of any third variable on the basis of the other two. Moreover, it is possible to estimate the limits within which the score is likely to lie. Such a technique was used with a randomly selected control group of 9 to 11 year old children to derive a measure of specific reading retardation (Rutter *et al.* 1970, Yule 1967).

The mean age of the control group was 10 years 1 month (S.D.=6·9 m) so that most of the children lay in the age range 8 years 11 months to 11 years 3 months, the range in which the measure of reading is most sensitive. However, the present study of neurological handicap is concerned with children of a wider age range, and care is needed in using such equations outside the range on which they were standardised. The procedure has been found useful in studying reading handicaps, and no other equations are available across the complete age-range. Therefore, we decided to apply them to the present group with two provisos: (1) any child who was reading at or above the 11 year level on both the Accuracy and Comprehension sub-tests of the Neale Reading Test would be regarded as an adequate reader, irrespective of his predicted reading age, and (2) children who were younger than 8 years of age when tested would be excluded from the analysis since the predicted reading age, particularly for the duller children, would be too low to allow the child to be identified as being retarded by two or more years. This latter proviso raises the problem that retardation is a comparative concept, and two years of retardation in a teenager is, perhaps, less disabling than two years' retardation in a nine-year-old. There is no easy way in which to deal with the developmental problem, but most authorities would agree that a retardation of two years is a definite educational handicap for any child of school age.

Table 55 shows the average reading ages in the groups, although these are difficult to interpret when there are age and IQ differences between groups. Attainment can be more meaningfully assessed from Table 56 which shows the degree of specific reading retardation in the three major groups of neuro-epileptic children—those with uncomplicated epilepsy, those with cerebral palsy and those with other brain disorders.

TABLE 55
Reading attainment of neuro-epileptic children

Group	*Age in months*		*Accuracy*		*Comprehension*	
	Mean	*S.D.*	*Mean*	*S.D.*	*Mean*	*S.D.*
Cerebral palsy	139·8	28·9	101·8	26·1	102·4	32·3
Other brain disorder	119·6	36·9	89·8	21·5	89·0	20·1
Epilepsy	127·8	30·2	116·4	27·1	115·0	27·7
Below brain stem	131·2	29·4	116·0	20·4	118·2	22·7
Deaf	133·1	36·3	109·8	26·0	108·2	31·0
Developmental language disorder	92·6	19·2		Non-readers		

TABLE 56
Specific reading retardation (children aged 8 years or more only)

Reading comprehension	*Uncomplicated epilepsy*		*Other brain disorder*		*Cerebral palsy*	
	No.	%	*No.*	%	*No.*	%
Not retarded	22		1		7	
Retarded by 1-11 mths.	9		2		3	
12-23 mths.	10		2		3	
24 mths. or more	9	18	3	38	9	41
Total	50		8		22	

Whilst half the epileptic children were reading adequately, 9 of the 50 (18 per cent) aged over 8 years were at least two years retarded on reading comprehension. Similarly, of the 22 cerebral palsied children aged over 8 years who were tested, 9 (41 per cent) were at least two years retarded, as were 3 of the 8 children with other brain disorders. Combining the last two groups, 12 of the 30 children (40 per cent) were at least two years retarded in their reading.

In the random control group of 147 on whom the prediction equations were based, only 10 (6·8 per cent) were retarded by two years or more on either the Accuracy or Comprehension parts of the Neale test. The difference between the epileptics and the controls is statistically significant at the 5 per cent level and that between the cerebral palsied group and the control group is significant at the 0·1 per cent level. Thus, the general backwardness in reading attainment shown in Table 55 cannot be explained simply by the lower intelligence of the cerebral palsied and other brain disorder children. Even when this important factor is partialled out statistically, these children and those suffering from uncomplicated epilepsy who were, on average, of normal intelligence, had specific handicaps in reading.

It is possible that the poor scholastic attainment was in part due to poor school attendance, rather than to any direct effect of brain dysfunction. From our studies of reading retardation in the general population, we know that school absence is not a crucial factor in reading attainment, but it may be of greater importance in a group of brain disordered children. Unfortunately, records of school attendance were not available over the complete age range studied. The only evidence we have relates to the 9 and 12 year olds, where it was found that children with brain disorder were indeed absent from school significantly more often than were a randomly selected control group (Rutter *et al.* 1970). Furthermore, within the neurological group, those with reading retardation had more absences than the remainder. However, while this is likely to have been one factor in the children's reading failure, it cannot be taken as a sufficient explanation, for two reasons. In the first place, the children with uncomplicated epilepsy were, on average, off school on 37·4 occasions, only marginally higher than the control group's 33·9 absences. Yet, in spite of normal intelligence and a near-normal school absence rate, the epileptic children had a high rate of reading retardation. Secondly, the school absence rate was similar for children whose physical disorders did not involve the brain (48·1 per cent) and for children with brain disorders (48·7 per cent), yet the rate of reading retardation was nearly twice as high (26·5 per cent compared with 14·3 per cent) in the latter group. It seems probable that the poor reading of the brain disorder group was in part due to the direct effects of brain dysfunction (see chapter 5 of Rutter *et al.* 1970).

Discussion

WISC Verbal-performance Discrepancies

Much of the psychological literature has been concerned with discussing the diagnostic use of intelligence scales and other instruments. Where groups of children with a variety of neurological dysfunction have been studied, they have been treated as a group of 'brain-damaged' children and little attempt has been made to examine clinically homogeneous sub-groups. The fallacy of expecting a characteristic psychometric result from a heterogeneous sample is now well recognised (Herbert 1964, Meyer 1957, Piercy 1964, Yates 1954). Nonetheless, patterns of intellectual test scores still occupy a large place in descriptions of the characteristic features of the child with 'brain damage' (Clements and Peters 1962, Hatton 1966, Paine 1962) and the view that a WISC performance score well below the verbal score is a sound indicator of brain disorder has come to be accepted by many clinicians. Data to support this view are lacking (Herbert 1964, Hopkins 1964) and it is worth considering how this belief has arisen.

In the first place, as far as work using the WISC is concerned, clinical findings with adult patients have been extended downwards and applied to children. Early work with the Wechsler-Bellevue scales gave rise to the hypothesis that higher verbal than performance IQs tend to be characteristic of brain-damaged adults (Allen 1947, Patterson 1953, Wechsler 1958). The concept of verbal-performance discrepancies as diagnostic indices has not been adequately considered in relation to the WISC (Wechsler 1949) but yet a new test extending the same concept to still lower ages has now appeared (Wechsler 1967, Yule *et al.* 1969).

Apart from the problems of working with highly selected clinical material and discussing 'brain-damage' as if it were a unitary phenomenon, it is clearly wrong to conclude that because damage to a mature adult brain tends to result in a particular, characteristic cognitive pattern, a similar pattern will result from damage to an immature brain (see chapter 1). The question of patterns of cognitive abilities following various types of brain dysfunction in children is a matter for empirical investigation, not deductive reasoning.

Much of the work examining behavioural indices of brain injury in school children has centred on the child's visuo-perceptive and visuo-motor performances (Benton 1962). The clinical expectation and consensus is that brain-injured children tend to have greater visuo-motor and perceptional difficulties than language difficulties. Bakwin and Bakwin (1960) stated that 'Children with cerebral damage, from whatever cause—anoxia at birth, trauma, infection—usually score less in performance. The WISC is an excellent aid in differentiating this group'. Commenting on this statement, Hopkins (1964) noted that 'One is usually unsuccessful, however, in locating research corroborating such statements'.

In his review of researches with brain-injured children in which the WISC had been used, Hopkins found that all but three of the sub-tests (Information, Vocabulary and Picture Completion) had been cited as diagnostic of brain damage when a low score was achieved. This use of single sub-tests as diagnostic indices, as opposed to the two sub-scales, is generally most unsatisfactory. Individual sub-tests are less reliable than the composite sub-scales, and their low reliability does not warrant their use in such a manner (Littell 1960).

Most findings leading to the use of verbal-performance discrepancies as diagnostic indices of brain damage stem from studies of groups of children. Typically such studies compare the average verbal IQ with the average performance IQ of a group of children suffering some brain dysfunction. Young and Pitts (1951) found that in a group of 40 negro children with congenital syphilis, the average verbal IQ was higher than the average performance IQ. This was also the case in Beck and Lam's study (1955) of 75 children with IQs below 80. They further reported that the lower the IQ, the greater the possibility of 'organicity'. This latter finding is certainly in agreement with studies of severely subnormal children (Crome 1960).

However, studies of groups of children with low IQs do not agree on this matter of cognitive patterning. Newman and Loos (1955) found that children with 'familial mental deficiency' scored significantly higher on the performance scale of the WISC than did a group of 'brain damaged' mental defectives. They were at pains to caution readers about interpreting small differences in individual results. On the other hand, Horne and Justiss (1967) failed to find more signs of neurological dysfunction (such as EEG abnormalities) among mentally retarded children whose verbal IQs exceeded their performance IQs by at least 15 points than among a control group matched for sex, age and full scale IQ, but not having such discrepancies. Likewise, Birch *et al.* (1967) concluded that WISC patterning is not systematically associated with the presence of brain damage or factors of risk among educable mentally subnormal children. Their study is the only one reported based on a total population survey, and it avoids many of the methodological errors of others cited above.

In dealing with groups of brain disordered children regardless of their IQ, there is a consensus that the group's mean verbal IQ will exceed its mean performance IQ. As regards children in the educable mentally subnormal range, the evidence is conflicting. Even accepting the consensus, the difficulty remains—what implication does a statistically significant difference based on group results carry for an individual child's score? The larger the group studies, the smaller need be the difference between the means of the verbal and performance scales before they are statistically significant. Small differences are not only unreliable, they are also very frequent and, consequently, they can have no diagnostic significance.

To sum up, the history of the use of verbal-performance discrepancies on the WISC as diagnostic indicators of 'brain damage' is beset with not only all the common faults of studying atypical and highly selected groups of children, but also two other main fallacies: firstly, the unwarranted generalisation of tentative hypothesis based on studies of adults and, secondly, the confusion between statistical and clinical significance in applying group results to the study of the individual.

A few studies have attempted to look at the verbal-performance discrepancies in individuals within groups. Clements and Peters (1962) claimed that if the verbal IQ exceeded the performance IQ by at least 15 points, this was a sign of brain damage. On the other hand, noting that some children have a performance IQ which exceeds the verbal IQ by at least 10 points, they state that, 'In our experience, the child with WISC Pattern III (*i.e.* higher performance IQ) invariably has dyslexia'. As Paine *et al.* (1968) point out, had Clements and Peters consulted the normative data published by Field (1960), they would have seen that their cut-off would diagnose some 25 per cent of children in the general population as having 'minimal cerebral dysfunction'. This reinforces the absurdity of assessing such isolated signs without considering how frequently they can be expected to occur in the general population.

Paine *et al.* (1968) did find that of 34 children whom they diagnosed as showing 'minimal cerebral dysfunction', 21 had higher verbal IQs on the WISC and that nearly twice as many cases as expected had discrepancies in excess of 22 points. In a follow-up study of the sequelae of meningitis, Lawson *et al.* (1965) reported that 18 out of 65 children had discrepancies of at least 15 points. This is not greatly above the expected level (though the direction of the discrepancy was not mentioned). In their series of severely clumsy children, Walton (Walton *et al.* 1962) and Gubbay (Gubbay *et al.* 1965) noted that in all but 3 out of 21 children the verbal score was higher. 'It is still apparent that a discrepancy between the verbal and performance IQ scores of the WISC is the single most useful test in recognising such cases . . .'

These studies are cited as examples where clinicians made determined efforts to utilize psychometric results in a diagnostic fashion. Where they largely fail (apart from Paine *et al.* 1968) is in not recognising the error of measurement inherent in the test results, and, therefore, in ignoring discrepancies which fall into the range of such error. As stated earlier, a difference of 9 scaled points between the verbal and performance scales is necessary before the discrepancy can be considered abnormal. In normal intelligence test scoring systems, this is equivalent to a difference of 25 points between the verbal scale IQ and the performance scale IQ on the WISC. Even then, about 6 per cent of the population have discrepancies of this magnitude.

Norris (1960) and Holroyd and Wright (1965) are among the very few workers to have looked at verbal-performance discrepancies in terms of each individual's results, at the same time defining a discrepancy sufficiently large to be statistically abnormal and reliable. Comparing the records of 15 children diagnosed in the children's department of a psychiatric teaching hospital as having neurological disorders with 183 records of cases of 'non-organic' psychiatric disorder, Norris found that only 14 children had verbal IQs significantly higher than performance IQs at the 10 per cent level of abnormality (one tail test). Of these 14, only 3 were diagnosed as having neuro-epileptic disorder. In other words, at this level of statistical abnormality, approximately one fifth of the children identified had a brain condition, but four fifths of the children with a neuro-epileptic disorder remained undetected. The brain-disordered children differed from other children only to a small extent in the proportion with verbal IQ abnormally higher than performance IQ.

Holroyd and Wright (1965) used the opposite strategy. From a psychiatric hospital population, they selected 20 children with at least a 25 point verbal-performance discrepancy and compared them with controls matched for age, sex and full scale IQ, on medical records, neurological examination (done without knowledge of whether the child was a 'case' or 'control'), EEG and various psychological tests. Of the 20 children with large discrepancies, 14 showed definite or possible abnormalities on neurological examination compared with 6 of the controls, on the EEG the comparison was 9 to 6 abnormal and on the medical history 12 to 4 abnormal. Taking all 3 measures, 16 of the 20 children with 25 point V-P discrepancies showed some evidence of possible or probable brain disorder as against 10 of the controls.

In both studies, referral biases could well have upset the results. It is possible, for instance, that only equivocal cases are sent for opinion to a psychiatric unit, whilst more clear-cut cases go to neurology clinics. The present population based study, following essentially similar techniques, is in a better position to clarify the situation, even though the numbers are still rather small.

Our findings offer modest support for the view that a performance score much below the verbal score shows some association with brain disorder. However, the clinical significance must be interpreted in the light of the strength of the association, which is not a strong one—only 14·0 per cent of the children with brain disorder had a significant verbal-performance discrepancy (13 out of 84 cases) and 7·5 per cent of the control group had a similar discrepancy. This means that somewhere between 550 and 800 children in the total population of 11,865 could be expected to show equally large discrepancies. Proportionately twice as many brain-disordered children as controls exhibited abnormally high verbal-performance discrepancies but, since brain disorder is so much rarer than normality, a child who has a large V-P discrepancy is still more likely to be normal than brain-disordered. We can only conclude that a large verbal-performance discrepancy is of little use as a sign of brain disorder.

Wide scatter across the sub-tests in the WISC has also been suggested as an index of brain disorder. Although this is allied to the verbal-performance discrepancy concept, the issue could not be examined in the present study as only four sub-tests were used. Previous studies suggest that although scatter may be somewhat greater in children with brain damage, the difference from normal children is not great enough for scatter to be of use as an indicator of brain damage (Birch *et al.* 1967). In addition, it has sometimes been said that children with brain disorder are less consistent in their scores from one occasion to the next than are normal children. Again this could not be tested in this study as the children were tested on one occasion only.

Level of Intelligence

Brain damage can, and frequently does, cause a global reduction in intelligence level. This is shown by the IQ distribution of children with cerebral palsy and other brain disorders which is heavily skewed to the lower end, as found in numerous other investigations. The effect of brain damage on IQ may be either very slight or quite severe, as shown by studies of monozygotic twins, only one of whom has a brain disorder (Bradway 1937, Jenkins 1935).

An IQ which is significantly below that 'expected' may indicate brain damage (Benton 1962). Paine *et al.* (1968) in a study of children with possible minimal brain dysfunction found a mean IQ of 96. As the children were predominantly upper middle class, the mean IQ of the group might be expected to be some 10 or 20 points higher. Although this might indicate brain disorder, some perfectly normal middle class children have IQs of 96. There are rarely any adequate means of assessing what an individual child's IQ should be, and it is rarely possible to be sure that anyone's IQ is significantly below expectation. In any case, there are many causes of depression of intelligence other than brain damage and some children with undoubted brain disorder are of superior intelligence. Except for very low levels of intelligence or for children who can be shown to have deteriorated in intelligence, the IQ is but a poor indicator of brain disorder.

It was notable that the children with uncomplicated epilepsy in this study, as in others (Cooper 1965, Halstead 1957), showed a normal level of intelligence. As a rule, it is only when epilepsy is associated with other neurological disorder or with status epilepticus that the IQ is depressed (Lindsay 1966, Ounsted *et al.* 1966). Epileptiform activity in the brain can certainly interfere with cognitive function (Hutt 1967; Morrell 1956; Stamm and Pribram 1960, 1961; Tizard and Margerison 1963) but only rarely is there a persisting effect on IQ. Very occasionally mental deterioration is seen in epileptic children (Chaudhry and Pond 1961) but it is likely that this is often associated with a structural brain lesion.

Reading Retardation

There was a very high rate of reading retardation in children with all kinds of neuro-epileptic disorders. Although most marked in the children of low intelligence, reading difficulties were common even in those of normal or above normal intelligence. Because of the cross-sectional nature of the study, the wide age-range of the children and the small numbers involved, it was not possible to determine the relative importance of the different factors causing reading failure. Nevertheless, it is likely that abnormalities of brain function were in part directly responsible. The kinds of language and perceptual abnormalities shown to be associated with specific reading retardation in the general population (Rutter *et al.* 1970) are also associated with brain disorder and probably played a part in the children's reading difficulties. Recurrent absence from school is another factor which is held in common with children with other physical handicaps not involving the brain. Whatever its cause, reading retardation in children with neuro-epileptic disorders constituted one of the most important of their handicaps. This emphasises the importance of paediatricians having close links with the school health service so that the educational implications of chronic physical handicap can be adequately considered.

Most epileptic children and many cerebral palsied children can cope perfectly well in the ordinary school, provided that the situation is properly handled. It is largely when there are severe intellectual or behavioural problems in addition that special schooling is required (Ministry of Education 1962). Unfortunately, owing to a singular lack of research into the education of children with neuro-epileptic disorders, little is known about the relative efficacy of different methods of teaching or of providing schooling for handicapped children (Tizard 1965). Studies in this area are much needed.

CHAPTER 10

Social Aspects of Neuro-epileptic Disorders

Social Background of Children

The family background of the children with neuro-epileptic disorders was broadly similar to that of the children in the randomly selected general population control group. The father's occupation, graded on the Registrar-General's classification (Table 57), the degree of over-crowding and the families' facilities (running hot water, bath, toilet, separate kitchen) were all closely comparable. These findings are in agreement with those of previous studies of cerebral palsied (Henderson 1961, Illingworth *et al.* 1961, Ingram 1964) and epileptic children (Cooper 1965).

TABLE 57
Social class

Diagnostic groups	*Non-manual* %	*Skilled manual* %	*Unskilled/ semi-skilled* %	*Total known* %
Controls	35	45	20	145
Uncomplicated epilepsy	34	38	28	61
Cerebral palsy	47	30	23	30
Other brain disorder	50	22	28	18
Lesion below brain stem	33	40	27	15
Severe intellectual retardation	34	50	16	32

The children with cerebral palsy, other brain disorders and epilepsy tended to come from somewhat smaller families than the control children, suggesting a lower fertility rate (Ingram and Russell 1961) or that there may have been some restriction on having further children when one was known to be handicapped. However, the finding must be accepted with some reserve in view of the fact that the neuro-epileptic groups had a wider age range than the control group. The family size difference did not apply to the intellectually retarded children with cerebral palsy who tended to be only children, or to those with Down's syndrome who generally came from large families. Presumably, this was because cerebral palsy is more common in first births and Down's syndrome is more frequent in children born to elderly mothers. The number of children with a developmental language disorder was too small for findings on family size to be reliable, but, although the children were considerably younger than those in other groups, five out of the nine came from families where there were at least four children.

Impact of the Child's Disorder on the Family

A handicap in a child has an effect not only on the child himself but on others, and in particular on other members of his family. Although more attention has usually been paid to the effects on the child, the way in which a family copes with handicap in one member must be considered in any provision of services.

The manner in which an ordinary family (in which no-one is handicapped) responds to crises and problems is influenced by many factors such as its size, its social and material circumstances and the mental and physical characteristics of family members (Clausen 1966, Hill 1949). When one of the children is handicapped, additional forces are brought to bear on the family. These will vary with the child's age and sex, the nature and severity of the handicap, the demands that treatment makes on the child and family and the services available to them (Curran *et al.* 1964, Farber 1959, Tizard and Grad 1961). Elsewhere (Rutter *et al.* 1970) we have considered the effects on families of a variety of psychiatric and physical disorders in children. Here we are concerned only with the effects of a neuro-epileptic disorder.

The Parental Interview

Our principal source of information on family life was an interview with a parent, usually the mother; supplementary information was obtained from questionnaires filled in by teachers and parents and from medical and social sources. The fathers were not usually seen.

The parent was seen in her own home by a social scientist or a doctor for an interview which lasted on average 1½ hours. Information was obtained on the composition of the household and the family, the health of family members, the health and behaviour of the child, and any medical or other help the family had had in dealing with the child's handicap. All parents were asked whether their child had any emotional or behaviour problems and were systematically questioned about this aspect of the child's development. There was a section covering the amenities of the home, followed by questions on the occupation of the parents and their physical and mental health. Questions were also asked about the family's financial position, about changes in the organization of routine tasks and in family relationships which might have come about as a consequence of the child's condition and about contacts they had had with services during the preceding twelve months. Mothers were also asked to fill in a 24 item 'malaise inventory' concerning their own health (see page 159).

The chief purpose of the interview was to obtain data about the child's handicap, and in this respect it proved very useful. As a technique for gaining information about family dynamics or the impact of the handicap on the family it was more limited, partly because it was not primarily designed with this end in view and partly because of the difficulty in getting this kind of information in a single interview in which only a brief time could be devoted to it.

Methods of Analysis

The questions in the family interview which referred to the impact of the child's handicap upon the family were divided into three groups. The first seven items dealt with patterns of daily living, from which we tried to assess the extent to which disorganization of routine, or inconvenience to or alterations in the established patterns of family life were judged to have followed from the child's handicap. The second group of five questions covered family relations and the extent to which the child's handicap was thought to be responsible for impaired social relations among members of the family. From the third group of eight questions, we attempted to assess the amount of dissatisfaction with services.

In the first two sections we divided replies into three categories: no problem, a minor problem or a major problem. In the section on services, the information collected was too sparse to allow us to grade the replies and they were categorised simply into 'no problem' or 'problem'. To gain an idea of the severity of the family's problems, items in each category were summed to give an overall score, on the assumption that, in general, families who report many problems are likely to be more affected by a child's handicap than are those who report few (Sainsbury and Grad 1966, Tizard and Grad 1961).

Results

In general, the proportion of families with problems in each section tended to increase with the severity of the child's handicap. However, the association was quite slight (and statistically insignificant) so that the impact on the family was clearly influenced by other factors. The nature of the child's handicap also bore little relationship to the proportion of families with problems in any section.

Impact was also assessed by examining the average problem score in each section according to diagnosis. Again, there was little association between the diagnosis of the child's condition and the degree of impact on the family, except in so far as there was less disorganization of routine in the families of epileptic children (mean score 1·9) and most in those with severe intellectual retardation or a lesion below the brain stem (mean scores of 4·4 and 4·5 respectively). The mean score for families with a cerebral palsied child was 3·7 and for those with a child having some other brain disorder it was 3·2. Similar differences are found if severe problems only are considered.

In the intellectually retarded children the disorganisation often stemmed from behaviour difficulties. For example, housing was a problem with a 7 year old severely subnormal boy who attended the junior training centre. He was so destructive that the parents had to arrange the house carefully to avoid damage, purchasing robust furniture and hiding ornaments and antiques. They rarely took him out because of the disturbance he caused but, equally, going out without him was a problem in that he could only be left with one or other parent. The mother had to organise her day so that all the housework was completed by the time he arrived home.

In the children with lesions below the brain stem, difficulties usually arose from the child's physical incapacity. Although some of the children (particularly those with pareses following poliomyelitis) were only slightly handicapped, this group also included some of the most severely handicapped children. One family with a 9 year old boy with muscular dystrophy had to move from a three storey house to a ground floor flat in which the council had had a ramp fitted to take the boy's wheelchair. Another family, with a 13 year old son who had muscular dystrophy had also had to move to a house without steps and the father had to return home from work during the day in order to lift him, dress him and take him to the toilet. They had had to buy a larger car in order to accommodate his wheelchair when they took him out and had been unable to go away for a holiday for some years because of their son's physical incapacity. Another family had had to buy a van in order to take the wheelchair. Transport, housing and holidays were all a considerable problem for families with children who were unable to walk.

Impaired social relations were less frequently reported and their rate was approximately the same in all diagnostic groups. Most families in all groups were dissatisfied with services.

Disorganisation of Routine (Table 58)

Difficulties or Inconvenience in taking a Child to a Hospital or Clinic

Many children attended hospital for regular check-ups or for treatment. In most cases out-patient attendance did not cause any difficulties for either the child or the parents. However, where the child was severely handicapped it was sometimes necessary for the father to take time off work to help lift the child into a car or in other ways to help with transport. When both parents were at work, hospital attendance also necessitated one or other parent taking time off. In a few cases hospital attendance presented a problem because the child was afraid or otherwise reluctant to go.

Time taken by Outpatient Attendance

We asked how long visits usually took and arbitrarily classified those which took more than two hours as constituting a minor problem and those which took more than three hours a major problem. Altogether about a third of the families had a problem in the time taken for hospital attendance, 15 per cent a minor problem

TABLE 58
Problems involving disorganisation of routine

Problem	*Uncomplicated epilepsy* %	*Cerebral palsy* %	*Other brain disorder* %	*Lesion below brain stem* %	*Severe intellectual retardation* %
Visiting clinics	5	3	16	19	7
Time taken for visits	29	31	32	50	21
Going out with child	19	58	26	44	61
Going out without child	21	45	42	38	64
Holidays	6	14	26	25	29
Housing	13	28	16	28	43
Other	8	34	26	25	46
Total cases known	62	29	19	16	28

and 19 per cent a major problem. Hospital services were centered at Newport and Ryde and quite a time could be spent in getting there from the more distant parts of the Island. The length of time which was spent waiting in outpatient departments was mentioned as a problem by only very few parents. This is a common complaint about hospitals in the country generally so that in this respect the Island hospital services appeared better organised than most.

Going out with the Child

There was considerable variability between the groups in the proportion of families who had difficulties taking the child out, the highest rate being in the intellectually retarded (61 per cent) and the lowest in the epileptic (19 per cent). In most cases the difficulties came from the child's disturbed behaviour or from gross physical incapacity. One retarded deaf girl screamed and fought and her mother had to pull her along whenever she went out. A cerebral palsied boy behaved so badly in front of other people that his family had ceased going out together. Several families had found going out much easier since they got a car. However, where the child could walk with assistance and where the wheelchair was folding, travel by bus sometimes proved only a minor problem.

Going out without the Child

Difficulties in going out without the child occurred in roughly the same proportion of families, again being most frequent in the intellectually retarded and least frequent in the epileptics. Where the child showed very disturbed behaviour or was severely handicapped many parents felt they could not use a 'baby-sitter'. The parents of one intellectually retarded girl with cerebral palsy had never been out together without the child since she had been born. The parents of a retarded child with muscular dystrophy only went out for short periods, leaving the child in bed and hoping for the best. They worried greatly while out, particularly as the boy was fascinated by fire and matches.

Holidays

If the family had to make special arrangements to meet the child's needs this was classed as a 'minor' problem; where families had felt unable to go away because of the child's handicap this was graded a 'major' problem. Difficulties in holiday arrangements occurred in much the same families as those who had difficulty taking the child out. Incontinence was a special problem in going to hotels.

Housing

Changes in sleeping or other arrangements were classed as a 'minor' problem and a change of house as 'major'. Most frequently changes were necessary because the child's physical disability prevented him climbing stairs. In some cases this was met by the child sleeping downstairs, but where a wheelchair was required it was necessary for there to be a ramp up to the house. In some children, particularly the intellectually retarded, destructive or hyperkinetic behaviour required the parents to take special precautions to avoid damage to furniture or ornaments.

Other Changes in Household Routine

In about a quarter of the families (a third in the case of the cerebral palsied and nearly half of the intellectually retarded) the child's handicap had led to changes in household routine which were not covered by the previous categories. For example, special arrangements sometimes had to be made to take the child to and from school. Where the mother was unable to leave the child, all food had to be delivered. In the case of a few of the most handicapped children who remained at home, virtually the whole of the mother's life was spent catering to the child's needs.

Controlled studies of the effects of a handicapped child on family life are few and far between (Jordan 1962), but what evidence there is suggests that severe handicap sometimes has a considerable impact on family routine. Hewett *et al.* (1970), comparing young cerebral palsied children with the Newsons' general population sample of four year olds (Newson and Newson 1968), also found appreciable effects. Half the parents whose children had special equipment found difficulty in using it. Twice as many cerebral palsied children had daily temper tantrums, but a third of the parents (compared with 3 per cent of the controls) never smacked their child. Twice as many of the handicapped children shared their parents' bedroom.

Most obviously, physical and mental handicap restricts the range of the child's activities outside the home. Hewett *et al.* found that, in families without a car, 11 out of 26 severely handicapped children rarely went out compared with only 4 out of 40 mildly handicapped children. Similarly, among those with a car, 23 out of 36 severely handicapped children had a narrow range of outings compared with 7 out of 37 of the mildly handicapped. Even so, it was striking that in many respects the activities in families of *young* cerebral palsied children were substantially similar to those of the families of normal children. Whether the restriction of family activities is greater when the handicapped children are older is not known.

Impaired Social Relations

Parents were asked about five aspects of social relations which might have been impaired by the child's condition: (a) whether they had quarrelled about how to look after the child or what he should be allowed to do, (b) whether there had been any restriction on their entertaining friends in the home, (c) whether other children in the family had to limit the amount of entertaining they did, (d) how relatives behaved towards the child, and (e) how neighbours and other people outside the family responded to him. In each case, codings referred only to impairment thought to have resulted from the child's handicap.

An increase in parental quarrelling was much the most common complaint and occurred in about a fifth of the families. Often this centred on how to manage behaviour problems, the mother arguing that the father was too strict and the father complaining that the mother was not firm enough, or vice-versa. In a few families, particularly of the older children, there was a state of chronic tension, the parents feeling tired and worn-out by the constant need to care for the child and the inability to get a break or go out without him. In a few cases conflict arose because one parent had given up everything to look after the handicapped child and the other was unwilling to drop all leisure pursuits and social activities.

Family entertaining was restricted in a fifth of the families with intellectually retarded children and a similar proportion of those with some brain disorder other than cerebral palsy. Usually the problems in entertaining were due to gross behavioural disturbances in the child or to his undue dependance on his parents. Only 5 per cent of the parents of epileptic children and 10 per cent of the parents of cerebral palsied children reported difficulties of this kind.

One pleasing finding was the comparative infrequency (about one in 20 families) of reports of hostility on the part of relatives or the general public. No parent of an intellectually retarded child reported negative responses from relatives although three mentioned difficulties with neighbours. On the whole, there seems to have been a reasonable tolerance of difficulties in other people's children.

Whether the extent of impaired social relations in these families should be regarded as 'high' or 'low' obviously depends on the findings in other groups. In this connection, comparisons with children having other physical handicaps may be informative. Asthmatics were studied in the same way in a parallel study (Rutter *et al.* 1970). In most respects the families of neuro-epileptic children reported more social difficulties. Whereas only 8 per cent of the parents of asthmatics reported an increase in parental quarrelling, 28 per cent of the parents of cerebral palsied children and 21 per cent of the parents of epileptics did so.

On the other hand, we found, as did Hewett *et al.* (1970) that the great majority of parents of handicapped children coped remarkably well with their difficulties, in spite of the strain involved.

Dissatisfaction with Services

Three questions in this section related directly to medical services and a further question was asked on whether the parents were worried about the cause of the child's condition. There were three questions on schooling and a final enquiry about whether the parents felt a need for additional services. There were no sizeable differences between the diagnostic groups in the numbers of problems reported.

Medical Problems

Parents were asked whether they had found any difficulties or inconvenience in doing what the doctors had advised, whether there was any way in which they felt their doctor could have been of more help, and whether they thought that doctors had done everything possible.

About a quarter of the families said that they had had difficulties in following medical advice. In many cases this concerned a failure to get specific advice on how to deal with some problem, particularly where this concerned behaviour difficulties. The parents of retarded children sometimes felt that no-one had told them what to do and they had just been left to find out for themselves. Other parents felt that advice had been impractical.

Worries about the cause of the child's condition were expressed by one in four parents. These were most frequent among the parents of retarded children who were often concerned that something that had happened during the pregnancy might be to blame. Parents also frequently found it hard to accept that the cause of the child's handicap was not known. In some cases worries concerned realistic fears such as the genetic risk to younger sibs in the case of children with muscular dystrophy. Some parents felt that they had not had an adequate opportunity to discuss aetiology with the doctors looking after their child.

School Problems

Parents were usually more forthcoming in their criticism of schools than they had been of medical services. Over a third expressed some complaint or dissatisfaction about education. It is difficult to assess the significance of this in that we have no data on the level of dissatisfaction in the general population. Naturally, parents were frequently concerned about their child being backward at school. They felt frustrated in not knowing the cause of the backwardness and sometimes thought that the teachers were not doing enough to help. In other cases difficulties arose because parents disagreed with the assessment they had been given on their child's abilities. Some of the parents of children at schools for the physically handicapped said that there was not enough basic teaching. A frequent complaint was the lack of special help for children with reading difficulties.

Only a few parents (less than 10 per cent) complained of teachers' attitudes. About one in ten thought their child was at the wrong sort of school.

Additional Services

About a third of the parents expressed a wish for additional services of some kind, particularly the parents of children with intellectual retardation (57 per cent). They tended to repeat specific points made earlier in the interview, such as the need for better transport to and from hospital, special clinics for children with their child's particular problem or help with housing. The most frequent suggestion was special provision for the children to have holidays. Several mentioned the continuous strain in looking after a severely handicapped child and suggested that tempers might get less frayed if parents could be given a break from time to time. A few pressed for a child-minding service so that husband and wife might go out together on occasions. Others felt that parents needed more advice on how to care for the children. The need for a laundering service when children were incontinent was mentioned by several parents, as was the lack of adequate facilities for the long-term hospital care of mentally retarded children. Some felt that some kind of emergency provision of care for the child if the parent fell ill was needed.

Many of the complaints referred to deficiencies in services which are well recognised. However, the most striking feature of the comments was that often parents referred to the need for services which already existed. For example, children can be admitted to hospital or to a Children's Home or a Home Help may be provided at times of parental illness, and there *are* holiday homes for handicapped children. Such provision is not as plentiful as it needs to be but parents were often totally unaware that anything at all existed. Psychiatrists and paediatricians seemed to have fallen down in discussing available services with the parents and parents had not always felt able to ask about these things. It is possible, too, that doctors themselves were not always aware of what social and educational services there were. Whatever the reason, clearly many families were facing formidable difficulties at home for which they were not receiving sufficient help.

The associations between the severity of the child's physical handicap and the different types of impact on the family are shown in Table 59. There was a highly significant association between the severity of the child's handicap and the extent of disorganisation of family routine, the rate of disorganisation going up markedly when the child had a severe or very severe handicap. There was a similar but less marked trend with impairment of social relations which fell just short of the 5 per cent level of statistical significance. The pattern in relation to dissatisfaction with services was more complicated in that there was little association with the severity of handicap apart from a much higher rate of dissatisfaction in the parents of children with severe (but not very severe) physical handicaps. The meaning of this finding is obscure. It may be that an association between severity of handicap and amount of dissatisfaction has been concealed by the fact that the most handicapped children have better services or have their needs met more successfully.

TABLE 59

One-way analyses of variance of impact scores by severity ratings over total group of children

		Mean scores			
Severity of physical handicap	*No. of children*	*Disorganisation of routine*	*Impairment of social relations*	*Dissatisfaction with services*	*Total*
0	41	1·9	0·6	1·5	4·0
1	68	2·1	0·5	1·6	4·2
2	30	2·8	0·5	1·6	4·8
3	19	6·2	1·3	2·8	9·6
4	8	6·9	1·4	1·4	9·0
Degrees of freedom		4/161	4/162	4/163	4/163
F ratio		19·91	2·27	3·54	10·79
Significance level		p. < 0·001	p. almost 0·05	p. < 0·01	p. < 0·001

Parental Health

The quality of family life and the ability of the family to cope with additional stresses are likely to be influenced by the parents' health, both physical and mental (Rutter 1966). Two assessments of the physical and mental health of the parents were carried out. First, an overall rating of the parent's general physical health during the previous 12 months was made on the basis of systematic questioning on illnesses, ill-health, attendance at hospital, contacts with the family doctor and time off work. A rating of physical illness was made when the parent had been handicapped in his/her job or housework for at least one month during the preceding year. Illnesses in which handicap had lasted for a year or longer were separately noted but their number was too small to warrant separate analysis.

An assessment was also made of the mother's mental well-being. This took the form of a standardised questionnaire which was filled in by the mother at the end of the interview. The questionnaire (or 'malaise inventory') was largely adapted from the Cornell Medical Index Health Questionnaire (the C.M.I.) which originally contained 195 questions (Brodman *et al.* 1949, 1952). Fourteen questions in the malaise inventory were identical with ones in the C.M.I. and a further 10 items were added (by MR and PG), making a questionnaire of 24 items using simple language and designed to tap the different types of emotional disturbance commonly seen in adults.

The items referred to the emotions ('are you easily upset or irritated?'; 'do you often feel miserable or depressed?') and to physical matters which have important psychological components ('do you feel tired most of the time?'; 'is your appetite poor?'). The respondent had to circle 'yes' or 'no' to each of the questions (see below).

HEALTH QUESTIONNAIRE

PLEASE RING THE CORRECT ANSWER

1.	Do you often have back-ache?	Yes	No
2.	Do you feel tired most of the time?	Yes	No
3.	Do you often feel miserable or depressed?	Yes	No
4.	Do you often have bad headaches?	Yes	No
5.	Do you often get worried about things?	Yes	No
6.	Do you usually have great difficulty in falling asleep or staying asleep?	Yes	No
7.	Do you usually wake unnecessarily early in the morning?	Yes	No
8.	Do you wear yourself out worrying about your health?	Yes	No
9.	Do you often get into a violent rage?	Yes	No
10.	Do people often annoy and irritate you?	Yes	No
11.	Have you at times had a twitching of the face, head or shoulders?	Yes	No
12.	Do you often suddenly become scared for no good reason?	Yes	No
13.	Are you scared to be alone when there are no friends near you?	Yes	No
14.	Are you easily upset or irritated?	Yes	No
15.	Are you frightened of going out alone or of meeting people?	Yes	No
16.	Are you constantly keyed up and jittery?	Yes	No
17.	Do you suffer from indigestion?	Yes	No
18.	Do you often suffer from an upset stomach?	Yes	No
19.	Is your appetite poor?	Yes	No
20.	Does every little thing get on your nerves and wear you out?	Yes	No
21.	Does your heart often race like mad?	Yes	No
22.	Do you often have bad pains in your eyes?	Yes	No
23.	Are you troubled with rheumatism or fibrositis?	Yes	No
24.	Have you ever had a nervous breakdown?	Yes	No

Questionnaire completed by Mr/Mrs. ....

Questionnaire applies to Mother/Father

Several studies have shown that the total score (the number of questions answered 'yes') on the C.M.I. (both in its original version and in short forms) is a useful indicator of emotional disturbance which agrees fairly well with independent psychiatric assessments (Culpan *et al.* 1960, Gibson *et al.* 1967, Hamilton *et al.* 1962, Rawnsley 1966).

During the course of the study, 36 mothers were re-interviewed about their children's behaviour, 35 of whom also completed the malaise inventory on both occasions. Although they tended to acknowledge slightly fewer symptoms on the second occasion (Rutter *et al.* 1970), there was a very high correlation (0·91) between the scores, indicating that the pattern of results was very reliable. In other studies undertaken by one of us (MR), it has been found that the inventory differentiates moderately well between parents with and without psychiatric disorder. This, together with the findings of earlier studies, argues for the validity of the shortened scale.

Mother's Malaise Score, Child's Handicap and Social Class

The correlations between the malaise score and social class within each diagnostic group and in the total group were low and statistically insignificant (Tables 60 and 61), as found also in other samples (Rutter *et al.* 1970). However, the malaise score and total impact scores correlated positively and relatively highly, indicating that mothers who perceived their child's handicap as impinging greatly on family life were also more likely to report more symptoms of malaise in themselves. The differences in malaise score in relation to the diagnosis of the child were for the most

TABLE 60
Average malaise scores for mothers by diagnosis of child

Diagnostic group	*Malaise score* *No.*	*Mean*	*S.D.*	*Correlation between malaise score and* *social class*	*total impact*
Uncomplicated epilepsy	58	4·8	3·5	0·16	0·45***
Cerebral palsy	30	3·0	3·1	−0·04	0·46**
Other brain disorder	20	2·9	2·4	−0·18	0·52*
Lesion below brain stem	15	3·5	3·0	0·11	0·77***
Severe intellectual retardation	30	2·5	2·8	−0·35	0·29
General population control group†	162	3·1	2·6		

Significantly different: * p. < 0·05; ** p. < 0·01; *** p. < 0·001.
†*This control group is comparable to but different from the control group used for other measures.*

TABLE 61
Social class and malaise scores over total group

	Non-manual *No.*	*Mean*	*S.D.*	*Manual* *No.*	*Mean*	*S.D.*	*t*	*p.*
Malaise score	57	3·30	2·69	103	3·83	3·39	1·03	N.S.
Total impact score	61	5·31	4·59	103	5·17	4·25	0·21	N.S.

part small and insignificant. However, the malaise scores of the mothers of epileptic children were appreciably higher than those of the mothers in any of the other groups, and only the mothers of epileptics differed in malaise scores from mothers of children in the general population.

Altogether a fifth of the children with a neuro-epileptic or sensory disorder had a parent who had been physically ill for at least one month during the previous year. There was no association between parental illness and the degree of impact on the family made by the child's condition (Table 62), but there was a tendency (significant at the 5 per cent level) for the ill mothers to have a slightly higher malaise score than the healthy mothers. Nevertheless, the mean score of the physically ill mothers (4·89) was well below that of an unselected sample of psychiatrically ill mothers (10·5) obtained in another study (Rutter, unpublished data) and also well below that of the mothers of children with psychiatric disorder (6·09) on the Isle of Wight (Rutter *et al.* 1970).

TABLE 62

Mother's illness and malaise and impact scores over total group

		Ill			*Well*			
	No.	*Mean*	*S.D.*	*No.*	*Mean*	*S.D.*	*t*	*p.*
Malaise score	34	4·59	3·12	129	3·40	3·11	1·99	$<0·05$
Impact score	34	5·85	5·77	132	5·06	3·89	0·95	N.S.

Although severe physical handicap in the child was sometimes associated with disorganisation of family routine and disturbed family relations, in only a few cases was the effect associated with malaise in the mother. Other studies (Cummings *et al.* 1966) have also shown that although chronic physical illness is a source of family strain it is generally less so than chronic mental handicap or psychiatric disorder.

Nevertheless, the findings do show that a neuro-epileptic disorder in the child may have widespread repercussions both in other aspects of his own development (see chapters 9 and 12) and on the life of his family. If these matters are to be effectively dealt with, it is essential that the paediatrician, psychiatrist or other doctors looking after the child should be aware of these implications and take active steps to remedy the difficulties. Time must be spent with the child and his parents considering the practical difficulties they face in adjusting to his handicap. Adequate social provision must be sought to assist with problems of housing, transport, holidays and other issues of this kind. It is particularly important that the parents be helped to strike a balance between caring for their handicapped child and maintaining their own social life. The needs of the other non handicapped children in the family have also to be considered. Although there are several papers on the topic (Caldwell and Guze 1960, Kaplan 1969) surprisingly little is known about the impact on the brothers and sisters of handicapped children.

Now that many of the killing infectious diseases of childhood are no longer the problem they were earlier in this century, the problems of the chronically handicapped child stand out more clearly. Adequate medical care for this group requires that doctors maintain a continuous interest in the child throughout his development and that social, educational, and psychological needs are considered carefully in relation to the physical aspects of his disability.

PART IV

Psychiatric Aspects of Neuro-epileptic Disorders

CHAPTER 11

Definition and Measurement of Psychiatric Disorder

Definition of Psychiatric Disorder

What is meant by the term 'psychiatric disorder'? Most disorders of emotions and behaviour in childhood do not constitute 'diseases' or 'illnesses' which are qualitatively different from the normal, so that there are problems in defining 'psychiatric disorder'. These have been much discussed in the literature (Bower 1960, Freud 1966, Lapouse 1965, Ministry of Education 1955, Rogers 1942, Ullman 1952) without any entirely satisfactory resolution of the difficulties.

The approach used in the present study may be termed 'clinical-diagnostic' in that psychiatric disorder was judged to be present when there was an abnormality of behaviour, emotions or relationships which was sufficiently marked and sufficiently prolonged to cause handicap to the child himself and/or distress or disturbance in the family or community, and which was continuing up to the time of assessment. This was a developmental assessment rather than a static description; the child's function was assessed in relation to what was normal for his age and in relation to the process of psychic development. As Freud has emphasised (1945, 1966), a child's level of performance fluctuates considerably and transient phases of inefficiency of functioning may be quite normal. For psychiatric disorder to be considered present, the disorder had to be abnormal in the broader context of the child's development, it had to be persistent and there had to be handicap which involved either the family/community or the child himself. Many pathological manifestations in childhood are successful in avoiding suffering for the child himself, and the restrictions and disturbances stemming from the pathology may be more upsetting to other people.

Two further features require emphasis. First, there was no necessary implication of persisting abnormality of personality (although undoubtedly this was present in some cases). In all but a few children the disorder had been present at least one year and in most cases had lasted several years, but it is likely that many will recover from their disorders. Second, there was no assumption about the need for psychiatric treatment. While the presence of persistent abnormality accompanied by handicap in most cases implies that the child needs help, it is possible that adequate treatment could be provided by professionals other than the psychiatrist. To what extent this would be possible would depend on the experience and training of the general practitioner, school medical officer, teacher, paediatrician and others looking after the child.

Diagnosis of Psychiatric Disorder

When psychiatric disorder was considered present, it was diagnosed according to a descriptive or phenomenological scheme based on the outline given by Rutter

(1965), but closely similar to the type of classification used in most child psychiatric clinics in this country (Ministry of Education 1955). Although there are theoretical disadvantages in the use of a descriptive classification (Freud 1966), its main justification lies in the power of its predictions. In the present state of knowledge, a classification based on descriptions of behaviour most easily conveys in a succinct form clinically useful information (Zigler and Phillips 1961).

In the past, disorders have often been considered under the general term of 'maladjustment' without further attempts at subdivision. However, the need for differentiation is shown by the major differences between diagnostic groups with respect to response to treatment, long term prognosis, aetiology, age and sex trends, and other epidemiological associations. (Robins 1966, Rutter 1965, Rutter *et al.* 1970).

For the purposes of the present study, six main diagnostic categories were used: neurotic disorder, antisocial or conduct disorder, mixed conduct and neurotic disorder, hyperkinetic syndrome, child psychosis and 'other'.

The category of *neurotic disorder* was used for disorders in which there was an abnormality of the emotions which was not accompanied by a loss of reality-sense (as in psychosis). Emotional disorders in this category included states of disproportionate anxiety or depression as well as obsessions, compulsions, phobias (which were abnormal in their developmental context), hypochondriasis and 'conversion hysteria'.

The term *conduct or anti-social disorder* was used to denote abnormal behaviour which gave rise to social disapproval but which was not part of any other psychiatric condition (such as psychosis). The category included some types of legally defined delinquency but it also included non-delinquent disorders of conduct (*e.g.* fighting, bullying and destructive behaviour). The mere fact that a child had committed a delinquent act was not sufficient for the diagnosis of conduct disorder; it was necessary for the behaviour to be abnormal in its socio-cultural context as judged by the frequency, severity and type of behaviour, and by its association with other symptoms such as abnormal interpersonal relationships. Fixed sexual perversion would be included in this category.

The category of *mixed conduct and neurotic disorder* was used for conditions in which both neurotic and antisocial symptoms were present, but in which neither type of syndrome predominated over the other. An analysis of the associations with other variables showed that the mixed group had much in common with the 'pure' antisocial disorders and much less in common with the 'pure' neurotic disorders (Rutter *et al.* 1970).

The *hyperkinetic syndrome* was used for disorders in which poorly organised and poorly regulated extreme overactivity, distractibility, short attention span and impulsiveness were the chief characteristics, and in which the disorder was not secondary to any other psychiatric syndrome. Marked mood fluctuations, aggressive and destructive behaviour commonly occur with the hyperkinetic syndrome.

Psychosis was diagnosed in terms of the clinical picture regardless of the presence or absence of associated organic brain disorder or intellectual retardation (Rutter 1968, 1969*b*). In planning the study, psychoses were subdivided into four categories:

infantile psychosis (beginning during the first two and a half years of life); regressive psychoses in which the child develops normally for the first few years of life and then, usually about the age of three or four, shows a severe disintegration of behaviour, emotions and relationships and a regression in development of speech and other functions; schizophrenia of later childhood and adult life; and manic-depressive psychosis (Rutter 1967*a*). As it happened, the only psychoses which were found were of the infantile variety which, apart from the age of onset, are characterised by an autistic type of disturbance in interpersonal relationships together with delayed or distorted language development, ritualistic or compulsive features with a resistance to change, irregular intellectual development and, often, motor stereotypes or mannerisms.

For present purposes, nocturnal enuresis (when it occurred in isolation) and other developmental deviations were not included as psychiatric disorders. Children with enuresis were rated as having psychiatric disorder only if there were other abnormalities of behaviour, emotions or relationships of sufficient severity to justify the diagnosis.

The '*other*' category was used only when conditions could not be included under one of these five headings.

Other Classifications of Psychiatric Disorder

Various other approaches to the definition, diagnosis and classification of psychiatric disorders have been employed in previous studies. The reasons why these approaches were rejected will be briefly considered.

For survey purposes, psychiatric disorder could be defined operationally in terms of children under psychiatric care. This definition was not used because of the very large geographical differences in rates of psychiatric clinic attendance and because of the evidence showing that clinic children are unrepresentative of children in the community with psychiatric disorder (Shepherd *et al.* 1966 *a* and *b*).

Alternatively, an assessment of need for psychiatric treatment could be used to define disorder. The chief difficulty with this method is the great variety of views on which children require psychiatric services. Such an assessment is a complex matter requiring consideration of many factors (Rutter and Graham 1966) and is unsuitable as the sole criterion of psychiatric disorder.

It has sometimes been suggested that the problems in the designation of psychiatric disorder are best avoided entirely by a simple reliance on 'deviant' behaviour defined in terms of its rarity and without any implication of pathology. This approach avoids conceptual problems, is easy to handle statistically and satisfactory reliability can usually be obtained. It is also suitable for use with questionnaires which makes it easy to study very large numbers of children. For these reasons we used this method in our initial screening of the total population. However, the use of the rarity of a behaviour to define its abnormality is a dubious procedure and an exclusive reliance on this approach allows no consideration of the context of behaviour, the degree of handicap or the course of psychological development—features which most psychiatrists would consider essential in diagnosis. Questionnaires based on a 'deviance' approach are very useful but they must be supplemented by more clinically orientated methods.

Some psychiatrists would consider an assessment of a child's internal 'conflict' over instinctual drives and his use of defence mechanisms as essential elements in diagnosis (Committee on Child Psychiatry 1966). However, these are not the sole criteria by which normality and pathology are assessed even by psychoanalysts (Freud 1966). The examination of the way in which a child copes with his problems is an indispensable part of a diagnostic formulation, but classifications based on judgements about intra-psychic mechanisms are of unproven value and suffer from the severe limitation that they cannot be communicated meaningfully between psychiatrists who hold different theoretical views.

For these reasons, a 'clinical-diagnostic' approach was used, but elements of the alternative approaches have played an important part in different stages of the investigation.

General Plan and Definition of Groups

In this section of the book, which is concerned with psychiatric aspects of neurological disorders, comparisons will be made between various groups of Isle of Wight children as described below.

General Population

Certain information was obtained on all the 3,300 children resident on the Island in 1964 who were born between September 1st 1952 and August 31st 1955 inclusive (aged 9 to 11 years at the time of the study). The children chosen for study were all those in this age group whose homes were on the Isle of Wight regardless of where they went to school (except that children attending private schools—5·8 per cent of the population in this age group—were excluded).

The information obtained on these children included group tests of verbal and non-verbal intelligence, reading and arithmetic, completion of behavioural scales by the child's teacher and the child's parents (see pages 169, 170) and information on social class and size of family.

Random Control Group

For a more detailed comparison of handicapped children and children in the general population a control group was selected by taking a random sample of 9 and 10 year old children (described in chapter 4). The group was intensively investigated in the same way as those children suspected of being handicapped.

Neurological Disorders

The identification and method of study of children with neurological disorders were fully described in chapter 6. For the purposes of psychiatric study the children with neurological conditions were subdivided as follows: (a) children with uncomplicated epilepsy, (b) children with a definite structural lesion above the brain stem but no fits (*i.e.* with cerebral palsy or some other pathological condition of the brain),

(c) children with a lesion above the brain stem (defined as above) and also fits, (d) children with a lesion at or below the brain stem.

Blindness or Deafness

The methods used to identify these children were described in chapter 6. Like those with neurological disorders, the blind and deaf children comprised all those with the handicap aged 5 to 14 years inclusive.

Chronic Physical Disorders (of a non-neurological kind)

This group consisted of all children born between September 1st 1952 and August 31st 1955 (aged 10 to 12 years at the time of study) who had a chronic currently handicapping physical disorder not involving the central or peripheral nervous system (*e.g.* asthma, diabetes, heart disease, talipes). These children were selected in the same manner (total population screening and individual study of possible cases) as that used for children with neuro-epileptic disorders (Rutter *et al.* 1970). Individual interviews with parents about the behaviour of the children and parental questionnaires together with questionnaires and other information from teachers were used in the same way as for the neuro-epileptic children to study the prevalence of psychiatric disorder in this group.

Psychiatric Disorders

The prevalence of psychiatric disorder in the general population of school age children was assessed in relation to the 2,193 children resident on the Isle of Wight in 1965 who were born between September 1st 1953 and August 31st 1955 inclusive (aged 10 and 11 years at the time of the study). The methods used to study psychiatric disorder are described more fully below.

Methods of Identification of Children with Psychiatric Disorder

I *Screening Procedures*

In June 1965 the first stage of the procedure used in the identification of children with psychiatric disorder was carried out. This consisted of a screening of the total population of children in the 10 to 11 year age group by means of behavioural questionnaires completed by parents and by teachers, and an identification of children in certain administrative groups. These are briefly described here but a fuller account is given in Rutter *et al.* (1970).

(*a*) *Teachers' questionnaire* The teachers' questionnaire (Rutter 1967*b*) was in the form of 26 descriptions of behaviour against which the teacher was asked to indicate whether each description 'does not apply', 'applies somewhat' or 'definitely applies' to the child in question (see Appendix H). It was found that using this scale, two teachers agreed well with each other when they completed the questionnaire independently about the same child (inter-rater reliability: r=0·72). Retest reliability with the same teacher filling in the form twice with a three month interval between completions was also high (r=0·89). The value of the teachers' questionnaire was shown by its efficiency in discriminating between children attending

Child Guidance Clinics and those in the general population. When a score of 2 was given for each statement marked 'definitely applies' and a score of 1 for each statement marked 'applies somewhat' it was found that a total score of 9 or more selected 72-88 per cent of boys attending a Child Guidance Clinic but only 9-11 per cent of boys in the general population. Similarly, 50-70 per cent of clinic girls scored 9 or more compared with only 3-5 per cent in the general population. The questionnaire, when scored to do so, has also been shown to discriminate well between different types of psychiatric disorder (Rutter 1967*b*).

These findings were further validated in the Isle of Wight study, although the discrimination was not quite as sharp. Of the children finally diagnosed as showing psychiatric disorder (most of these did not attend any clinic), 53·0 per cent scored 9 or more, compared with 7·1 per cent of the general population.

Teachers' questionnaires were obtained for 99·8 per cent of the children in the age group.

(*b*) *Parental questionnaire* The parental questionnaire (Rutter *et al.* 1970) had 31 items, 23 of which were identical to those on the teachers' questionnaire. When fathers and mothers were asked to complete forms independently for their children, agreement between them was quite good (inter-rater reliability: $r=0{\cdot}64$), and when mothers were asked to rate their children twice at an interval of three months, there was again quite good agreement between the two scores (retest reliability: $r=0{\cdot}74$).

As with the teachers' questionnaire, the parental scale discriminated well between children attending Child Guidance Clinics and children in the general population, and when individual items were scored to produce 'neurotic' and 'antisocial' scores, the scale differentiated well between those with neurotic disorders and those with antisocial disorders (agreement with findings based on examination of clinical records varied between 72 per cent and 92 per cent).

The findings were further validated in the Isle of Wight study with similar but less clear-cut results. Of the children finally diagnosed as showing psychiatric disorder, 54·5 per cent scored 13 or more compared with 6·0 per cent in the general population.

Parental questionnaires were obtained for 88·5 per cent of the children in the age group. A summary of the questionnaire items is given in Appendix G.

(*c*) *Administrative groups* In addition to children selected for individual study on the basis of questionnaire scores, all children in various administrative groups were also selected for study if they were thought to be at special risk for the presence of psychiatric disorder. These comprised three groups of children: those who had attended the Child Guidance Clinic during the previous year, those who had been charged at a Juvenile Court or who had been on probation during the previous year, and those who had been in the long-term residential care of the Children's Department for part or all of this time.

II *Selection of Children for Individual Study*

Children in the 10 to 11 year age group were selected for individual study if they scored above the cut-off points set for the behaviour scales (9 for the teachers' scale and 13 for the parental scale). The cut-off points were established in the validity studies of the scales mentioned above and described in more detail in Rutter (1967*b*) and Rutter *et al.* (1970).

In all, 271 children (172 boys and 99 girls) were selected for intensive individual study on the basis of their scores on either behavioural scale and a further 15 children (10 boys and 5 girls) were selected on administrative grounds alone, a total of 286 children.

III *Methods used in Intensive Individual Examinations*

The intensive study of the selected children consisted of a psychiatric interview with the child, an interview with the parents and a further report and completed questionnaire from the child's class teacher at school.

(*a*) *Psychiatric interview with the child.* The interview lasted half an hour and was carried out in the schools by psychiatrists who had had at least 6 months' special experience in child psychiatry. In brief (the interview is described fully in Rutter and Graham 1968), the child was seen on his own in a room with a minimum of (specified) toys. The first part of the interview was unstructured, the aim being to get the child relaxed and talking freely. The psychiatrist was expected to adapt the interview to the needs of each individual child, to convey to the child his interest in him and his ideas, feelings and activities, but also to maintain enough neutrality and objectivity to observe the child effectively. It was usually possible to make the interview a gratifying experience for the child, and most children appeared to enjoy it.

After the psychiatrist had spent about a quarter of an hour getting to know the child with a relatively informal approach, the child was asked more systematically about possible worries and anxieties, things he was afraid of, feelings of depression or unhappiness, frightening dreams, what sort of things made him angry, how he got on with other children and whether he was teased or picked on at school. The areas to be covered were specified and the codings categorised, but the exact wording of the questions was left to the individual psychiatrists. The child's persistence in carrying out mental tasks near to the limits of his abilities and his degree of distractibility were also noted. At the time of the interview, 21 individual ratings of the child's behaviour, emotions and relationships were made and there was also an overall assessment of psychiatric abnormality rated on a 3 point scale.

The reliability and validity of the interview with the child as a measure of psychiatric disorder have been examined in a series of four studies (Rutter and Graham 1968). The overall judgement of psychiatric disorder proved to be highly reliable. Two psychiatrists independently interviewed the same children (knowing only the child's name and age) on separate occasions with an average interval of 12 days between interviews. When one psychiatrist considered that the child had a 'definite and marked abnormality' the other agreed in 90 per cent of cases, and the product-moment correlation between ratings was 0·84. The agreement on the intermediate point 'some abnormality' was less good (51 per cent). Agreement on individual items of behaviour varied with the type of abnormality being rated but, on the whole, it was less good than agreement on the overall rating.

The validity of the interview was tested by comparing the ratings based on the interview with the child with ratings based on independent information from parents and from teachers. The agreement between the different ratings on the overall assessment of abnormality was good. It was concluded that a short psychiatric interview with a child was a reasonably sensitive diagnostic instrument which could give rise to reliable and valid judgements on whether the child exhibited any psychiatric disorder.

(*b*) *Interview with the parent.* One or both parents (in most cases the mother alone) was interviewed by a psychiatrist or by a graduate in one of the social sciences using a standard interview which lasted, on average, about one and a quarter hours. Complete interviews were obtained for 94 per cent of the selected children. The qualities of the interview are fully described in Graham and Rutter (1968) and only a brief account will be given here. Initially, the parent was asked whether she felt her child had any problems of behaviour or any nervous troubles. If she said not, the interviewer then went on to the second part of the schedule. If she mentioned some difficulties, her perceptions of them were explored and a detailed description was obtained on the symptoms she had reported.

In the second part of the interview the parent was systematically asked about 36 aspects of the child's behaviour, emotions and social relationships, the aim being to cover all the chief areas of clinical importance. For each 'symptom' mentioned, information was sought about when the behaviour began, what exactly happened when it was manifest, what made it better and what made it worse, how often it occurred, whether it was showing improvement or deterioration, in what situations it arose and under what conditions it did not appear. The exact nature of these probes was left to the interviewer but it was made clear that a comprehensive description of the aspect of behaviour in question was required. Interviewers were warned against accepting generalisations or inferences about what might be going on in the child's mind. Rather, they were asked to concentrate on obtaining factual accounts of what the child said or did and how he did it.

On completion, the interview schedule was rated by two psychiatrists on individual items of behaviour and on an overall assessment of psychiatric state. To test the reliability of ratings, 36 schedules were rated independently by the two psychiatrists. There was 76 per cent agreement on the diagnosis of 'definite psychiatric disorder' and 60 per cent agreement on 'no disorder'. Agreement on the intermediate rating of 'trivial or dubious abnormality' was less good (22 per cent). The inter-rater correlation was 0·81.

To examine the reliability of the parents as informants, 36 parents were re-interviewed by a different interviewer ten to thirty days after the first interview. The interviews were also rated by different psychiatrists so that both information gathered and rating were done completely independently on the two occasions. Agreement was again high, 76 per cent on 'definite disorder' and 56 per cent on 'no disorder'; the inter-rater correlation was 0·64. The reliability of individual symptoms was also high where strict behavioural criteria could be met, but items where inferences had to be drawn or where relationships were being judged proved less satisfactory. The parental interview was shown to be a most useful and reliable clinical tool in the assessment of psychiatric disorder.

During this interview with the parent, information was also obtained on the family and social situation (as described in chapter 10).

(*c*) *Information from teachers.* In November 1965 at the time of the individual examinations, the teachers of the selected children completed a questionnaire identical to that completed by a different teacher in June. In addition, on a form similar to that used in local authority Child Guidance Clinics, the teacher added comments under a number of headings including behaviour in and out of class, attitudes to teachers and to other children, any problems in school and elsewhere, and a heading asking for free comments on any other aspects which might be relevant in an assessment of the child's adjustment. Inter-rater reliability of judgements on psychiatric state, based on this information, was high (r=0·85).

IV *Diagnosis of Psychiatric Disorder*

On the basis of this detailed information from parents, teacher and child, an overall assessment was made on the child's psychiatric state. The inter-rater reliability for 80 cases rated independently by two psychiatrists was 0·89 using a 4 point scale. Diagnostic distinctions were made reliably at every level of enquiry. Complete agreement between two raters on diagnosis varied between 67 per cent and 74 per cent. The two largest diagnostic groups were neurotic disorder and antisocial or conduct disorder. When diagnosis was made on different parental interviews and rated by different psychiatrists, no children were placed in the neurotic category by one rater who were diagnosed antisocial by the other. Thus, it was shown that two psychiatrists could agree quite well on the diagnosis of children's psychiatric disorders.

Of the 286 children selected for individual study, 118 (excluding those with enuresis alone) were diagnosed as having some variety of psychiatric disorder—a prevalence rate of 5·4 per cent which does not include those children with psychiatric disorder who were missed by all the screening procedures. However, it was possible to estimate how many children were missed and so give a corrected prevalence rate.

This opportunity was provided by the psychiatric study of the children with neurological disorders or other chronic physical handicaps: 108 of these physically handicapped children fell into the same age group as the psychiatric group. They went through exactly the same screening procedures but *all* of them were studied individually regardless of whether or not they were picked up on any of the screening procedures. Of the 108 there were 24 who were finally diagnosed as showing psychiatric disorder and for 20 of these 24 there was questionnaire information available on the teacher and parent questionnaires*. In 16 (80 per cent) the questionnaire scores were above the cut-off point on one or other of the questionnaires. Thus, for every 16 children correctly identified by the group screening procedures 4 children were missed.

*There were special reasons, not applicable to the general population, why the other 4 did not have questionnaires.

The observed prevalence rate may therefore be corrected by multiplying by 5/4 to give a rate of 6·8 per cent. In all comparisons between handicapped groups and the general population, this corrected rate will be used throughout.

Method of Diagnosis within the Neuro-epileptic Group

In diagnosing psychiatric disorder in neuro-epileptic children, exactly the same information was available as that used in the diagnosis of psychiatric disorder in the general population; parent and teacher questionnaires were completed and there were the same interviews with parent and child. The only difference, as noted above, was that *all* the children were seen individually regardless of their scores on the screening questionnaires.

The correction factor obtained in relation to 10 and 11 year old physically handicapped children was found to be equally applicable in relation to 5 to 14 year old children with neuro-epileptic disorders. Of 36 finally diagnosed as showing psychiatric disorder, 7 had not been picked up on the screening questionnaires—again a correction factor of 5/4.

In the group of children with non-neurological physical disorders, the same methods were used to diagnose psychiatric disorder, except that the interview with the child was not included. Among the 126 children with psychiatric disorder identified for the general population, only 2 (less than 2 per cent) were identified as abnormal solely on the basis of the interview with the child (Rutter *et al.* 1970). The agreement between the interview with the child and the other methods of assessment was sufficiently high for the omission of the interview to make a negligible difference to estimates of prevalence of psychiatric disorder. Accordingly, the findings of the prevalence of psychiatric disorder in the physically handicapped group will be treated as comparable to that of the other groups.

It should be added that the psychiatric diagnosis did not take into account any aspect of the child's physical state, nor were his educational performance or his family and social situation considered. The records of each child were deliberately arranged so that information on these areas was unavailable to the psychiatrist making the diagnosis. Obviously, these factors would ordinarily form part of the clinical assessment of any child referred to a psychiatrist. However, if the psychiatrist had had knowledge of these factors when he made his diagnosis, there would have been the possibility of a bias inherent in the method of investigation which could have invalidated any examination of inter-relationships between psychiatric disorder and such factors as physical handicap, type of fit, family characteristics and educational attainment.

CHAPTER 12

The Prevalence of Psychiatric Disorder in Neuro-epileptic Children

In this chapter the prevalence of psychiatric disorder in children with neuro-epileptic conditions will be considered with particular reference to the question of whether the child's physical handicap or the presence of a lesion of the brain as such was more important as a causal factor in the development of emotional and behavioural problems.

Children who had been excluded from the educational system because of mental subnormality (*i.e.* were at home, at a junior training centre or in a mental subnormality hospital) were omitted throughout. If they had been included, IQ differences would have invalidated group comparisons; also, psychiatric disorders in the severely retarded are more frequent and differ in some important respects from those in children of normal intelligence (see chapter 13). Psychiatric disorder was very common in neuro-epileptic children with severe intellectual retardation, the rate being 50 per cent (19 out of 38). In addition, the lower the level of cognitive function the more difficult is the assessment of mental state.

Prevalence of Psychiatric Disorder (see Table 63)

The rate of psychiatric disorder in the general population of 10 and 11 year old children resident on the Isle of Wight was 6·8 per cent, or 6·6 per cent when children

TABLE 63

Prevalence of psychiatric disorder in neuro-epileptic children aged 5 - 14 years attending school

Groups	*No. with psychiatric disorder*	*%*	*Total known*
General population			
(10 and 11 year old children)	144	6·6	2,189
Physical disorders not involving the brain:	16*	11·6	138
Blind only	1	16·6	6
Deaf only	2	15·4	13
Lesion at or below brain stem	2	13·3	15
Miscellaneous other physical			
disorders (10 - 12 year old children)†	11	10·3	106
Brain disorder:	34***	34·3	99
Uncomplicated epilepsy	18***	28·6	63
Lesion above brain stem (but no fits)	9***	37·5	24
Lesion above brain stem (with fits)	7***	58·3	12

†*This group includes 2 children who also had a lesion below the brain stem.*
*Significantly different from general population: *at better than the 5 per cent level; ***at better than the 0·1 per cent level.*

not attending school by reason of mental subnormality were excluded. Psychiatric disorder was nearly twice as common (11·6 per cent) among children with chronic physical disorders not involving the brain. No differences in the rate of psychiatric disorder were found in relation to the diagnosis of the physical condition. The numbers were too small for comparisons to be reliable but it appeared that the rate of psychiatric disorder was much the same in blind children (16·6 per cent), deaf children (15·4 per cent), children with lesions at or below the brain stem (13·3 per cent) and children with other chronic physical disorders not involving the brain (10·3 per cent).

While non-cerebral disorders were accompanied by some increase in psychiatric disability, the rate of psychiatric disorder among children with neuro-epileptic conditions was very much higher. Over a third (34·3 per cent) showed psychiatric disorder, a rate 5 times that in the general population (p. < ·001) and 3 times that in children with physical disorders not involving the brain (p. < ·001). The rate was highest in children with neurological disorders accompanied by fits (58·3 per cent) and least high in those with uncomplicated or 'idiopathic' epilepsy (28·6 per cent) but these differences fell well short of statistical significance. The rate of psychiatric disorder was similar in children with cerebral palsy and in those with other pathological brain disorders.

The diagnosis of psychiatric disorder was a judgement by a psychiatrist based on all available information from an interview with the parent, a report from the child's class teacher and a psychiatric interview with the child himself. The prevalence of deviant behaviour may also be assessed by considering the proportion of children in each of the diagnostic groups who obtained 'high' scores on the parent questionnaire or on the teacher questionnaire. High scores were defined in terms of the cut-off points used in screening for psychiatric disorder, namely 9 or more on the teacher scale and 13 or more on the parent scale. The results are shown in Table 64 and it can be seen that the findings are closely comparable.

In the general population of 10 and 11 year old children, 6·8 per cent scored 13 or more on the parent questionnaire and again the rate was somewhat higher (10·0 per cent) among the children with chronic physical disorders not involving the brain. However, the rate among neuro-epileptic children (25·0 per cent) was much higher, nearly 4 times that in the general population (p. < ·001) and over twice that in the group of children with physical disorders not involving the brain (p. < ·01).

Similarly, the proportion of neuro-epileptic children with scores of 9 or more on the teacher questionnaire (32·0 per cent) was over 4 times that in the general population (p. < ·001) where the rate was 7·1 per cent, and nearly 3 times that in the other physical disorder group (p. < ·001), 11·9 per cent of whom scored 9 or more. Thus whatever method of assessment was used, the rate of emotional and behaviour problems in children with brain disorder was several times higher than that in the general population and over twice that in children whose chronic physical handicaps did not involve the brain.

Age and Sex Distribution

Before concluding that there was a real difference in the rate of psychiatric disorder between the groups it is necessary to examine the possible effects of the age

TABLE 64

Prevalence of deviant behaviour on parental and teachers' questionnaires in neuro-epileptic children aged 5-14 years attending school

Group	Parental questionnaire No. with score of 13 or more	%	Total known	Teachers' questionnaire No. with score of 9 or more	%	Total known
General population (10 and 11 year old children)	133	6·8	1,940	155	7·1	2,190
Physical disorders not involving the brain:	14	9·9	142	19*	11·9	160
Blind or deaf	3	18·8	16	2	10·5	19
Lesion at or below the brain stem	0	0·0	13	1	6·3	16
Miscellaneous other physical disorders† (10-12 year old children)	11	9·6	113	16*	12·6	127
Brain disorders:	21***	25·0	84	31***	32·0	97
Uncomplicated epilepsy	13***	24·5	53	16***	26·7	60
Lesion above brain stem (but no fits)	5**	23·8	21	10***	41·7	24
Lesion above brain stem (with fits)	3*	30·0	10	5***	38·5	13

†*This group includes 2 children who also had lesions below the brain stem.*
*Significantly different from general population: *at better than 5 per cent level; **at better than 1 per cent level; ***at better than 0·1 per cent level.*

TABLE 65

Age distribution of children according to diagnosis

(*children attending school only*)

Age	Brain disorder No.	%	Epilepsy No.	%	Blind or deaf No.	%	Lesion below brain stem No.	%	Other physical disorders No.	%
8 years or less	10	27·8	18	28·1	5	26·3	3	20·0	–	
9-12 years	17	47·2	33	51·6	7	36·8	7	46·7	127	(100·0)
13 years or more	9	25·0	13	20·3	7	36·8	5	33·3	–	
Total	36		64		19		15		127	

and sex differences between the groups. Whereas the neuro-epileptic group consisted of children aged 5 to 14 years inclusive, the other physical disorder children were aged 10 to 12 years, and the children in the general population 10 to 11 years. There was no difference in the age distributions of epileptic children, children with lesions above the brain stem, blind or deaf children, and children with lesions at or below the brain stem (Table 65).

There were no appreciable or statistically significant sex differences between any of the groups. Apart from the children with lesions at or below the brain stem, where there was a slight excess of girls, all the groups showed a slight male preponderance (brain disorder 61 per cent, epilepsy 53 per cent, blind or deaf 53 per cent, lesion below brain stem 40 per cent, other physical disorder 51 per cent).

Whether these large age differences and minor sex differences between groups could account for the inter-group differences in psychiatric disorder may be determined by examining the associations of age and of sex with the diagnosis of psychiatric disorder. In the general population, there is a considerable excess of boys among children with psychiatric disorder (Rutter *et al.* 1970). The lack of significant sex difference in relation to psychiatric disorder within the neuro-epileptic group is, therefore, all the more striking. The proportion of boys among the epileptic children with psychiatric disorder (55·6 per cent) was almost identical with that among the epileptic children without psychiatric disorder (51·1 per cent). Also, there was no significant difference between the proportion of boys among the brain disorder children with a psychiatric disability (68·7 per cent) and the behaviourally normal brain disorder children (55·0 per cent).

There was no relationship between age and the diagnosis of psychiatric disorder in either the epileptic group or the brain disorder group (Table 66). The inter-group differences in the rate of psychiatric disorder can therefore not be accounted for by the age differences between groups, nor are the findings explicable in terms of the trivial sex differences between the groups. There are real and large differences between the rates of psychiatric disorder found in the general population or children with chronic physical disorders which do not involve the brain and in children with neuro-epileptic disorders. What are the reasons for these differences?

TABLE 66
Age and psychiatric disorder within the neuro-epileptic group
(children attending school only)

Age	*Epilepsy*				*Brain disorder*			
	Psychiatric disorder		*No psychiatric disorder*		*Psychiatric disorder*		*No psychiatric disorder*	
	No.	*%*	*No.*	*%*	*No.*	*%*	*No.*	*%*
8 years or less	4	22·2	13	28·9	5	31·3	5	25·0
9 to 12 years	10	55·6	23	51·1	9	56·3	8	40·0
13 years or more	4	22·2	9	20·0	2	12·5	7	35·0
Total	18		45		16		20	

Physical Handicap or Lesion of the Brain as Cause of the High Rate of Psychiatric Disorder

The finding that psychiatric disorder was much more common when the physical condition involved the brain than when it affected some other organ or some other part of the body suggests that the very high rate of psychiatric disorder in children with neuro-epileptic disorders was associated specifically with a lesion of the brain rather than with the presence of physical handicap as such. Although the difference in the organ which was damaged is one obvious difference between the children with non-cerebral disorder and those with neuro-epileptic conditions, there are other differences and it is necessary to take these into consideration.

A wide variety of reasons have been previously suggested for such an increased rate of psychiatric disorder in neuro-epileptic children. These include the presence of a visible disability, the frustrations inherent in physical restrictions, adverse parental reaction to the child's handicap, perceptual abnormalities, poor speech and language resulting in the child being unable to express his wants adequately, visual defects, low intelligence, effect of drugs, community prejudices in relation to the disorder, the child's reactions to his disability and impaired emotional control produced by direct brain dysfunction (Bradley 1951, 1955; Bridge 1949; Cruickshank and Raus 1955; Gibbs 1958; Oswin 1967). While some of these factors are shared by children with other physical handicaps (Barker *et al.* 1953, Pringle 1964) others are unique to organic disorders of the brain.

Severity of Physical Handicap

The severity of physical handicap varied somewhat according to diagnosis (Table 67), being most marked in the structural brain disorder groups (both above and below the brain stem) and being least evident in the epilepsy group. The blind and deaf children and the children with other physical disorders were intermediate in this respect. It is obvious from these findings alone that differences in the severity of physical handicap cannot account for the differences in the rate of psychiatric disorder between the children with cerebral and non-cerebral physical disorders. While it is possible that the handicap difference might be responsible for differences between the brain disorder children and the children with other physical

TABLE 67
Chronic physical handicap and diagnosis
(*children attending school only*)

Physical handicap	*Brain disorder*	*Epilepsy*	*Blind or deaf*	*Lesion below brain stem*	*Other physical disorder*
None	1	40	0	0	51
Slight	16	23	14	6	41
Moderate	16	1	5	5	9
Severe	2	0	0	3	1
Total or almost total incapacity	1	0	0	1	0
Total	36	64	19	15	102
Not known	0	0	0	0	25*

**This number includes* 21 *children for whom parental interviews were not carried out due to the late identification of cases* (*Rutter et al.* 1970).

disorders, it could not account for the difference in psychiatric state between children with lesions above and below the brain stem. Furthermore, the epileptic children had a rate of psychiatric disorder several times that in the other physical disorder group in spite of the fact that they were less handicapped.

The matter may be taken one stage further by direct examination of the association between severity of physical handicap and psychiatric disorder. Although there was a slight tendency for the most handicapped children to show psychiatric disorder more often, the association fell well short of statistical significance in both the brain disorder group and the epileptic group. Among the brain disorder children with psychiatric disorder, 69 per cent (11/16) had a chronic handicap of at least moderate severity compared with 40 per cent (8/20) of the children without psychiatric disorder. What the presence of a moderate handicap meant in practical terms may be judged from the fact that to make this rating, there had to be difficulty or discomfort in the performance of ordinary activities or these activities had to be restricted or impaired. This would apply, for example, if the child used crutches, walked with a marked limp, could walk only short distances, was very slow in self-care or needed help with activities such as bathing or brushing hair.

Among the epileptic children with psychiatric disorder 50 per cent (9/18) had some measure of handicap compared with 33 per cent (15/45) of those without psychiatric disorder. In virtually all cases where there was handicap this consisted of a prohibition on swimming, sport, physical education at school or some other activity considered by the parent or doctor to constitute a danger to the child.

Psychiatric disorder among the least handicapped neuro-epileptic children was still considerably more common than in the group of children with non-cerebral disorders. Nine of the 39 non-handicapped epileptic children (26 per cent) and 5 of the 17 brain disorder children with only a slight handicap (29 per cent) had psychiatric disorder compared with only 12 per cent of the children with non-cerebral disorders.

Visibility of Handicap

It has been suggested (Cruickshank and Raus 1955) that the visibility of a handicap may influence society's reactions to the handicapped child. Children with cardiac lesions (where there is a non-visible physical disability) have been found to function better and to view themselves more favourably than do cerebral palsied children who have an obvious handicap which can be seen by everyone. The findings of the present study are consonant with this view in that cerebral palsied children showed more psychiatric disorder than did asthmatic children and children with other types of chronic lung and heart disease. However, the visibility of the handicap may not be the relevant variable. Most of the 'other physical disorder' group (in which there was a low rate of psychiatric disability) had non-visible lesions. Yet psychiatric disorder was no more common among the children with orthopaedic or other visible defects than among those with non-visible conditions. Furthermore, the children with lesions below the brain stem all had visible (and usually quite obvious) handicaps, yet their rate of psychiatric disorder was well below that in the children with lesions above the brain stem. The visibility or non-visibility of the lesion was not therefore the factor chiefly responsible for the high rate of disorder in the neuro-epileptic children.

While the visibility of the lesion cannot account for the inter-group differences in psychiatric disorder, nevertheless it may have played some part in the development of the child's difficulties. An unsightly deformity is likely to influence both the child's image of himself as a desirable person with positive attributes and also other people's reactions to him. Ogden (1959) suggested that the cosmetic correction of disfigurements in young criminals increased their chances of reformation. It is of some interest in this connection to consider the evidence on children's reactions to different forms of physical handicap. It might be supposed that the most severe disabilities would be the most unacceptable, but this does not seem to be the case, at least as measured by children's responses to pictures (Goodman *et al.* 1963, Richardson *et al.* 1961, Richardson and Royce 1968). Pictures of children with a slight facial disfigurement or obesity were less liked than those of a youngster with crutches and a leg brace.

Community Prejudice and Social Acceptance

There is now considerable evidence (Soldwedel and Terrill 1957) that children with a wide variety of physical disabilities (including deafness, speech difficulties, mental retardation, orthopaedic disabilities, cardiac lesions, poliomyelitis and cerebral palsy) tend to be less often chosen as friends compared with non-handicapped children (Baldwin 1958, Elser 1959, Force 1956, Woods and Carrow 1959). Surprisingly, there have been few attempts to compare different types of handicap in this respect, but there is some suggestion that severely mentally retarded children are least acceptable (Jones *et al.* 1966) and that, as judged by sociometric techniques, cerebral palsied children tend to be rejected more than children with other forms of handicap (Force 1956). This effect may sometimes be increased by the stereotypical negative attributes associated by the general public with the diagnostic label of cerebral palsy (Combs and Harper 1967).

However, the relationship between social rejection and psychological development is a complex interaction in that, although social rejection may well adversely affect a child's emotional adjustment, it also seems that children may be rejected *because* of their undesirable behavioural characteristics (Jacobs and Pierce 1968). It is difficult to determine which usually leads to which.

In the past, community prejudice has been most evident with respect to epilepsy (Whildin 1947), but the situation now, at least in Britain, is much more enlightened (Pond and Burden 1963, Ministry of Education 1962) and to what extent prejudice still exists is uncertain (Rose *et al.* 1955). Many writers have emphasised the family and social rejection experienced by the epileptic child (see de Haas 1962 for review of these) and there can be little doubt that when this occurs it may have severely deleterious effects on the child's psychological development. How often it occurs is unknown, and how social prejudice in relation to epilepsy compares with that in relation to cerebral palsy or poliomyelitis has been remarkably little studied.

The matter can be taken very little further in relation to the Isle of Wight findings. That the rate of psychiatric disorder was slightly (but not significantly) higher among the epileptics whose physical activities had been restricted is consistent with the concept of the influence of social prejudice in so far as prohibiting a child from taking part in, for example, school sports automatically labels the child as 'different' and may draw attention to the fact that he suffers from epilepsy. On the other hand, the finding that the difference was quite small also suggests that prejudice probably played little part in the development of psychiatric disorder. In many cases the children had only infrequent nocturnal fits and the school teachers (and probably other people outside the children's family) were unaware of the epilepsy. The exact extent of other people's knowledge of the child's fits was not determined. However, the school teachers of all physically handicapped children (epileptic and non-epileptic) were asked if, to their knowledge, the child had had a fit in the last year. In the majority of cases of epilepsy the teacher reported that no fit had occurred and there was no significant association between this and the presence of psychiatric disorder, although there was a slight tendency for more of the children with psychiatric disorder to have been reported by the teacher as having a fit in the last year (33 per cent) than among the children without psychiatric disorder (19 per cent).

The children on the Isle of Wight were not asked systematically about friendship patterns but on both the teacher questionnaire and the parent questionnaire there were items on this topic. While the responses of outsiders on children's friendships may not be quite the same as the replies which would be given by the children themselves, it has been shown in previous studies that teachers' ratings agree quite well with sociometric ratings (*i.e.* ratings made by the children) in this respect (Gronlund 1959). The findings are shown in Table 68 for children with brain disorder and epileptic children as compared to the figures for asthmatic children given in Rutter *et al.* (1970), which have been shown to be closely similar to those for other non-cerebral physical disorders. The differences are not great but it may be seen that, compared with asthmatics, neuro-epileptic children were slightly more often reported as 'not much liked by other children' and 'rather solitary'.

The differences found were too small to give much support to the concept of the importance of social prejudice. Furthermore, the interpretation of even these small differences is complicated by the finding that the differences in these items was

TABLE 68

Peer relationships in children with brain disorder, epilepsy and asthma

Questionnaire item	*Brain disorder*		*Epilepsy*		*Asthma*	
	No.	*%*	*No.*	*%*	*No.*	*%*
Teacher scale						
'Not much liked by other children'	10	27·8	17	28·3	16	23·7
'Tends to do things on his own—rather solitary'	11	30·6	19	31·7	13	18·7
Parent scale						
'Not much liked by other children'	5	16·7	10	18·9	8	9·9
'Tends to do things on his own—rather solitary'	14	48·3	23	44·2	20	29·4

N.B. Percentages have been calculated on the number of cases for which a response to the item has been available. For this reason the total number of cases is not the same as the two scales, and occasionally the number differs from item to item. This applies to all tables. Teacher scales were available for 99·8 *per cent of the children and parent scales for* 88·5 *per cent.*

much greater in relation to the presence or absence of psychiatric disorder than it was in relation to physical diagnosis (Table 69). Whereas there was only a small difference between asthmatic children and neuro-epileptic children with regard to the frequency of social rejection, there were large differences between the children with and the children without psychiatric disorder. The question of which comes first—the rejection or the psychiatric disorder—is raised again. In so far as the ratings of teachers and parents can be taken as valid measures of the children's social acceptance, the relative size of the differences between groups suggests that the children are more likely to be rejected because they exhibit psychiatric disorder than because they have cerebral palsy or epilepsy. Thus, social rejection was somewhat greater for asthmatic children than for neuro-epileptic children without psychiatric disorder.

Social prejudice is most unlikely to have been the reason for the rate of psychiatric disorder being more than twice as high in the children with lesions above the brain stem as in the children with lesions below the brain stem. It would be an unusually sophisticated child who could make the differential diagnosis between cerebral palsy and muscular dystrophy! Probably both will be known to their schoolmates as 'spastics'. It is unfortunate in relation to the importance of this comparison that the group of below brain stem disorders was so small in the present study. It would be well worthwhile to make a systematic comparison of much larger groups of children with below and above brain stem disorders.

The extent of the influence of social prejudice in the development of emotional behaviour difficulties remains largely a matter for further research, but the present findings suggest that the inter-group differences in rate of psychiatric disorder are not easily explicable in terms of diagnostic differences in social acceptance and rejection.

TABLE 69
Peer relationships and psychiatric disorder in neuro-epileptic children

Questionnaire item	*No psychiatric disorder*		*Psychiatric disorder*	
	No.	*%*	*No.*	*%*
Teacher scale				
'Not much liked by other children'	8	13·1	19	55·9
'Tends to do things on his own—rather solitary'	12	19·7	19	55·9
Parent scale				
'Not much liked by other children'	7	13·5	8	26·7
'Tends to do things on his own—rather solitary'	19	38·0	17	56·7

Intellectual Differences

It was important to determine if the group differences in relation to psychiatric disorder were explicable in terms of intellectual differences between neuro-epileptic children and children with chronic non-cerebral physical disorders. The groups differed in terms of their IQ distribution in that the above brain stem group had a mean IQ well below average (see chapter 9) whereas all the other groups (including the epileptic children) showed a normal level of intelligence. This is likely to have influenced the findings to some extent in that both within the neuro-epileptic group (see chapter 14) and within the general population (Rutter *et al.* 1970) low IQ has been shown to be associated with a higher rate of psychiatric disability.

Whether the diagnostic differences in relation to rate of psychiatric disorder were due to IQ differences between the groups may be assessed by a comparison between groups confined to children whose IQ was at least 86, *i.e.* not more than 1 standard deviation below the mean. When attention was restricted in this way, the rate of psychiatric disorder in the neuro-epileptic group as a whole (24 per cent) was still over twice that in the group of children with physical disorders not involving the brain (9 per cent of psychiatric disorder) and four times that in the general population (6 per cent), both differences being statistically significant ($p. < \cdot 001$ and $p. < \cdot 001$ respectively in relation to other physical disorders and to the general population).

The findings were the same when parent and teacher scale scores were examined for children whose IQ was 86 or more. On the parent questionnaire, 24 per cent of the neuro-epileptic children scored above the cut-off point of 13 compared with 11 per cent of the children with physical disorders not involving the brain and 6 per cent of children in the general population. On the teacher questionnaire, the differences were closely similar; 23 per cent of neuro-epileptic children, 9 per cent of children with other physical disorders and 6 per cent of the general population scored above the cut-off point of 9. It may be concluded that low IQ could *not* account for the high rate of psychiatric disorder among children with neuro-epileptic disorders.

Discussion

The present findings clearly showed that, compared with the general population or children with chronic physical disorders not involving the brain, there was a much increased rate of psychiatric disability in children with neuro-epileptic conditions, and this difference could not be accounted for in terms of age or sex differences between the groups.

The presence of a chronic physical handicap *per se* was not a crucial factor in that psychiatric disorder was three times as common in the neuro-epileptic group as it was in the group of other physical disorders. The *severity* of the physical handicap might have been a factor in the psychiatric differences between children with cerebral palsy and similar disorders, and those with asthma, diabetes, heart disease, etc. (the latter group being on average less handicapped). However, it could not account for the difference between the cerebral palsied children and the children who were blind or who had lesions below the brain stem (such as muscular dystrophy or paralyses following poliomyelitis), nor could it account for the high rate of psychiatric disorder among the epileptic children, many of whom were very little handicapped. Furthermore, it was found that within the neuro-epileptic group there was no significant association between the severity of handicap and the likelihood of psychiatric disorder. The visibility of the handicap was also not a major factor in that psychiatric disorder was no more frequent in the children with lesions below the brain stem (who had visible disabilities) than in the children with miscellaneous non-neurological disorders (very few of whom had visible disabilities). The rate of disorder in both these groups was only a third of that in the neuro-epileptic group.

Community prejudice against epilepsy, and possibly also against cerebral palsy, may have been one adverse factor in the neuro-epileptic child's development. This is suggested by the slightly higher rate of psychiatric disorder in the epileptics whose condition was publicly identified by a restriction on physical activities. On the other hand, the fact that the difference was so small (and statistically insignificant) suggested that the influence of social prejudice was likely to have been small when assessed in relation to the influence of other factors.

Low intelligence was one important feature in relation to the frequent psychiatric abnormalities shown by children with lesions above the brain stem, but low IQ could not account for the high rate of disorder in the epileptic children. Furthermore, even when comparisons were restricted to children whose IQ was 86 or more, the rate of psychiatric disorder in the neuro-epileptic children was still more than double that in the group of children with other chronic physical handicaps.

Thus, it appeared that the most important feature in relation to the much higher rate of psychiatric disorder in the neuro-epileptic children, compared with other physically handicapped children, was the presence of dysfunction *specifically* of the brain. That is not to say that other factors were unimportant (indeed, as we shall see in chapter 14, several other features were strongly associated with the development of psychiatric disorder), but rather that the presence of organic brain dysfunction was the main feature associated with the finding that the rate of psychiatric disorder was higher for children with neuro-epileptic disorders than it was for children with other types of physical handicap.

CHAPTER 13

Organic Brain Dysfunction: Association with a Specific Type of Psychiatric Disorder?

As the high rate of psychiatric disorder in neuro-epileptic children was particularly associated with the effects of dysfunction of the brain (see chapter 12), it might also be expected that brain disorders would be associated with specific *types* of psychiatric problems.

Diagnosis of Psychiatric Disorder in Neuro-epileptic Children Attending School

Eighteen of the 63 children with uncomplicated epilepsy and 16 of the 36 children with a lesion above the brain stem had psychiatric disorder. As in the general population (Table 70), the majority of the neuro-epileptic children with psychiatric disorder suffered from neurotic or antisocial conditions.

TABLE 70
Diagnosis of psychiatric disorder in children attending school

Diagnosis	*General population (excluding neuro-epileptic children)*	*Neuro-epileptic children*	
		(i) with uncomplicated epilepsy	*(ii) with lesions above brain stem (with or without fits)*
	No. of cases	*No. of cases*	*No. of cases*
Neurotic disorder	42	8	4
Antisocial or conduct disorder	41	6	3
Mixed disorder	26	3	4
Hyperkinetic syndrome	1	1	3
Psychosis	0	0	1
Other	1	0	1
Total cases	111	18	16
Total population in each group	2,189	63	36

Case 1*

This 12 year old girl, who began to have major epileptic attacks at the age of 2 years, showed a neurotic disorder. Her epileptic attacks began with twitching of the

*All illustrated cases are chosen at random. Brown *et al.* (1966) have emphasised the importance of this. Specially selected 'typical' cases are given by most writers, but the selection of particularly striking cases can be seriously misleading. The cases described in this chapter, being randomly selected, are therefore not necessarily the most severe or the most striking cases in the category.

right side of her face and then right arm, followed by generalised convulsions with a total duration of unconsciousness of about 5 to 10 minutes. In the last 2 years she had also had petit mal. Every Thursday morning during term time she had stomach-ache and nausea associated with worry over a particular lesson; sometimes on these and other days she was reluctant to go to school. Particularly when worried, she tended to over-eat. Although she usually played on her own, her parents thought that she mixed quite well with other children. Since going to secondary school she had bitten her nails very severely. She had always been highly meticulous. At school she seldom mixed with other children and she appeared worried, fearful and unhappy. Her concentration was noted to be very poor. At interview she appeared markedly depressed and somewhat unresponsive. She said that she often wanted to run away from home and she described how other children picked on her and called her a 'fatso'. Sometimes she thought of killing herself and she had considered that she might use a knife; the last time she had these thoughts was a week before the interview.

This disorder was rated of 'slight' severity and was somewhat unusual in that it was diagnosed almost entirely on the basis of the school report and the interview with the child. The parents' descriptions of her behaviour, emotions and relationships were rated as showing only a dubious abnormality.

Case 2

This 14 year old boy with a spastic diplegia (most marked on the left and associated with dysarthria) is an example of a child with a 'conduct or antisocial disorder'. He had had cyanotic attacks in infancy and major fits (which were followed by a left facial paralysis lasting up to 2 hours after the attack) began at the age of 6 years. Status epilepticus led to admission to hospital a year before the survey. He was a very lonely boy who did not make friends with other children. Often he lied and blamed other people for his own misdeeds. He was reported to be rather quick tempered and very fidgety, and to scratch and pick at himself a great deal. Twice shortly before the survey he had stopped little girls in the street and tried to get them to pull down their knickers; on the second occasion his mother reported him to the Police. The school said that he had no friends and tended to quarrel and fight in a childish way. He was excitable and found an informal unstructured atmosphere difficult to cope with. His concentration was very poor. At school he explored the girls physically, lifting their skirts and touching them. At interview he was friendly and talked freely of fishing, boating and the TV programmes which he watched. He said he had not many friends and he showed poor concentration.

This disorder was rated 'severe'. The boy was one of the very few with any sort of overtly sexual disorder. He showed no significant anxiety, fears or depression, but such associated emotional disturbances were common in children with antisocial or conduct disorders (as they were also in the general population, see Rutter *et al.* 1970).

Case 3

This 12 year old boy with craniostenosis had a mixed disorder of severe degree. His early motor development was normal but there was some delay in speech development and articulation was poor. Major fits started in infancy. At the age of 4 years craniotomy was performed, following the discovery of papilloedema. Psychomotor attacks began at the age of 5 years and at the time of the survey he was having them about twice a year. Nocturnal enuresis occurred twice a week. He had truanted from school several times two years ago but not since. He frequently tormented and provoked other children, including his sibs; this often led to arguments and fights. He wanted to join in with other children but did not know how to do so. He was irritable and easily upset and there was much sucking and biting of his fingers and handkerchief, as well as chewing of his cuffs and the corners of toys. Since he choked on a fish bone at 4 years he had refused to eat fish. Although he went to bed at 8 p.m., he kept going downstairs and was not asleep until 10.30 p.m. He tended to take things apart and sometimes destroyed them. At school he tormented other children and was irritated by them, but got on well with his class teacher. He was unable to play properly, was disobedient and got into many fights. There was a lot of trouble with him on the school bus. His teacher noted that he had interests of his own, including fanciful and enjoyable blank verse. At interview he was markedly distractible and appeared worried and severely depressed. He spoke of his lack of friends and described running away from home twice. The Police had twice cautioned him for misbehaviour.

The hyperkinetic syndrome (4 cases) and child psychosis (1 case) were diagnosed rather more frequently than expected on the basis of the diagnostic distribution of psychiatric disorders in the general population, but the numbers were far too small for this finding to be reliable. Furthermore, at least in neuro-epileptic children attending school, these conditions accounted for only a small proportion of psychiatric disorders. Thus, while organic brain dysfunction had important associations with psychiatric disorder, the results of this study suggest that the association was not with any specific type of disorder. The varieties of psychiatric problems in neuro-epileptic children were similar on the whole to these found in any group of children with psychiatric disorder (and no known organic brain condition). Neurotic and antisocial disorders formed the bulk of the cases found.

These conclusions apply only to neuro-epileptic children who had remained within the educational system (in effect this meant that their IQ was above about 50). In these comparisons, and in those made in the previous chapter, children outside the educational system were excluded on the grounds that psychiatric disorder in children of very low IQ differs in some important respects from that in children of normal intelligence. We shall now consider to what extent this assumption was justified.

Psychiatric Disorder in Children Excluded from School

Table 71 shows psychiatric disorder according to diagnosis among the children excluded from school by reason of severe mental subnormality. For this purpose all children with severe intellectual retardation who were not attending school were included regardless of their neurological state, on the grounds that practically all children of IQ below 50 have structural brain pathology (Crome 1960, Penrose 1963). Of the 38 children, 10 had cerebral palsy, 10 had other neurological disorders involving definite lesion above the brain stem, 11 had Down's syndrome and 7 had some other condition.

In marked contrast to the type of psychiatric disorder seen in children of normal (or only slightly subnormal) intelligence, just over half of the children with psychiatric disorder (among those excluded from school) showed either the hyperkinetic syndrome or psychosis. Neurotic and antisocial disorders also occurred, but were less frequent. In five children, no rating of psychiatric state could be made because of the severity of handicap and the consequent marked limitation of the children's behavioural and emotional repertoire. For example, one girl had a very gross bilateral hemiplegia, was blind, without speech, was doubly incontinent and spent her time lying curled up in a hospital bed; a boy who was dying of cerebral lipoidosis was almost continuously in coma from recurrent fits.

TABLE 71
Diagnosis of psychiatric disorder in children outside educational system

Diagnosis		*No. of cases*
Not designated		5
No psychiatric disorder		14
Psychiatric disorder:		
Neurotic disorder	5	
Antisocial or conduct disorder	1	
Mixed disorder	1	
Hyperkinetic syndrome	5	19
Psychosis	5	
Other	2	
Total no. of children		38

Case 4

This 8 year old girl* with a right hemiplegia (but some weakness in the other side) is an example of a child with the hyperkinetic syndrome. She tormented and upset her sibs so that there was frequent squabbling and fighting, she constantly wanted attention and was always coming to her parents for loving and kissing. She could never stay still and was always running around all over the place, often tearing things up or breaking them. She never stayed on one task or game for longer than five minutes. Although she liked to be with other children they excluded her from their games. If told to do something, she usually refused and rebelled although eventually she complied. With her teacher she was very friendly and responsive, but she was extremely erratic in class with a very limited attention span. Both in and out of class she was noisy and excitable, difficult to control but also likeable and affectionate. At interview she was extremely disinhibited and distractible, talking all the time but difficult to engage in conversation because she tended to jump from topic to topic and activity to activity. In an offhand way she said she had few friends and was frequently picked on and teased.

*This child was chosen at random from the total number of hyperkinetic children and, as it happened, she was not in the group excluded from school (although she had been when younger).

Case 5

This boy of 12 years, who is now in a mental subnormality hospital, is an example of a psychotic child. As an infant he had sucked poorly and was noted to have had a constant blank expression. He was said to have spoken a few words when younger but at the time of the survey he was completely without speech. As a young child he paid no attention to other people and pushed his mother away when she made a fuss of him. When seen during the survey he still did not join in with other children and had very limited relationships with adults, often appearing detached and aloof, although he came for a cuddle at other times. Since early childhood he had always taken a piece of string with him wherever he went, getting upset if it was taken away from him. Whenever he went outside he had a short but complicated set route which he always followed, repeating it time and time again. When young he was markedly overactive but also agile and nimble. He rarely cried and never laughed but there was frequent grimacing. He played with puzzles but did very little else constructive. The EEG had shown a constant spike and wave focus in the left Sylvian region, and major fits began at the age of 10 years. There was some inequality of the deep tendon reflexes and both plantar responses were probably extensor, the right definitely so.

The extent to which the hyperkinetic syndrome and child psychosis are specifically associated with organic brain pathology cannot be determined from the present study in view of the very small number of cases of this kind which were found. To some extent, the small number of cases of the hyperkinetic syndrome may be a function of the difficulties in the diagnosis of the syndrome in later childhood. Overactivity in the young child generally diminishes as the child grows older and is quite often replaced by an inert underactivity (see chapter 1). Nevertheless, on the criteria used in this study the hyperkinetic syndrome is a decidedly uncommon disorder.

The fact that the disorders are so much more frequent in children with severe intellectual retardation might reflect an association with profound cognitive impairment (or mental immaturity) but equally it might reflect an association with generalised cerebral damage or dysfunction. Nearly all children with an IQ below 50 have demonstrable brain pathology, but whether the association is primarily with mental age or with organic damage can only be determined satisfactorily by an investigation of these disorders in children of normal intelligence. The evidence both in relation to the hyperkinetic syndrome (see chapter 1) and in relation to child psychosis (Rutter 1967) is far from conclusive. It seems that, although both conditions are associated with a low mental age, they are also often associated with organic cerebral dysfunction even in children of normal intelligence. In other cases, however, no evidence of such organic dysfunction can be found, so that it is far from an invariable relationship. Furthermore, in so far as it constitutes a specific relationship, it is a relationship not just with organic brain dysfunction but with organic dysfunction in an *immature* and developing brain. Whether there is a weak or a strong association between these disorders and neurologic dysfunction remains a question for further research.

It should also be emphasised that, regardless of what may be discovered in relation to these two rare syndromes, the great majority of psychiatric disturbances in normally intelligent children with neurological disorder do *not* take this form. In these children there was nothing specific or characteristic about the *type* of psychiatric abnormality; the distribution of diagnoses was much the same as that found in any group of children with psychiatric disorders. A knowledge of the type of emotional and behavioural disturbance tells one little or nothing about the possible existence of organic brain pathology.

Individual Items of Behaviour in Neuro-epileptic Children

It could reasonably be argued that the diagnostic groupings represent very broad categories of disorder and that, if individual symptoms or signs were examined, brain disorders might still be found to be associated with specific types of psychiatric abnormality. The fact that a child was rated as having no psychiatric disorder does not exclude the possibility of his having had various minor oddities of behaviour which might be specific to organic brain dysfunction.

Case 6

This 11 year old boy was rated as having no psychiatric disorder. He had a mild right hemiparesis but fairly marked dyspraxia which had developed following encephalitis at 7 months. A major fit occurred at the age of 3 years and he was on anti-convulsants until shortly after starting school. In the mornings he frequently said that he did not want to go to school but in fact he always went happily and without difficulty. On the whole he got on well with his brothers but there were mild arguments most days. He was a good mixer and made friends easily. He tended to get irritable if he did not get things right first time; about once a fortnight he lost his temper and threw whatever he was doing on the ground. He was still frightened of storms and when it thundered he went into his parents' room. The school commented on his poor physical co-ordination and his tendency to squabble, but they said that he was a friendly and co-operative boy who mixed fairly well with other children. At interview he was cheerful, friendly, mildly disinhibited and rather fidgety.

The question of whether or not organic brain disorders are characterised by particular individual items of behaviour will now be considered in relation to the individual ratings obtained on the parental questionnaire, the teachers' questionnaire and the interview with the child.

Table 72 shows certain items of behaviour which have frequently been specifically associated with brain damage. It may be seen that the teachers reported more restlessness, more fidgetiness, poorer concentration, greater irritability and more fighting among neuro-epileptic children than they did for children in the general population*. However, these items were equally common in children with neurotic and antisocial disorders but *no* neurological abnormality. The findings based on parental reports were substantially the same.

In the psychiatric interview with the child, there was a systematic assessment of many different aspects of behaviour, emotions and relationships as well as a global

*In order to eliminate possible age differences, attention was confined in this Table, and in Tables 73 to 76, to children aged 9 to 12 years.

TABLE 72
Behaviour as judged from questionnaires and psychiatric interview with child
(9-12 *year age group*)

	Brain disorder %	*Epileptic* %	*General population* %	*Neurotic* %	*Antisocial* %
(*a*) **Teachers' questionnaire**					
Very restless	24	28*	11	31*	63*
Squirmy, fidgety	30	37*	15	34*	61*
Poor concentration	68*	50*	30	67*	86*
Irritable	24	22*	7	21*	37*
Fights	30*	15	7	24*	61*
Total no. of cases	17	32	2,163	41	39
(*b*) **Parental questionnaire**					
Very restless	57*	45	31	60*	66*
Squirmy, fidgety	36*	35*	12	43*	38*
Poor concentration	64*	41*	22	48*	63*
Irritable	50	45	30	70*	69*
Fights	29	38*	10	35*	56*
Total no. of cases	14	29	1,919	40	32
(*c*) **Interview with child**			(*Control group*)		
Activity: high	12	3	1	7	8
low	18	12	5	0	0
Fidgetiness	47	48	51	63	71*
Poor attention span	30*	16	4	34*	43*
Distractibility	30*	12	10	22	23
Disinhibition	12	18	12	10	33*
Total no. of cases	17	33	147	41	39

**Significantly different from general population/control group at better than the 5 per cent level.*

rating of psychiatric disorder (Rutter and Graham 1968). As may be seen from Table 72*c*, motor and cognitive abnormalities were again more common in the neuro-epileptic children than in children chosen at random from the general population (the control group), but they were not more frequent than in the groups of children with neurotic or antisocial disorders.

In view of the high rate of these conditions in the neuro-epileptic group, it was possible that the motor, cognitive and aggressive abnormalities were associated less with the brain disorder itself than with the psychiatric disorder from which so many of the epileptic and cerebral palsied children suffered.

Thus, comparisons were made again after controlling for the presence of psychiatric disorder. In order to avoid unduly small numbers, the two neuro-epileptic groups were combined into one category. Table 73 *a*, *b* and *c* shows motor behaviour and relationships in neuro-epileptic children with and without psychiatric disorder. As in the general population, most of the items were more common in the neuro-epileptic children with, than in those without, psychiatric disorder. In general, motor

TABLE 73
Motor behaviour and relationships in groups controlled for presence of psychiatric disorder (9-12 *year age group*)

	Neuro-epileptic (non-psychiatric) %	*General population (excluding psychiatric group)* %	*Neuro-epileptic (psychiatric)* %	*Psychiatric* %
(*a*) **Teachers' questionnaire**				
Restlessness	13	11	47	50
Fidgetiness	20	15	58	52
Twitches/tics	3	3	27	18
Poor concentration	50**	30	69	76
Irritability	7	7	47	33
Not much liked	13	12	53	48
Solitary	20	14	63*	30
Total no. of cases	30	2,163	19	113
(*b*) **Parental questionnaire**				
Restlessness	27	31	82*	64
Fidgetiness	19	12	59	45
Twitches/tics	8	4	24	18
Poor concentration	35	22	71	59
Irritability	39	30	59	72
Tempers	39	18	59	59
Not much liked	15	5	29	20
Solitary	31	23	59	45
Total no. of cases	26	1,919	17	95
(*c*) **Interview with child**		*Control group*		
Activity: high	6	1	5	7
low	10	5	21*	3
Fidgetiness	42	51	58	74
Poor attention span	7	4	37	43
Distractibility	13	10	26	27
Disinhibition	16	12	16	23
Startle	10	5	11	25
Poor emotional responsiveness	19	15	47	33
Poor relationship with examiner	10	9	32	28
Total no. of cases	31	147	19	108

**Significantly different from general population at better than the 5 per cent level.*
***Significantly different from psychiatric groups at better than the 5 per cent level.*

and relationship abnormalities were associated with psychiatric disorder rather than with organic brain dysfunction as such. An exception to this was reduced motor activity which was found in 21 per cent of the neuro-epileptic children with psychiatric disorder but in only 3 per cent of the psychiatrically abnormal children in the general population. Although only a minority of neuro-epileptic children showed reduced motor activity, it does appear from the present findings and from those of other investigations (Schulman *et al.* 1965) that there is a significant (but not strong) association between hypoactivity and organic brain dysfunction.

There was also a tendency (significant only on the teacher questionnaire) for poor concentration to be found more frequently among neuro-epileptic children without psychiatric disorder than among children in the general population—probably a reflection of the well documented effect of brain damage on intellectual development. The only other difference between groups was the higher frequency with which neuro-epileptic children were described by teachers (and to a lesser extent by the parents) as 'solitary'.

Table 74 *a*, *b* and *c*, shows neurotic items and Table 75 *a* and *b* shows antisocial behaviour in the same groups of children. Neuro-epileptic children were more often

TABLE 74

Neurotic items in groups controlled for presence of psychiatric disorder

(9-12 *year age group*)

	Neuro-epileptic (non-psychiatric) %	*General population (excluding psychiatric group)* %	*Neuro-epileptic (psychiatric)* %	*Psychiatric* %
(*a*) **Teachers' questionnaire**				
Tears on arrival at school	0	1	5	3
Worried	27	23	58*	31
Miserable	7	7	47	23
Fearful	37	19	47	33
Fussy	13	8	32*	11
Total no. of cases	30	2,163	19	113
(*b*) **Parental questionnaire**				
Tears on arrival at school	8	1	6	4
Worried	62	39	65	64
Miserable	23	11	53	47
Fearful	39	27	59	43
Fussy	4	16	18	30
Total no. of cases	26	1,919	17	95
(*c*) **Interview with child**		*Control group*		
Preoccupation with anxiety topics	32	20	33	48
Preoccupation with depressive topics	13	9	22	44
Anxious expression	23	23	47	44
Sad expression	16	14	37	42
Depressed or sad mood	23	13	42	39
Anxiety	29	36	53	45
Total no. of cases	31	147	19	108

**Significantly different from psychiatric group at better than the 5 per cent level.*

rated as fussy, worried and disobedient, but the parent and teacher scales did not agree in these findings. As only 3 significant differences were found in 60 comparisons (*i.e.* the number expected by chance alone) these differences are probably without meaning.

TABLE 75

Antisocial behaviour in groups controlled for presence of psychiatric disorder

(9-12 *year age group*)

	Neuro-epileptic (non-psychiatric) %	*General population (excluding psychiatric group)* %	*Neuro-epileptic (psychiatric)* %	*Psychiatric* %
(*a*) **Teachers' questionnaire**				
Truants	0	1	5	10
Steals	0	2	21	27
Destructive	0	1	21	18
Disobedient	3	7	37	50
Lies	3	5	32	40
Bullies	0	4	32	31
Fights	7	7	42	44
Total no. of cases	30	2,163	19	113
(*b*) **Parental questionnaire**				
Truants	0	0	0	3
Steals	0	3	6	24
Destructive	4	4	41	27
Disobedient	50*	26	71	65
Lies	19	11	35	44
Bullies	8	5	41	30
Fights	23	10	53	45
Total no. of cases	26	1,919	17	95

**Significantly different from general population at better than the 5 per cent level.*

Table 76 *a* and *b* shows developmental and other items of behaviour; again, no differences were found between neuro-epileptic children and other children, once the groups had been controlled for the presence of psychiatric disorder. The consideration of individual items confirmed that there were few features of behaviour, emotions or relationships that could be said to be characteristic of organic brain disorders. There was a slight tendency for neuro-epileptic children without psychiatric disorder to show poor concentration more often than children in the general population, and there was some evidence to suggest a significant but weak association between a low level of motor activity and neuro-epileptic disorder. While many types of deviant behaviour were more frequent in neuro-epileptic children than in the general population, it was found that this was a function of the high rate of psychiatric disorder in the group and (apart from the slight exception noted above) in no way

TABLE 76
Developmental and other phenomena in groups controlled for presence of psychiatric disorder
(9-12 *year age group*)

	Neuro-epileptic (non-psychiatric) %	*General population (excluding psychiatric group)* %	*Neuro-epileptic (psychiatric)* %	*Psychiatric* %
(*a*) **Teachers' questionnaire**				
Wets/soils	0	1	11	5
Stutter	0	2	0	7
Other speech disorders	3	3	23	11
Sucks thumb	7	5	11	13
Bites nails	13	19	26	27
Total no. of cases	30	2,163	19	113
(*b*) **Parental questionnaire**				
Enuresis	8	6	12	28
Encopresis	4	2	12	11
Stutter	0	2	30	7
Other speech disorders	8	5	35	11
Sucks thumb	12	11	24	8
Bites nails	35	30	35	45
Total no. of cases	26	1,919	17	95

specific to organic brain dysfunction. These negative findings agree with those of other systematic controlled studies in the literature (see chapter 11), and it appears that the concept of a specific behaviour syndrome for children with cerebral damage is incorrect. The contrary findings in the literature are mostly explicable in terms of bias in the judgements made and the highly selected nature of the samples studied.

However, while not all brain-damaged children show the same behavioural pattern, it could still be that some *rare* psychiatric disorders are usually due to brain damage. As discussed already, this may apply to infantile psychosis, disintegrative psychosis and the hyperkinetic syndrome. It certainly applies to dementia, and confusional states are also 'organic' in origin although the cause may be a toxin or drug intoxication rather than actual damage to the brain.

Age Differences in Relation to Behaviour

The discussion has been restricted so far to the findings in relation to children aged 9 to 12 years, as this was the only age-group for which there were comparable data on children in the general population. Without such comparable data very little can be concluded concerning age differences in relation to behaviour. However, all ratings were examined for possible age trends. Few sizeable age differences were found and in general the findings in relation to older and younger neuro-epileptic children were closely similar to those for the 9 to 12 year olds. At all ages a considerable

TABLE 77
Motor items in neuro-epileptic children according to age

	No psychiatric disorder Less than 9 years %	9-12 years %	13 years or more %	*Psychiatric disorder* Less than 9 years %	9-12 years %	13 years or more %
(*a*) **Teachers' questionnaire**						
Restlessness	28	13	15	89	47	50
Fidgetiness	22	20	15	78	58	33
Poor concentration	50	50	31	78	68	83
Total no. of cases	18	31	13	9	19	6
(*b*) **Interview with child**						
Overactivity	0	7	0	33	5	17
Underactivity	6	10	0	0	21	0
Fidgetiness	71	42	13	67	58	0
Short attention span	12	7	25	56	37	33
Distractibility	24	13	13	56	26	0
Total no. of cases	17	31	16	9	19	6

heterogeneity of deviant behaviour was found, and there was nothing at any age to support a behavioural stereotype of the 'brain-damaged' child. There was a tendency for restlessness, fidgetiness and poor concentration to be more common in the younger children (Table 77). Whether or not the differences between neuro-epileptic and other children might have been greater on these items in early childhood is not known. However these items, in any case, are also more common in early childhood in children without organic brain dysfunction (Grant 1958, Macfarlane *et al.* 1954).

CHAPTER 14

The Pathogenesis of Psychiatric Disorder in Neuro-epileptic Children

In this chapter we shall attempt to determine what factors were responsible for the development of psychiatric disorder in children with neuro-epileptic conditions by comparing the children with psychiatric disorder with those who did not have psychiatric disorder. The factors discussed in previous chapters in terms of their association with *neuro-epileptic* disorder were re-examined in terms of their association with *psychiatric* disorder within the neuro-epileptic group. Only a limited range of variables was measured so that this can only be a preliminary consideration of the problem. Moreover, it will only be possible to find out what factors were *associated* with the development of psychiatric disorder. Nevertheless, a study of associations may provide powerful pointers to items likely to have constituted pathogenic influences. Aetiological hypotheses can derive from such a study, and can then be further investigated by longitudinal studies and tested by experimental methods (Robins 1970). The present study can only take us on the first step of that course but it could be an important step.

Epileptic Children

There were 63 children with uncomplicated epilepsy for whom psychiatric ratings were available; 18 showed psychiatric disorder and 45 did not. These two groups were compared with regard to the nature and treatment of the epilepsy, intellectual and educational factors, social background, sex of the child and family characteristics.

Nature and Treatment of Epilepsy (Table 78)

The frequency of fits bore no relationship to the presence of psychiatric disorder, but this finding must be treated with some caution as there were very few children who were having frequent attacks. The age of the child at the time fits first began also showed no association with psychiatric disorder, though this does not mean that the time of life when fits start is an unimportant variable. It has been shown previously that fits beginning in the neonatal period are commonly a symptom of structural brain disease and carry a poor prognosis (Schulte 1966). However, this would not be reflected in the present findings as children with brain disorders other than epilepsy were excluded from consideration. It is also known that children who develop convulsions during the six-month to three-year age period have a particularly good prognosis (Bower 1969, Cooper 1965, Costeff 1965). Fits are very common at this age, occurring in at least 2 or 3 per cent of children and probably as many as 6 or 7 per cent (Cooper 1965, Miller *et al.* 1960, Pond *et al.* 1960). Most of these children cease to have fits before they start school and only a very small minority develop chronic epilepsy. Again, the good prognosis of this group would not be reflected in the present findings as the 63 children studied only included children who were continuing to have fits (or who were still on anticonvulsants).

As previously noted, epileptic children who were handicapped in their activities were no more likely to have psychiatric disorder than were non-handicapped children.

With the important exception of the high rate of psychiatric disorder in children with psychomotor fits, the types of fits were generally similar in the two groups of children. The frequency of focal fits was also much the same, as was the frequency of major fits unaccompanied by any other type of attack. Pure petit mal was too rare a condition for its association with psychiatric disorder to be examined.

TABLE 78
Epileptic factors associated with psychiatric disorder in 5-15 year old epileptic children attending school

	Psychiatric disorder		*No psychiatric disorder*		
	No.	*%*	*No.*	*%*	*Total*
Psychomotor attacks	6	33**	2	4	8
Other focal attacks	4	22	6	13	10
Onset of fits before 2 years	5	28	10	22	15
More than 10 attacks (other than psychomotor) in last year	2	11	3	7	5
Activities restricted or handicapped	9	50	15	33	24
Total no. of cases	18		45		63

***Difference between groups significant at 1 per cent level.*

Electroencephalographic findings were only available for some of the children so that the diagnosis of type of fit was based solely on the clinical characteristics of attacks.

Although there were just 8 children with psychomotor attacks, there was a marked and statistically significant association between fits of this type and psychiatric disorder. Six of the 8 children with psychomotor fits showed psychiatric disorder compared with 12 out of 55 children with other kinds of fits, or, put another way, 33 per cent of the 18 children with psychiatric disorder had psychomotor fits compared with 4 per cent of the 45 children without psychiatric disorder. There were too few children to determine whether psychomotor fits were associated with any particular type of psychiatric disorder. No specific type of disorder was apparent: the 6 children with psychiatric disorder consisted of 3 with neurotic conditions and 3 with antisocial disturbances.

As psychomotor fits have previously been found to be more common in children of low IQ, it was possible that low IQ rather than psychomotor fits was the relevant factor in the development of psychiatric disorder. However, the intelligence of the 8 children with psychomotor fits followed a normal distribution (one child of IQ 71-85, two of IQ 86-100, four of IQ 116-130, and one of IQ over 131), probably accounted for by the exclusion from the group of all epileptic children with any other neurological disorder. It may be concluded that psychiatric disorder is considerably more common in children with psychomotor fits than in children with other varieties of epilepsy.

No association was found between anticonvulsant medication and psychiatric disorder (Table 79). The clinical significance of the finding is limited by the fact that the great majority of children were taking phenobarbitone, usually on its own but sometimes in conjunction with another drug.

TABLE 79
Anti-convulsant medication and psychiatric disorder in 5-15 year old epileptic children attending school

Medication	*Psychiatric disorder*		*No psychiatric disorder*		
	No.	*%*	*No.*	*%*	*Total*
None in last year	4	22	3	7	7
Phenobarbitone	10	56	27	60	37
Other than phenobarbitone	0	–	6	13	6
Phenobarbitone plus other	4	22	8	18	12
Medication (nature not known)	0	–	1	2	1
Total no. of cases	18		45		63

Intellectual and Educational Factors

Low intelligence (IQ 85 or less) was more than twice as common in the epileptic children with psychiatric disorder (28 per cent) as in other epileptic children (12 per cent), and a level of reading which was at least two years below that expected on the basis of the child's age and intelligence was over three times as common in the psychiatric group (36 per cent compared with 11 per cent). Because of the small numbers, neither difference quite reached the 5 per cent level of significance. Nevertheless, in view of the size of the difference and the fact that a similar association between intellectual/educational retardation and psychiatric abnormality was found in the other brain disorder children (see below) as well as in the general population (Rutter *et al.* 1970), it is likely that the findings in the epileptic children represent a meaningful association.

Social Factors

Psychiatric disorder was significantly less common in epileptic children whose fathers had a non-manual occupation (professional, managerial or clerical) but otherwise social factors were unassociated with psychiatric disorder (Table 80). Whether the mother had a job outside the home or was at work when the child returned home from school was unrelated to the presence of pspchiatric disorder. Family size (expressed as the number of children in the household) and overcrowding were also unrelated to psychiatric disorder.

The meaning of the association with social class is difficult to interpret as no association between social class and psychiatric disorder was found in either the general population or in the group of children with neurological disorders other than epilepsy. The issue requires further investigation.

TABLE 80
Social factors and psychiatric disorder in 5-15 year old epileptic children attending school

	Psychiatric disorder		*No psychiatric disorder*		
	No.	*%*	*No.*	*%*	*Total*
Non-manual occupation (father)	1	6*	15	34	16
Person/room ratio of 1·5 or more	6	33	8	18	14
Mother with part-time or full-time job	11	61	23	51	34
Mother at work when child returns from school	3	17	9	20	12
Number of children in household:					
1	2	11	8	18	10
2	4	22	15	33	41
3	9	50	13	39	
4 or more	3	17	9	20	12
Total no. of cases	18		45		63

* *Difference between groups significant at 5 per cent level.*

TABLE 81
Ordinal position and psychiatric disorder in 5-15 year old epileptic children attending school

	Psychiatric disorder		*No psychiatric disorder*		
	No.	*%*	*No.*	*%*	*Total*
Eldest	8	44	12	27	20
Youngest	7	39	14	31	21
Only child	2	11	8	18	10
Other	1	6	11	24	12
Total no. of cases	18		45		63

Sex and Ordinal Position

Although in the general population psychiatric disorder is considerably more common in boys than girls (Rutter *et al.* 1970) this was not found in epileptic childern. Ten of the 33 epileptic boys showed psychiatric disorder compared with 8 of the 30 epileptic girls. The numbers were too small to allow a detailed examination of sex differences within diagnostic groups. However, it was found that of the 8 neurotic children, 4 were boys and 4 girls; and of the 9 children with antisocial or mixed disorders 5 were boys and 4 girls. In the general population antisocial and mixed disorders are much more common in boys than in girls.

The epileptic child's ordinal position was unrelated to the presence of psychiatric disorder (Table 81).

Familial Factors

Psychiatric disorder was no more frequent in children whose parents had separated, divorced or been widowed than in children who were still living with both their natural parents.

Information on the psychiatric state of parents was restricted to the standardised 'malaise' inventory, described in chapter 10. Scores of 6 or more were more than twice as common in the mothers of the epileptic children who showed psychiatric disorder (Table 82), suggesting that when the children had psychiatric problems their mothers were also more likely to report emotional disturbance. The last item on the questionnaire asked if the mother had ever had a 'nervous breakdown'. Two-fifths of the mothers of the children with psychiatric disorder reported that they had, a proportion over three times as great as in the mothers of the epileptic children without psychiatric disorder.

The meaning of these findings will be considered after an examination of the differences between the children with psychiatric disorder and those without psychiatric disorder in the group with brain disorders other than uncomplicated epilepsy.

TABLE 82
Familial factors associated with psychiatric disorder in 5-15 year old epileptic children attending school

	Psychiatric disorder		*No psychiatric disorder*		
	No.	*%*	*No.*	*%*	*Total*
'Nervous breakdown' reported by mother	7	39*	5	12	12
Mother's 'malaise' score of 6 or more	12	67*	11	26	23
Broken home	4	22	9	20	13
Total no. of cases	18		45		63

**Difference between groups significant at 5 per cent level.*

Children with Brain Disorder

There were 36 children with a structural disorder of the brain who attended school and who had psychiatric ratings. Most of these children had cerebral palsy but the group included some with other brain conditions such as hydrocephalus and craniostenosis (see chapter 7). Sixteen of the children showed psychiatric disorder and 20 did not. These two groups will be compared with regard to neurological factors, intellectual and educational factors, social background, sex of the child and family characteristics in the same manner as used for epileptic children.

Neurological Factors (Table 83)

Psychiatric disorder was significantly more common when there was evidence of a bilateral brain disorder than when the disorder was strictly unilateral. For this purpose, a strict definition of unilateral disorder was followed: children with any *definite* signs on both sides were included in the bilateral disorders group. Thus, a child with a left hemiplegia but a bilateral positive Babinski response would be classed as having a bilateral disorder. Defined in this way only 7 children had a strictly unilateral disorder, none of whom showed psychiatric disorder. This suggests that the extent of the brain lesion is an important factor in the development of psychiatric disorder. The association between psychiatric disorder and the severity of physical handicap was slight and not significant, so that the importance of a bilateral brain lesion was *not* merely a reflection of the severity of physical handicap.

Psychiatric disorder was slightly more common in children who also had fits, but the difference fell short of statistical significance. However, strabismus and language retardation were significantly associated with the presence of psychiatric disorder. Both these features were to some extent associated with low IQ, but although the numbers were too small to assess the strength of the association after controlling for IQ, it was evident that the association could not be due solely to IQ effects.

TABLE 83
Neurological factors associated with psychiatric disorder in 5-15 year old children with brain disorder attending school

	Psychiatric disorder		*No psychiatric disorder*		
	No.	*%*	*No.*	*%*	*Total*
Strictly unilateral disorder	0	–**	7 (out of 19)	37	7
Presence of fits	7	44	5	26	12
Strabismus	8	50**	3	15	11
Articulation defect in speech	11	69	10	50	21
Retarded language	12	75**	6	30	18
At least moderate handicap	11	69	8	40	19
Total	16		20		36

***Difference between groups significant at 1 per cent level.*

Intellectual and Educational Factors

As in the epileptic group, both low IQ and reading retardation were strongly associated with psychiatric disorder. Of the 16 children with psychiatric disorder 13 (83 per cent) had an IQ of 85 or less compared with only 8 (40 per cent) of the 20 without psychiatric disorder. The proportion with at least 2 years' specific reading retardation (64 per cent) was nearly three times that in the group without psychiatric disorder (22 per cent). The measurement of reading retardation was made after partialling out IQ so that this difference can not be accounted for in terms of the IQ difference between the groups (see chapter 9).

It is notable that low IQ was associated with psychiatric disorder in both the epileptic and the other brain disorder groups, although the cause of the low level of intelligence was probably different in the two groups (Table 84). The distribution of intelligence in the children with uncomplicated epilepsy was closely similar to that in the general population, so that the presence of epilepsy did not appear to have affected the IQ level. Furthermore, within the epileptic group IQ was associated with the same kinds of variables as in the general population. Thus, there was a sizeable association between IQ and social class. Among the children from families where the father had a non-manual occupation, twice as many had an IQ of 116 or more as among the children from families where the father had a manual occupation; similarly the proportion with an IQ of 85 or less was less than a third of that in the children from families where the father had a manual occupation. The intelligence of the epileptic child was probably influenced by the same kinds of genetic and environmental factors as those influencing intelligence in any other child.

In contrast, it is probable that low IQ in the brain disorder group was largely a result of the brain disorder itself. The distribution of intelligence was abnormal, over half the children showing an IQ of 85 or less. In addition, unlike the situation with the epileptics and the general population, there was no association between IQ and social class. Genetic and environmental factors of a kind normally associated with social class may have played some part in the development of intelligence, but their influence was swamped by the much greater effect of brain damage.

Nevertheless, in spite of these differences in the factors leading to low intelligence, children of low IQ in both groups had an increased risk of developing psychiatric disorder.

TABLE 84
IQ and social class within epileptic and brain disorder groups

	Epileptic group				*Brain disorder group*			
IQ	*Non-manual*		*Manual*		*Non-manual*		*Manual*	
	No.	*%*	*No.*	*%*	*No.*	*%*	*No.*	*%*
85 or less	1	6	9	21	8	57	13	62
86-100	3	19	17	40	2	14	2	10
101-115	4	25	5	12	3	21	3	14
116 or more	8	50	11	26	1	7	3	14
Total	16		42		14		21	

Social Factors

None of the social factors which were examined showed any association with psychiatric disorder (Table 85). Social class, family size, whether or not the mother went out to work, and the degree of overcrowding were all unrelated.

TABLE 85
Social factors and psychiatric disorder in 5-15 year old children with brain disorder attending school

	Psychiatric disorder		*No psychiatric disorder*		
	No.	*%*	*No.*	*%*	*Total*
Non-manual occupation (father)	6	38	8	40	14
Person/room ratio of 1·5 or more	3	19	6	30	9
Mother with part-time or full-time job	8	50	12	60	20
Mother at work when child returns from school	1	6	3	15	4
Number of children in household:					
1	2	13	3	15	5
2	7	44	8	40	15
3	3	19	4	20	7
4 or more	4	25	5	25	9
Total no. of cases	16		20		36

TABLE 86
Ordinal position and psychiatric disorder in 5-15 year old children with brain disorder attending school

	Psychiatric disorder		*No psychiatric disorder*		
	No.	*%*	*No.*	*%*	*Total*
Eldest	4	25	4	20	8
Youngest	7	44	7	35	14
Only child	2	13	3	15	5
Other	3	19	6	30	9
Total no. of cases	16		20		36

Sex and Ordinal Position

Neither the sex of the child nor his position in the sibship (Table 86) was associated with the presence of psychiatric disorder. Of the 22 boys with a brain condition, 11 had psychiatric disorder compared with 5 of the 14 girls. Two boys and 2 girls showed the hyperkinetic syndrome or psychosis. Of the remaining 9 boys with psychiatric disorder, 3 had a neurotic disorder and 6 an antisocial or mixed disorder; of the 3 girls, one had a neurotic disorder, one a mixed disorder, and one a personality disorder. The numbers were too small to consider sex differences in relation to psychiatric diagnosis.

Familial Factors

The proportion of mothers with high scores on the malaise inventory was very much lower in the brain disorder group than in the epileptic group, and the association between the malaise score and psychiatric disorder was not significant. Nevertheless, of the 4 children whose mothers had a score of 6 or more, 3 showed psychiatric disorder. There was also a strong association between psychiatric disorder in the child and a 'broken home'.

TABLE 87
Familial factors associated with psychiatric disorder in 5-15 year old children with brain disorder attending school

	Psychiatric disorder		*No psychiatric disorder*		
	No.	*%*	*No.*	*%*	*Total*
'Nervous breakdown' reported by mother	0	–	0	–	0
Mother's 'malaise' score of 6 or more	3	20	1	5	4
'Broken home'	6	38**	0	–	6
Total no. of cases	16		20		36

***Difference between groups significant at 1 per cent level.*

Discussion

The finding that many variables were associated with psychiatric disorder in children with neuro-epileptic conditions makes it clear that psychiatric disorder can only rarely be viewed as a direct outcome of the brain abnormality. However, the associations with particular neurological features suggest that brain abnormalities play an important (although not exclusive) role in the development of the emotional and behavioural difficulties.

Although the extent of the physical handicap (as measured by the degree to which the child was impaired in his daily activities) was *not* associated with psychiatric disorder, the extent and activity of the brain lesion probably were important factors in the development of psychiatric disorder. This is suggested by the finding that psychiatric disorder was more frequent when there were bilateral neurological abnormalities than when the disorder was strictly unilateral. The relatively high rate of language retardation in the children with psychiatric disorder may also reflect the importance of bilateral brain dysfunction, since language is rarely affected by unilateral lesions which have occurred in early life. On the other hand, the association may also be important in its own right.

Speech and language defects have been mentioned by several writers (Floyer 1955, Gibbs 1958, Oswin 1967) as factors which are important in the pathogenesis of psychiatric disability in children with cerebral palsy. This is to be expected in that language plays a most important part in all aspects of development (Rutter 1969*b*).

Low intelligence and reading retardation were two of the variables most strongly associated with psychiatric disorder, and language is important for both intellectual and educational development. Intellectual processes which require symbolisation and abstraction are seriously impaired by a paucity of language (Lockyer and Rutter 1970). Language also aids the formation of concepts and the solving of problems (Luria 1957, Luria and Yudovich 1959, O'Connor and Hermelin 1963, Vygotsky 1962). A lack of language is associated with a poverty in the use of symbols and an impairment of logical thought. Reading is in large part a language skill and children who are retarded in their language development are also often retarded in reading (Rutter *et al.* 1970).

However, a specific intellectual defect of a verbal nature is not the only consequence of language failure. The use of language increases both the quantity and quality of interaction with other people and the child whose language is poor tends to have less contact with other children or adults and at a much more simple and crude level, without the richness of normal conversational interchange. Accordingly, the language retarded child not only has less opportunity for learning from other people but also his social and emotional development will be handicapped. The frequency of emotional and social difficulties in children with developmental language problems has often been noted (Ingram 1959*b*), although not systematically studied. In the present study there were only 9 children with a developmental language problem, but it was striking that 4 of these had a neurotic disorder. Speech and language difficulties are also important in the problems experienced by many deaf children in ordinary schools (Ministry of Education 1963), partly through the children's difficulties in joining in conversation and partly through the teasing brought about by a speech impediment.

Strabismus may also have been important through its tendency to lead to teasing. Personal oddities of this kind may impair a child's social acceptance, particularly if the child himself is self-conscious about the defect. Such factors in themselves are unlikely to lead to psychiatric disorder but they may be important as subsidiary causes which add to the child's difficulties and which, in the presence of other handicaps, may tip the balance.

Psychomotor epilepsy (defined in clinical terms rather than in terms of EEG findings) was strongly and significantly associated with a high rate of disorder, although the number of cases of this type of epilepsy was quite small. The result is in keeping with the systematic studies of temporal lobe epilepsy in children by Nuffield (1961) and Ounsted *et al.* (1966) as well as other less well controlled investigations, although there have also been some negative findings both in children (Wilson and Harris 1966) and in adults (Small *et al.* 1962, 1966). It is not possible to reconcile these differences entirely satisfactorily in view of substantial differences in definitions of cases and in determination of psychiatric disorder (see chapter 1), but it appears probable that psychomotor fits (but not necessarily temporal lobe spikes) are associated with a particularly high rate of psychiatric disorder.

Although the connections between the temporal lobe and rhinencephalic structures (important in motivation and effect) are well recognised, the actual mechanism of the association with psychiatric disorder is poorly understood. A neuro-physiological mechanism appears most likely, but states of partial consciousness may well be more psychologically threatening to a child than a total loss of consciousness. He may also encounter rejecting attitudes from those about him who have not recognised that he is unaware of what he is doing.

The elucidation of the neurophysiological components of the association between epilepsy and psychiatric disorder is hampered by the difficulties in the measurement of brain activity. The EEG provides at best a very crude measure of but a small segment of the brain's electrical activity. The relationship between the EEG and the other measures of neurological dysfunction has been found to be quite low in several independent studies (Paine *et al.* 1968, Schulman *et al.* 1965, Stevens *et al.* 1968). Furthermore, the interpretation of the EEG in children is complicated by the major changes associated with maturation (Gibbs *et al.* 1954, Pond 1963). The high rate of EEG abnormalities reported to be associated with psychiatric disorder in non-epileptic children (Stevens *et al.* 1968) may be in part a function of the delayed maturation of the children rather than a reflection of any structural brain pathology (Pond 1963). The very limited studies which have been carried out so far into the predictive value of the EEG in children with psychiatric disorder have shown it to be of little use (Pond 1951, Pond and Landucci 1954).

Although there is good evidence that epileptogenic lesions have behavioural and emotional effects over and above those found in overt fits (Pond 1961), very little is known about the physiology of the effect. The specific association of psychiatric disorder with psychomotor epilepsy provides a pointer to some of the possible mechanisms which may be involved, but the nature of the strong association between other sorts of epilepsy and psychiatric disorder may well be different.

The present study suggested that anticonvulsant medication played little part in the genesis of psychiatric disorder, although this negative finding may be related to the narrow range of drugs used with the Isle of Wight children. Most of the children were being treated with phenobarbitone which often makes epileptic children irritable. The dosage used was usually quite low and irritability was not the children's most prominent symptom, so that this drug effect was probably not very important. Interest in the possibly deleterious side-effects of anticonvulsant drugs has been revived by the recent finding that folic acid deficiency (which sometimes results from treatment with various antiepileptic drugs) may cause mental disturbances in the absence of megaloblastic anaemia (Gordon 1968, Reynolds 1968). The possible importance of this effect in the genesis of psychiatric disorder in epileptic children requires further study. However, the evidence to date suggests that folic acid deficiency is likely to be more relevant to the chronic deterioration seen in some severe epileptics than to the more everyday disorders seen in the children we studied.

Up to now, the factors discussed have been ones particularly associated with neuro-epileptic conditions and underline the finding (see chapter 12) that children with these conditions have a much increased rate of psychiatric disorder. The presence of organic brain dysfunction is associated with a high *susceptibility* to psychiatric disorder and this susceptibility must be taken into account in any plan of treatment for the child with psychiatric disorder. Nevertheless, the effect of brain dysfunction is largely to render the child more liable to react adversely to the stresses and strains which may impair the development of any child; many of the factors associated with the development of psychiatric disorder in the children with neuro-epileptic conditions were factors also important in the development of psychiatric disorder in other children.

Low intelligence was associated with psychiatric disorder in these children just as it was in children in the general population of the Isle of Wight (Rutter *et al.* 1970). This association was independent of social class differences and in the general population it applied across the whole range of IQ. Thus, it was *not* just an association with severe intellectual retardation; psychiatric disorder was more common in children of relatively lower IQ at all levels of intelligence. Psychiatric disorder generally has little effect on IQ so that the association cannot be explained in terms of a possibly depressing effect of emotional disorder on intellectual performance.

Why low IQ should be associated with psychiatric disorder is not known. It may be that temperamental attributes which tend to lead to psychiatric disorder are more frequent in the child of low IQ. Also, low IQ is associated with poor educational performance and scholastic failure may be more important in relation to the development of psychiatric disorder. Reading retardation was even more strongly associated with psychiatric disorder than was low IQ; a third of the epileptic children and two-thirds of the children with other brain conditions who had psychiatric disorder were at least two years retarded in reading. It appeared from an analysis of this association in children who did not have neuro-epileptic conditions that in some cases the behavioural difficulties (especially of an antisocial nature) may arise as a maladaptive response to educational failure (Rutter *et al.* 1970). The child who consistently fails in his school work and is thereby denied status and satisfaction, may rebel and seek satisfaction in antisocial activities which run counter to everything for which the school stands.

Social class was unrelated to psychiatric disorder in the general population and in children with a structural brain condition, but epileptic children whose fathers had a manual job were more likely to have psychiatric disorder. Whether or not this is a meaningful association can only be determined from further studies. In any investigation, some 'significant' associations are likely to arise by chance and this may be the explanation of this finding. On the other hand, social class may be important in epilepsy in a way that it is not in the general population. For example, if prejudices against epilepsy were stronger in the working class than in the middle class, this might lead to more working class epileptic children developing psychiatric disorder.

'Broken homes' and emotional disturbance in the mothers (as measured by the malaise inventory) were both associated with psychiatric disorder in neuro-epileptic children. There is a large literature on this association in children without neuro-epileptic conditions (Rutter 1966) and it seems likely that the same mechanisms are operative in children who do as in those who do not have organic brain conditions. Broken homes may have an adverse effect on a child's psychological development through the harmful consequences of a separation experience (Yarrow 1961, 1964) but in general it appears that the break-up of the home is usually less harmful than the preceding discord and tension.

Severe physical handicap or psychiatric disorder in a child may lead to emotional disturbance in a parent but also mental abnormalities in a parent may lead to psychiatric disorder in the children. In the case of the neuro-epileptic children, it is likely that the association is mainly accounted for by parental abnormalities leading to the children's emotional and behavioural difficulties. This is suggested by the finding that *across* diagnostic groups neither the severity of the child's physical handicap nor the presence of psychiatric disorder related to the frequency of parental pathology. Thus, children with intellectual retardation were the most handicapped of all groups but the average malaise scores of the mothers did not differ from the general population norms (see chapter 10). Similarly, although epileptic children had less physical handicap and less psychiatric disorder than children with other brain conditions, the mothers showed more emotional disturbance. A fifth of the mothers of epileptic children and none of the mothers of the children with cerebral palsy and similar conditions reported having a 'nervous breakdown'. Similarly, a third of the mothers of epileptic children had a score of 6 or more on the 'malaise inventory' compared with 1 in 9 of the mothers of children with other brain disorders.

The association between psychiatric disorder in the parent and in the child is probably due to many factors. In the epileptic group, the association may be mediated in part by the inheritance of electroencephalographic abnormalities. EEG abnormalities are more common in the relatives of epileptics than in the general population (Harvald 1954), and it is known that the rate of EEG abnormalities is increased in some types of personality disorder, perhaps because of maturation delays (Gibbens *et al.* 1959). To what extent EEG abnormalities and psychiatric disorder are found in the same relatives of epileptics is uncertain (Harvald 1954).

It is also clear that disorder in the child may often be due to the disturbed family relationships which are frequently (but far from always) associated with mental illness in parents. Where there is parental discord, tensions and quarrelling, the children run a much greater risk of developing psychiatric disorder (Craig and Glick 1965, McCord *et al.* 1959, Rutter 1970.) The type of home in which a child is reared has an important influence on his psychological development. This is true for the epileptic child or cerebral palsied child just as it is for any other child.

Psychiatric disorder in the child with a neuro-epileptic condition is multifactorially determined, with neurological features, intellectual and educational factors and socio-familial influences all playing a part in causation. The child with organic brain dysfunction has a much greater susceptibility to psychiatric disorder than other children in the general population. In addition, specifically neurological influences are to some extent responsible for the development of emotional and behavioural disorders. The factors associated with psychiatric disorder in the neuro-epileptic child, however, are largely the *same* as in other children and the mechanisms involved in the causation of disorder are probably similar.

CHAPTER 15

Conclusions

In the present state of knowledge, any study of neurological disorder in children is likely to raise more issues than it settles, and this study is no exception. Even at this stage, however, findings on the prevalence of different forms of handicap and on associations between them necessarily carry implications for the planning of services. Some of these implications will be considered here together with a few of the more urgent problems which require further research before the questions we have tackled can be answered.

Neurological Assessment

In common with almost all forms of clinical examination which have been studied, there are deficiencies in the reliability of some parts of the paediatric neurological examination, and some signs appear to have dubious validity. It is evident that clinicians should be cautious in diagnosing 'minimal cerebral dysfunction' on the basis of isolated slight abnormalities. Furthermore, deficiencies in the concept of 'minimal cerebral dysfunction' suggest the need to move from general categories of brain damage to the more detailed study and delineation of specific forms of brain dysfunction and disorder.

The lack of sophistication of some attempts by psychologists to develop global measures of 'brain damage' may owe much to their relative lack of collaboration with paediatric neurologists and developmental neurophysiologists. We have suggested that psychologists have an important role to play in the design and evaluation of standardised tests of developmental functions. If they are to do this successfully, psychologists working with children must have an adequate clinical training, which should include neurological as well as psychiatric practice. In this connection, as in others, the split between educational and clinical psychology is a hindrance; skills and training in both are required.

Equally, however, neurologists and paediatricians have much to learn from psychologists with respect to developmental evaluation. Many descriptions of the clinical assessment of, for example, motor co-ordination, speech or language in children suffer from a vagueness as to how the degree of impairment is to be judged in relation to the child's age. All too often criteria for abnormality are stated in terms of the 'average' age at which a child achieved some skill or the limits within which a delay *can* be normal. These are of very little help. What are needed are the range and spread as measured by standard deviations or percentile limits (Zdanska-Brincken and Wolanski 1969), together with the probability at any point that a finding indicates normality or pathology. In many cases these data are not yet available, particularly in the age-period after infancy. Further developmental studies of children aged three to five years would be valuable.

Prevalence of Neurological Disorder

Our estimates of the prevalence of cerebral palsy and epilepsy are not greatly different from those obtained from previous comprehensive general population studies. The knowledge on the epidemiology of these disorders, however, only serves to highlight our ignorance on the prevalence of other neurological or developmental disorders in childhood such as language retardation, severe clumsiness and perceptual disorders. Furthermore, our knowledge on the extent to which severe developmental delays are merely extreme variants of the normal, reflections of specific disorders in the maturation of certain parts of the brain, or consequences of some type of structural brain disease or damage is minimal. These are issues needing much further investigation.

Educational, Behavioural and Social Handicaps Accompanying Neuro-epileptic Disorder

The finding that children with a neuro-epileptic disorder have a one in three chance of having an additional psychiatric disability and an equal likelihood of intellectual or educational retardation makes it clear that paediatricians and neurologists dealing with such children need to have available considerable expertise on these related subjects. Our findings also show that the care of the child with a severe neuro-epileptic disorder (particularly if he is also intellectually retarded) can impose severe stresses on the family. To provide adequate medical care it is necessary to be well-informed on the child's family situation and social circumstances and to take all appropriate steps to provide suitable social and financial support for those looking after the child at home.

Training

The need for a broader training for the paediatrician and family doctor is becoming increasingly recognised. The establishment of courses in 'developmental paediatrics' is one sign of this trend (although we are unable to define an area which could reasonably be called *non*-developmental paediatrics). Now that there is effective treatment for so many acute illnesses, the problems of the chronically handicapped child are receiving more attention than in the past. Neurological disorders constitute a sizeable proportion of handicapping disorders in childhood and for this reason (as well as others) paediatricians in training require experience in paediatric neurology. In addition there is a need for far more systematic post-graduate training in child psychiatry and child psychology. Paediatricians in training will benefit from a period of attachment to a department of psychological medicine in order to gain insight into the scope and limitations of present day assessment and treatment of psychiatric and educational disorders. Without such a background he may well develop unreasonably high or low expectations of psychological treatment or he may miss the significance of handicapping emotional or behavioural symptoms present in his patients.

The obverse is just as true for the child psychiatrist in training, partly because of the frequency with which developmental problems are referred to psychiatric clinics and partly because of the importance of organic brain dysfunction in the pathogenesis of some psychiatric disorders. A period spent in a department of paediatric neurology could only be of benefit. Broadening the basis of training may well achieve more than the sharing of factual knowledge, highly important though this may be. Understanding the work of other disciplines should enable the trainee to appreciate the value of other approaches to his subject and so suggest alternative ways of tackling research problems or improvements in the provision of care and treatment.

The extent of school problems in physically handicapped children emphasises the need for hospital psychologists to have educational as well as clinical training. Both the educational and the clinical psychologists lack experience in developmental psychology, a deficiency most evident in the assessment of preschool children. In this country, there is no training in child psychology as such, and it is very evident that a course incorporating clinical, educational and developmental aspects of the subject should be provided.

Provision of Services

However broad his training, it is unlikely that the physician primarily concerned with the physical care of his patients will, or perhaps should, ever feel competent to deal with all aspects of the psychological and psychiatric care of his patients. He will need to have colleagues available to advise on emotional and learning problems if effective early treatment is to be provided. However, the argument for psychiatric and psychological services for neuro-epileptic children does not rest only on the curative efficacy of such services. Some of the psychological problems that arise in these children can be relieved by appropriate treatment but many, like many of the physical problems, are relatively intractable and not amenable to cure in the ordinary sense of the word. Nevertheless much can be done to alleviate suffering and to prevent the formation of secondary handicaps and this in itself is a worthwhile therapeutic goal.

If advice is to be translated into action, there will have to be improved communication between hospital departments, community services, doctors and schools. Many neuro-epileptic children have emotional, behavioural, and educational difficulties in the school situation. Yet all too often teachers know little about the conditions from which the children suffer and even less about the implications of medical findings for learning or behaviour in the classroom. It is important also for the doctor to be informed by the teacher what difficulties the children experience at school and if there are any effects of drugs on their performance. Schools need to be kept informed on the results of psychological testing carried out at hospital and teachers need to be able to turn to someone for advice about medical issues. All of this means that paediatricians and psychiatrists, too, should have close and effective links with schools. Perhaps the best way to achieve this is for the hospital consultant to spend some of his sessions with the local authority; this does occur in several local authorities, now including the Isle of Wight.

The mechanisms underlying the learning difficulties of many neuro-epileptic children are ill-understood, and advice to schools is necessarily limited by this. It is often impossible to determine whether the difficulties stem from interference by abnormal cortical activity or from impairment by short attention span (Ounsted 1968), from developmental disorders similar to those in specific reading retardation

(Rutter *et al.* 1970) or from the effects of drugs, either directly (Hutt *et al.* 1968) or indirectly via effects on folic acid metabolism (Reynolds 1968).

Assessment Centres

The multiplicity of handicaps in many children with neuro-epileptic disorder makes it highly likely that several specialists will be needed in the diagnostic evaluation and in the planning of treatment. The number of these children means that an expansion in services for them is needed. The specialised regional centre equipped to provide expert paediatric, neurological, psychiatric, psychological, audiological, opthalmological, speech and language assessment will have an important part to play in the study of children with developmental problems. The value of such centres is evident but it is also necessary to consider their limitations. It is obvious to everyone that children change as they grow older, but the implications of this are not always adequately taken into account in the planning of services. Because a child's neurological state alters with maturation, because hearing and vision may deteriorate or improve, because new psychological problems may emerge and others cease to handicap and also because assessments made in infancy may prove later to be mistaken, it is essential that the need for repeated assessment and re-evaluation be kept in mind by the doctor primarily responsible for continuing medical care. Although a team of specialists may be involved in different aspects of care, there must always be one individual who has the overall responsibility of integrating what is done and in seeing that fresh problems are not overlooked. This presents difficulties if that person is situated in some remote hospital centre (Whitmore 1969). He must function in the child's own community and have good liaison with community services.

The Intellectually Retarded Child

The problems of the child with severe intellectual retardation are considered more fully in relation to our other studies on the Isle of Wight (Rutter *et al.* 1970). Suffice it to say that a high proportion of severely retarded children have gross physical problems and prominent psychiatric disorders. Paediatricians, neurologists and psychiatrists all have a place in the assessment and care of these children. There is the same need for an ongoing assessment and for the alleviation of family problems (which are greatest of all in this group) as in the case of children with other neurological conditions.

The Association between Neuro-epileptic Disorder and Psychiatric Disability

The strong and important association between organic brain dysfunction and child psychiatric disorder and the resulting need for close collaboration between paediatricians and psychiatrists has been clearly shown by the present study. As psychiatric complications of neuro-epileptic disorders are affected by the extent and activity of the lesion and by the type of fit, psychiatrists must be able to evaluate neurological functions in relation to psychological development; to do this effectively, they must be suitably trained.

Similarly, the fact that there is no one 'brain-damage syndrome' but rather many different psychiatric disorders resulting from interaction between neurological dysfunction, family disturbance, and social circumstances means that paediatricians and neurologists must be aware of the complex nature of normal and abnormal psychological development and of the effects of parental illness and family discord.

The strength of the demonstrated association between neuro-epileptic disorder and psychiatric disability must not blind us, however, to the vast areas of ignorance still remaining on the nature of this association. Some of the most important questions outlined in the first chapter remain unanswered. Does the locus of the brain lesion influence the likelihood or the type of psychiatric disorder? To what extent are the psychiatric consequences affected by the child's age at the time of occurrence of the brain injury? How does the electrical activity of a brain lesion affect the development of psychiatric disorder? Is the nature of the brain pathology relevant in this context?

It appears that boys and girls with a neuro-epileptic condition are equally likely to develop psychiatric disorder. If this finding is confirmed in subsequent investigations, the question arises: why does the sex ratio differ from that for psychiatric disorder in the general population (where disorder is much more common in boys)?

It was found that the degree of physical handicap was not an important factor in the development of psychiatric disorder. This issue, too, requires further investigation in view of the small number of children with a severe handicap and yet normal intelligence. It may be that the factors leading to psychiatric disorder are different in the intelligent child with cerebral palsy. Our limited findings on the families of neuro-epileptic children showed that, as in any group of children, parental disturbances were associated with problems in the children; again, this is a matter requiring deeper exploration. We still know very little about which factors in the family influence the development of brain-injured children. Reading retardation was found to be strongly associated with psychiatric disorder, but the mechanisms underlying this association remain obscure. While it is known that physically handicapped children often experience social rejection, we know little about whether the likelihood of rejection differs with different forms of handicap, nor do we know the importance of this in the child's personality development.

These are but a few of the outstanding questions needing investigation with respect to the association between organic brain dysfunction and child psychiatric disorder. The question of whether brain injury increases the likelihood of psychiatric disorder has been clearly answered in the affirmative. While our findings have also rejected the behavioural stereotype of 'the brain-damaged child' they have emphasised the richness of this field of study and the value of the harvest still to be gathered.

One final point remains to be made. As we stated at the outset, we chose to clarify the issues by concentrating on a group of relatively well-defined neurological disorders about which quite a lot is known. We believe that our results have justified this strategy. However, our findings refer only to that small segment of the population with overt epilepsy, cerebral palsy or other discrete conditions. Others have used associations within this group to argue that beneath this tip lies the rest of the iceberg of brain damage which is not manifest in motor abnormalities or fits but which is still just as influential in distorting a child's development. Such ideas underlie, for example, Pasamanick and Knobloch's concept (1961) of a 'continuum of reproductive casualty'. Nelson (1968) has pointed out the weaknesses of this line in argument, but the question remains: to what extent is organic brain dysfunction a contributory factor in the pathogenesis of psychiatric disorder in children without fits or spasticity? Similarly the emotional problems of the child who is slow to speak have often been noted (Lewis 1963) but the importance of developmental delays in the pathogenesis of psychiatric disorder has yet to be determined. The collaboration of psychiatrists, psychologists and paediatric neurologists is needed to answer these questions, just as their co-operation is needed in the care of the neuro-epileptic child with multiple handicaps.

APPENDIX A

Brief Case Histories of Children with Neurological Disorders (other than Uncomplicated Epilepsy)

A. LESIONS BELOW THE BRAIN STEM

Poliomyelitis

1. *Male*—13 years. Poliomyelitis age 5 years with residual paralysis of left upper limb. Attends normal school.
2. *Female*—12 years. Febrile illness age 8 years associated with weakness and wasting of the right leg. Poliomeylitis diagnosed. Very slight residual weakness inversion and eversion of right ankle. Attends normal school.
3. *Female*—10 years. Poliomyelitis with paralysis of legs at age 3 years. Weakness, wasting, hypotonia and shortening of right leg. Wears orthopaedic boot. Attends normal school.
4. *Female*—14 years. Poliomyelitis with paralysis of both legs at age 18 months. Flail leg, amputated at 13 years. Some weakness and hyporeflexia in right leg. Attends normal school.
5. *Female*—9 years. Poliomyelitis age 6 months with residual weakness of left leg. Now normal power in all limbs except that left leg tires more easily after exertion. Hypotonia. Attends normal school.
6. *Male*—12 years. Poliomyelitis age 5 years with marked residual weakness and wasting of left leg. Attends normal school.
7. *Female*—11 years. Poliomyelitis aged 2 years with residual weakness of left arm and shoulder. Now only slight weakness and wasting, particularly of left deltoid. Attends normal school.

Muscular Dystrophy

8. *Male*—7 years. Facio-scapular-humeral muscular dystrophy diagnosed age 5 years. Winging of scapulae, very little movement of face or palate. Right ptosis. Attends normal school.
9. *Male*—10 years. Muscular dystrophy, Duchenne type, first noted at age 2 to 3 years. Attended spastics day unit since age 6 years. Now confined to a wheelchair. Generalised weakness, most marked proximally.
10. *Male*—9 years. Muscular dystrophy, Duchenne type, first noted at age 4 years. Now marked weakness in all four limbs. Confined to a wheelchair for last 6 months. Attends spastics day unit.
11. *Male*—13 years. Muscular dystrophy, Duchenne type. Onset in infancy. Marked wasting and weakness in all four limbs but most marked proximally. Confined to a wheelchair. Attends spastics day unit.
12. *Male*—14 years. Muscular dystrophy, Duchenne type. Onset about age 10 years. Apparently normal development in first 2 years and then regression with loss of speech. Now gross weakness and wasting in all four limbs but most marked in shoulder girdle. Confined to a wheelchair and has flexion deformity knees. Markedly retarded language development. Attends junior training centre.

Amyotonia Congenita

13. *Female*—6 years. Noticed to be very floppy in infancy. Amyotonia congenita diagnosed at age 2 years. Has not improved to any extent and now marked weakness and hypotonia in all four limbs. Reflexes all absent or greatly diminished. Attends normal school.

Spina Bifida

14. *Female*—8 years. Spina bifida. Marked flaccid weakness and wasting of left leg, for which she wears a support. Tendon transplant age 3 years. Attends normal school.

Syringomyelia

15. *Female*—13 years. Began to get back-ache associated with spinal scoliosis age 11 years, followed by loss of balance, weakness in legs, diplopia and difficulty in swallowing. Posterior column loss in legs. Hyporeflexia in arms and hyperreflexia in legs. Myelogram showed complete hold-up at T 12 and long cavitation of the cord extending from the lower dorsal region into the medulla. C.S.F. protein greatly raised. Syringomyelia diagnosed. Attends normal school.

Peripheral Nerve Palsy

16. *Female*—14 years. Erb's palsy partially corrected by tendon transplant age 8 years. Still has marked weakness of abduction and external rotation of left arm. Unable to straighten arm fully at elbow. Attends normal school.
17. *Male*—9 years. Psychomotor attacks began a year ago. Perthes' disease—caliper fitted eighteen months ago. In recent months found to have left sciatic nerve palsy due to pressure from caliper. Flexion and extension of foot very weak but just beginning to recover. Attends normal school.

Freidreich's Ataxia

18. *Female*—9 years. Freidreich's ataxia with some features of peroneal muscular atrophy. Onset age 4 years. Weakness in all limbs, most marked in lower limbs. High-stepping gait associated with posterior column deficit affecting lower limbs. Walks only with difficulty. Attends normal school.

Peroneal Muscular Atrophy

19. *Female*—14 years. Severely subnormal, an in-patient of mental subnormality hospital. Early history not known. Wasting of both forearms, both calves and the lowest third of both thighs. Minimal weakness. Upper limbs hypotonic and lower limbs hypertonic. Thought to have peroneal muscular atrophy.

B. SPINAL DEFICIT WITH ONLY DUBIOUS NEUROLOGICAL DEFECT

(*N.B. These two cases excluded from all analyses*)

20. *Female*—8 years. Multiple deformities. Imperforate anus, recto-vaginal fistula, hydronephrosis left kidney, absent right kidney and numerous vertebral deformities including spina bifida. Hyporeflexia but no definite neurological abnormality. Possible defect of pelvic nerves. Attends normal school.
21. *Male*—9 years. Spina bifida and hair lip—corrective operations for both soon after birth. Left leg shorter than right. Dubious mild degree of hydrocephalus and possible left extensor plantar response. However, no unequivocal neurological abnormality and child not examined in survey due to parental refusal.

C. CEREBRAL PALSY

Hemiplegia: Post-natal Cases

22. *Female*—8 years. Age 4 years fell out of a window, unconscious for three weeks followed by spastic quadriplegia which was most marked on the right, aphasia and double incontinence. Now right spastic hemiparesis with only very slight involvement of the left side, marked constructional apraxia and minimal language deficit. Fully continent. Attends spastics day unit.
23. *Male*—9 years. Encephalitis age 3 years followed by left hemiparesis, frequent major fits, and oculogyric crises. Normal intelligence but child kept at home by parents.
24. *Female*—9 years. Normal development until encephalitis age 6 years associated with epidural haematoma following head injury received during confused state. Followed by left spastic hemiparesis. Weakness now slight and confined to left hand but moderate apraxia. Attends normal school.
25. *Male*—11 years. Vaccinial encephalitis at 7 months with residual right hemiparesis. One major fit age 3 years. Now only very slight weakness but considerable dyspraxia right arm and leg. Attends special day school for educationally subnormal.

Hemiplegia: Congenital Cases

26. *Male*—10 years. Age 1 year noted not to be using right hand, found to be spastic. Marked weakness of right leg, and inco-ordination of fine finger movement in right hand. Bilateral extensor plantars. Operation to lengthen right tendo achilles age 7 years. Attends normal school.
27. *Male*—12 years. Birth weight 11 lb. Later noted that right arm and leg were shorter and smaller than left. Slight hypertonia on right but no weakness. Both plantars equivocal but right almost certainly extensor. Thought to have slight right hemiparesis. Attends normal school.
28. *Male*—13 years. Weakness of right hand noted at 6 months. Right spastic hemiplegia diagnosed at 9 months. Now has moderate weakness and slight spasticity of right arm and leg with mild dysarthria. Limps slightly. Attends normal school.
29. *Female*—8 years. Neonatal difficulties, in oxygen tent for 2 days. Delay in motor and language development. Very marked difficulties in co-ordination and in constructional tasks. Right facial palsy and right extensor plantar. Now normal level of language and speech. Attends normal school.
30. *Male*—13 years. Twin. Gait noted to be very abnormal about age 3 to 4 years. Found to have weakness and spasticity of left leg which was smaller than right. Weakness and spasticity now only slight with little in the way of handicap. Monoplegia. Attends normal school.
31. *Female*—11 years. Left spastic hemiparesis first noticed in infancy, weakness most marked in left hand. Major fits since age 6 years and psychomotor attacks since age 10 years. Attends normal school.
32. *Male*—12 years. Left spastic hemiparesis, first noticed in infancy. Weakness most marked in left leg. Some spasticity of right leg also. Major fits since age 10 years. Attends special day school for educationally subnormal.
33. *Male*—14 years. Cyanotic attacks in infancy. Left hemiparesis first noticed at 18 months. Spastic left hemiplegia with minimal signs on right. Spastic dysarthria. Major fits followed by transient paralysis of left side of face since age 6 years. EEG grossly abnormal with bilateral spikes and slow waves. Attends special day school for educationally subnormal.
34. *Male*—14 years. Development generally delayed. Marked general clumsiness. Spastic weakness left leg and to lesser extent left arm. Bilateral extensor plantars. Mild right hemiparesis. Attends special day school for educationally subnormal.

Diplegia

35. *Male*—10 years. Birth weight 3 lb. 4 oz. Spasticity diagnosed in infancy. Almost completely blind and quadriplegic but fair verbal skills. Weakness and spasticity much more marked in the lower limbs than in the upper limbs. Attends residential school for spastics.
36. *Female*—6 years. Some neonatal difficulties, did not cry properly and oxygen given for a while. Retardation of motor development and very floppy. Taken to hospital at age 2 years and diagnosed as benign congenital hypotonia. Now spastic quadriparesis more marked in the lower limbs, with bilateral extensor plantars. Clumsy, somewhat laboured gait. Mild spastic dysarthria and probably slightly retarded language development. Attends normal school.
37. *Female*—14 years. Twin. Considerable neonatal difficulties. Abnormality of gait noted when started to walk. Cerebral palsy diagnosed age 3 years. Some athetosis. Mild spastic quadriparesis with legs more affected than hands, but moderate difficulties in co-ordination of all four limbs. Mild spastic dysarthria. Attends normal school.
38. *Female*—12 years. First seen at hospital at age 4 years because kept falling; spasticity of lower limbs and bilateral extensor plantars noticed. Also language retardation. Slight hydrocephalus. Deprived child and early history not known. Age 11 years weakness of hip flexors and hypotonia also noticed. Normal knee jerks and absent ankle jerks but plantars remained extensor. Malnourished. Electromyogram showed no evidence of lower motor neurone lesion. Articulation defect. Attends special day school for educationally subnormal.
39. *Female*—10 years. Birth weight 2 lb. 13 oz., in oxygen tent for over a week. Almost completely blind, following retrolental fibroplasia. Spastic diplegia with now only slight weakness both legs. Major fits in last year. Attends junior training centre.

40. *Male*—12 years. Premature birth, one of 3 surviving children out of 10 pregnancies. Spastic diplegia first diagnosed age 3 years. Lengthening of tendo achilles at age 6 years. Clumsiness of upper limbs but spasticity and weakness confined to lower limbs. Attends normal school.
41. *Male*—7 years. Spasticity noted at 10 months. Now has gross spastic quadriplegia most marked in the legs, with spastic dysarthria. Near normal language development. Attends junior training centre.
42. *Female*—14 years. Motor development retarded. Spastic quadriplegia diagnosed at age 4 years. Some athetosis. Marked spasticity and slight weakness in all four limbs, but most marked in lower limbs. Marked spastic dysarthria. Attends spastic day unit.
43. *Male*—13 years. Spastic diplegia with marked athetosis first noticed at 10 months. Spastic dysarthria. Attends spastic day unit.
44. *Male*—12 years. Spastic quadriparesis, first noticed at age 18 months. Development generally delayed. Minor epileptic attacks since age 3 years. Now only mild weakness and hypertonia in all four limbs, slightly more marked in lower limbs. Articulation defect. Attends special day school for educationally subnormal.
45. *Male*—5 years. Mild spastic diplegia, most marked on the right. Major fits since age 3 years. Attends spastic day unit.
46. *Male*—11 years. Premature baby, birth weight 4 lb. Spastic weakness in both legs noted age 2 years. Spastic diplegia. Moderate weakness in both legs with only minimal clumsiness in hands. Attends spastics day unit.

Bilateral Hemiplegia

47. *Female*—11 years. All aspects of development grossly delayed. Spastic quadriplegia equally marked in all four limbs. First noted age 2 years. No speech. Unable to walk. Attends junior training centre.
48. *Female*—8 years. Spastic quadriparesis first diagnosed at 1 year. Now hypertonic but probably only slight weakness. Gross retardation of all aspects of development. Virtually no speech. In-patient of mental subnormality hospital.
49. *Female*—7 years. Birth weight 4 lb. In oxygen tent for 2 weeks. Partially blind due to retrolental fibroplasia. Gross spastic quadriplegia. No speech. Major fits, also petit mal attacks in past. In-patient mental subnormality hospital.
50. *Female*—12 years. Cyanotic attacks and feeding difficulties in neonatal period. Cerebral palsy diagnosed. Major fits between 1 and 9 years. These started as focal attacks involving left arm and followed by a Todd's paralysis of left arm. Generally very clumsy and marked constructional difficulties. Little useful speech. Mild spastic quadriparesis. Attends junior training centre.
51. *Male*—10 years. Cerebral palsy noted in infancy. General delay in development. Moderate spastic quadriparesis. No speech. Frequent major and minor fits. In-patient mental subnormality hospital since age 5 years.
52. *Male*—8 years. Convulsions in infancy. Cerebral palsy noted soon after birth. Now has athetosis and spastic quadriparesis. Marked constructional difficulties. Spastic dysarthria. Attends spastic day unit.
53. *Female*—11 years. Marked neonatal difficulties. Frequent convulsions from early infancy. Spasticity noted at 1 year. Gross spastic quadriplegia with very frequent major and minor fits. Little useful speech. Child at home.
54. *Female*—7 years. Microcephaly. Toxoplasmosis, diagnosed in infancy. Blind due to bilateral optic atrophy and choroido-retinal degeneration. Spastic quadriplegia. No speech. In-patient mental subnormality hospital.

Dyskinesia

55. *Male*—14 years. Abnormal movements first noted in infancy. Diagnosed as spastic at 18 months. Still falling frequently age 3 years. Motor development much delayed. Now generally clumsy with marked generalised choreo-athetoid movements. Hypotonia and diminished reflexes. Attends normal school.

Ataxia

56. *Male*—8 years. Major fits in early childhood, still on anticonvulsants. Gross retardation of all aspects of development, first diagnosed in infancy. Mild degree of hydrocephalus. Markedly ataxic. Minimal weakness in all four limbs. Very gross generalised hypotonia with increased tendon reflexes and bilateral extensor plantar reflexes. In-patient of mental subnormality hospital.

D. OTHER BRAIN DISORDERS

Craniostenosis

57. *Male*—12 years. Major fits and delayed development in early childhood. Papilloedema noted age 4 years and craniotomy performed for craniostenosis. Psychomotor attacks since age 5 years. Generalised clumsiness. Articulation defect. Very marked choreiform movements and mirror movements. Attends special day school for educationally subnormal.

Galactosaemia

58. *Female*—14 years. Galactosaemia. Gross constructional dyspraxia. Tremulous and generally clumsy. Gross disorder of articulation. Equivocal plantar responses. Has had operation for bilateral cataracts. Psychomotor epilepsy. Attends special day school for educationally subnormal.

Cerebral Lipoidosis

59. *Male*—6 years. Cerebral lipoidosis, onset age 4 years. Now in moribund state in mental subnormality hospital. Myoclonic status epilepticus.

Hydrocephalus

60. *Male*—7 years. Neonatal difficulties. Asphyxia. Said not to cry for 24 hours after birth. Convulsions in infancy. Did not walk until nearly 3 years. Strabismus. Mild hydrocephalus. Reflexes somewhat diminished but equivocal left plantar and extensor right plantar. Poor gait. Major fits age 3 years which began as a right sided focal fit. Attends normal school.
61. *Male*—6 years. Hydrocephalus. Development generally delayed. No speech. Ataxic; completely helpless. Marked hypotonia and weakness all four limbs. In-patient mental subnormality hospital.

Other

62. *Female*—11 years. Cerebral palsy noted in infancy at time when having recurrent convulsions. Odd facies. Small skull. Gross general clumsiness and constructional difficulties. No useful speech. Hypotonia and weakness all four limbs but slight hyperreflexia. Attends junior training centre.
63. *Male*—10 years. Delayed in motor and language development. Continued to be markedly clumsy. Attended ordinary school. Age 8 years diagnosed as mild cerebral palsy. Transferred to spastics day unit, largely because of extreme distractibility. Large asymmetrical head. Bilateral convergent strabismus and inco-ordinate eye movements. Some impairment of fine finger movements and gross impairment of co-ordination in lower limbs. Hypotonia and slight weakness in all four limbs.
64. *Male*—8 years. Abnormal posture and gait noted when started to walk. Wears out the toes of both shoes. Marked clumsiness in upper and lower limbs. Generalised hyperreflexia. Onset of major fits shortly after survey. Attends normal school.
65. *Female*—7 years. Motor development retarded from the start. First referred to hospital at 3 years. Did not talk until 3½ to 4 years of age. Odd shaped head with small low forehead. Marked clumsiness in relation to fine and gross movement. Unable to throw or catch a ball properly. Gross constructional difficulties. Considerable retardation of language with marked articulation defect. Hypotonia in upper limbs. Equivocal plantar responses. Attends normal school.

66. *Female*—14 years. Some general delay in development but particularly affecting language. Now gross constructional difficulties. Possible astereognosis. Clumsiness of fine finger movements. Marked language retardation and slight articulation defect. Equivocal left plantar response and right extensor plantar. Attends junior training centre.
67. *Female*—13 years. Major fits in early childhood. None for several years but still on anticonvulsants. General delay in development from infancy. No speech. Asymmetry of face. Marked abnormality of gait—walks with left foot inverted. Slightly increased reflexes in both legs and bilateral extensor plantars. In-patient mental subnormality hospital.
68. *Male*—11 years. Moderate neonatal difficulties. Development generally delayed. Generally very clumsy. Marked constructional difficulties. Marked articulation defect and considerable language retardation. Hypertonia in all limbs and hyperreflexia in lower limbs. Attends junior training centre.
69. *Male*—12 years. Moderate neonatal difficulties. General delay of development. Onset of major fits age 6 years. No fits for several years but still on anti-convulsants. No speech. General hyperreflexia. Right plantar equivocal and left extensor. Wave and spike focus in left Sylvian region on EEG. In-patient mental subnormality hospital.
70. *Female*—6 years. Minor fits since age 4 years. Strabismus. Facial asymmetry. Slight hypertonia in both lower limbs but no weakness and normal reflexes. Bilateral extensor plantar responses. Attends normal school.
71. *Male*—9 years. First seen at 5 months because eyes thought not to fixate. Generally delayed language development. First words at 4 to 5 years. First phrases at about 6 to 7 years. Comprehension very limited in early childhood. Language still markedly retarded. Moderate articulation defect. Major fits between 3 and 6 years of age. Autistic. Attends special day school for educationally subnormal.
72. *Female*—9 years. Epicanthic folds. Generalised hypotonia. Constructional dyspraxia. Articulation defect and severely retarded language development. Skin biopsy reported as showing chromatin configuration of male type. Low serum calcium. Attends junior training centre.
73. *Male* 5 years. Major fits since infancy. Moderate delay of general development. Hypertelorism Strabismus. Gross constructional difficulties. Marked general clumsiness. Equivocal plantar responses. Mild language retardation and articulation defect. Attends normal school.
74. *Female*—9 years. Moderate delay in language development. Major fits in last year. Gross constructional apraxia. Generally clumsy. Marked articulation defect. Equivocal plantar responses. Attends special day school for educationally subnormal.
75. *Male*—11 years. Early history not known except that had multiple eye operations. Gross clumsiness and gross constructional difficulties. Moderate language retardation and marked articulation defect. Vision severely impaired. Microcephaly. Attends junior training centre.
76. *Male*—14 years. General delay of development. Cerebral palsy first diagnosed age 5 years. Then had spastic lower limbs and athetosis. Now no speech and gross general clumsiness. Tends to drag feet when walking and has eversion of right foot. In-patient mental subnormality hospital.

E. SEVERE MENTAL SUBNORMALITY

Mongolism

77. *Female*—13 years. Mongol. Extreme hyporeflexia. Almost blind from lens opacities and also uveitis. Living at home.
78. *Female*—7 years. Mongol. Blind due to bilateral lens opacities. Marked hypotonia. In-patient mental subnormality hospital.
79. *Female*—5 years. Born 8 weeks before term, weight not known. Noted to be profoundly deaf at 12 months. Deafness confirmed at 2 years. Development generally delayed. Now slightly clumsy and without speech. Many psychotic features. Attends junior training centre.
80. *Female*—10 years. Mongol. Slight hypotonia and moderate constructional difficulties. Attends special day school for educationally subnormal.
81. *Female*—5 years. Mongol. Marked hypotonia. Generally very clumsy. Strabismus. Attends junior training centre.

82. *Female*—5 years. Mongol. Marked hypotonia. General clumsiness and probably slight weakness of both legs. Attends junior training centre.
83. *Female*—11 years. Mongol. Hypotonia, some clumsiness and possibly slight weakness of all limbs. Marked constructional difficulties. Attends special day school for educationally subnormal.
84. *Female*—7 years. Mongol. Marked hypotonia. In-patient mental subnormality hospital.
85. *Male*—7 years. Mongol. Very gross hypotonia, marked clumsiness and constructional difficulties. Possibly some weakness in lower limbs. Attends special day school for educationally subnormal.
86. *Male*—14 years. Mongol. Hypotonia, nystagmus and constructional dyspraxia. Attends junior training centre.
87. *Female*—7 years. Mongol. Slight hypotonia. Marked constructional difficulties. Fallot's tetralogy with congestive cardiac failure. Child at home.
88. *Female*—10 years. Mongol. Moderate hypotonia. Marked nystagmus with generally jerky and inco-ordinate eye movements. Strabismus. Generally clumsy. Moderate constructional difficulties. Attends junior training centre.
89. *Female*—9 years. Mongol. Coarse pendular nystagmus. Slight hypotonia. Clumsy. In-patient mental subnormality hospital.

Other

90. *Male*—5 years. Birth weight 2 lb. 12 oz. Development generally delayed. Said to have spasticity in lower limbs at an earlier examination, but this not found on survey examination. Severely subnormal child without speech. Attends junior training centre.
91. *Female*—9 years. Infantile spasms up to age 2 years. Major fits since age 4 years, and petit mal since age 9 years. Severely subnormal. In-patient mental subnormality hospital.
92. *Female*—8 years. Microcephaly. Generally very clumsy and marked constructional difficulties. Markedly retarded language development. Attends junior training centre.
93. *Male*—7 years. Normal development until age 4 years when developed mild febrile illness followed by convulsions lasting 1 hour and stuporose state for 2 to 3 days. Severe regression in behaviour with incontinence and loss of speech associated with destructive and hyperactive behaviour. Gradual improvement since. Now echolalia and slight retardation of language. Shoe tips unevenly worn, with severe wear outer tip left shoe but no detectable abnormality on formal neurological examination. Psychotic. Attends junior training centre.
94. *Female*—5 years. Generally delayed development. Severely subnormal and psychotic. No speech. In-patient mental subnormality hospital.

Also cerebral palsy cases 39, 41, 47, 48, 49, 50, 51, 53, 54 and 56; other brain disorder cases 59, 61, 62, 66, 67, 68, 69, 72, 75 and 76; lesion below the brain stem cases 12 and 19.

F. BLINDNESS

Retrolental Fibroplasia

95. *Female*—13 years. Almost totally blind following retrolental fibroplasia. Birth weight 3 lb. 12 oz. In oxygen tent for 2 weeks. Attends residential school for the blind.

Also cerebral palsy cases 35, 39 and 49

Lens Opacities

96. *Female*—6 years. Partially blind due to congenital cataract first diagnosed at 4 months. Attends residential school for the blind.
97. *Female*—13 years. Bilateral congenital cataract diagnosed age 1 year. Multiple operations age 7 years. Now partially blind and attends residential school for the blind.

Also severe mental subnormality cases 77 and 78; other brain disorder case 58.

Optic Atrophy

98. *Male*—12 years. Craniopharyngioma treated with irradiation at age 4 years. Now has optic

atrophy but no other neurological abnormality. Almost completely blind and attends residential school for the blind.

99. *Female*—13 years. Partially blind because of hereditary optic atrophy. First noted at age 1 year. Attends residential school for the blind.
Also cerebral palsy case 54; other brain disorder case 59.

Congenital Glaucoma

100. *Male*—15 years. Almost completely blind due to bilateral congenital glaucoma. Attends residential school for the blind.

Other

Other brain disorder case 75.

G. DEAFNESS

Nerve Deafness

101. *Male*—12 years. Severe congenital nerve deafness. Attends residential school for the deaf.
102. *Male*—7 years. High frequency deafness first noted at 2½ years. Wears hearing aid. Attends normal school.
103. *Female*—6 years. Premature birth. Some general retardation of development. Moderately severe perceptive deafness most marked in high frequencies. Wears hearing aid. Attends normal school.
104. *Male*—15 years. Partially deaf with possible additional central defect in comprehension of language. Moderate language retardation with marked articulation defect. Wears hearing aid and attends normal school.
105. *Female*—5 years. Partial nerve deafness. Little speech until age 4 years but now only slight language retardation with mild articulation defect. Wears hearing aid and attends normal school.
106. *Male*—10 years. Bilateral high tone deafness first noted about age 4 years. Mother and sister have similar disability. Wears hearing aid. Now has normal language ability but very mild articulation defect. Attends normal school.
107. *Male*—12 years. Deafness queried by parents in infancy but not diagnosed until age 5 years. Nerve deafness. Wears hearing aid but also lip reads. Normal speech and language. Attends normal school.
Also severe mental subnormality case 79.

Conductive Deafness

108. *Male*—14 years. Partial conductive deafness following recurrent otitis media. Wears hearing aid. Attends normal school.
109. *Female*—Partial conductive deafness following recurrent otitis media. Wears hearing aid. Attends normal school.
110. *Female*—14 years. Partial conductive deafness. Wears hearing aid. Attends normal school.
111. *Female*—10 years. Recurrent otitis media in early childhood. Deafness first diagnosed at age 6 years. Wears hearing aid and attends ordinary school. Normal speech and language.
112. *Male*—12 years. Noted to be partially deaf about age 9 years. Conductive deafness. Wears hearing aid but hearing improving and now gradually discontinuing its use. Normal speech and language. Attends normal school.

Mixed Deafness

113. *Male*—8 years. No speech until 3 years. Several middle ear infections with residual drum perforation. Partial deafness first noted at age 5 years. Mixed perceptive and conductive deafness diagnosed. Wore hearing aid. Also had speech therapy from age 6 years. Now has normal or near normal language but mild articulation defect. Hearing now much improved and has just discontinued hearing aid.

114. *Male*—9 years. First words about 4 years, not speaking in sentences until age 6 or 7 years. Language development still markedly retarded. Mild articulation defect. Attends normal school. Strong family history of speech delay.
115. *Male*—9 years. First words about age 2½ years and no phrased speech until some time later (exact age not known). Now only slight language retardation but very gross articulation defect so that most speech quite incomprehensible. Poor co-ordination of fine finger movements. Attends special day school for educationally subnormal.
116. *Male*—6 years. First words age 5 years. Still moderate language retardation with articulation defect. Some constructional difficulties. Attends normal school.
117. *Male*—7 years. Severe language retardation. Speaks only in single words or very short phrases. Echolalia. Attends normal school.
118. *Male*—8 years. Marked retardation and moderate general clumsiness with severe constructional difficulties. Somewhat odd appearance. Attends special day school for educationally subnormal.
119. *Male*—9 years. Did not walk until 3 years and did not talk until 4 years. Generally clumsy, especially fine finger movements. Grossly retarded language development and gross articulation defect. Very dubious minimal weakness in right leg with doubtful increase in reflexes and equivocal plantar responses.
120. *Male*—7 years. Up to 3 or 4 years seemed not to understand anything said to him. First words about age 5 years. Now language greatly retarded and talks only at home. Anxious and socially withdrawn. Attends special day school for educationally subnormal.
121. *Male*—5 years. Started saying words about age 3 years but sentences only in last year. Now only moderate retardation of language, but very gross articulation defect so that speech almost incomprehensible. Attends normal school.
122. *Female*—5 years. Repaired cleft palate with residual palatal element to speech. In addition, some delay in language development. Now language probably only very slightly retarded but very gross articulation defect so that most of speech almost entirely incomprehensible. Misses off beginnings and ends of most words. Attends normal school.

APPENDIX B

Brief Case Histories of Children with Minor Fits

Psychomotor Fits

(a) *Male*—14 years. Major fits from 18 months to $4\frac{1}{2}$ years. Since 5 years has had attacks in which he screams at night, then lies unconscious with his eyes open, usually having wet himself. No convulsions, still having attacks of this kind. Also episodes in which he goes tense, clenches his hands, looks distant and then attacks someone, throws something or behaves oddly. No memory of these episodes. On regular anticonvulsants until 1 year ago.

(b) *Female*—14 years. Major fits from 3 years to 7 years. Since 6 years has had attacks in which she has headache and dizziness, appears blank, and is unable to answer for a few minutes; occasionally she falls down. These occur about once every 2 months. On regular anticonvulsants. EEGs have shown high voltage atypical spike and wave.

(c) *Male*—9 years. Fits began one year ago and has had 7 fits since then. During the fit he stares ahead and remains motionless with his eyes open, very occasionally falling. He remains in this state for anything from 1 to 30 minutes. On recovery he is unsteady and feels peculiar for a few minutes. On regular phenobarbitone.

(d) *Female*—11 years. Fits began one year ago and has had 3 fits since then. The fit starts with headache and then a feeling of pins and needles, spreading up the right arm from the fingers. She vomits and sweats, becomes confused and then sleeps for several hours. In one fit she had a prolonged period in which she behaved oddly and appeared confused, disoriented, and to a considerable extent unaware of her surroundings.

(e) *Male*—13 years. Major fits and petit mal since age 7 years. In the last few months began to have a different sort of attack in which he feels peculiar and partially loses touch with his surroundings. He looks odd and doesn't seem to know what he is doing; he wanders about in a semi-automatic way for periods of some minutes up to 2-3 hours. Several EEGs have shown bilateral high voltage slow waves with some spikes together with a spike focus in the left (and sometimes the right) mid-temporal regions. On regular primidone, phenytoin sodium and ethosuximide.

(f) *Male*—8 years. Fits started at age 18 months. These now consist of jerking movements of his shoulders and grunting noises. He is unaware of his surroundings for several minutes and is sleepy afterwards. Attacks occur once every few days. Was previously on phenobarbitone but his mother stopped this a year ago.

(g) *Female*—10 years. Major fits began when child aged 8 years. Shortly afterwards began also to have attacks in which she would complain of feeling unwell and then lose touch with her surroundings, remaining unresponsive and staring for 20-30 minutes during which time she clenched and unclenched her hands. On regular phenobarbitone.

(h) *Male*—11 years. In the last 3 years has had attacks in which he feels dizzy, has headache and is then unable to swallow or speak for 1 to 15 minutes. He stands with saliva running from his mouth but does not fall. On regular phenobarbitone. An EEG showed a persistent right anterior temporal focus.

(i) *Male*—12 years (case 57). Craniostenosis, 4 or 5 convulsions at 1 to 4 years. Age 5 years began to have attacks which begin with his gasping and swallowing repeatedly, looking very frightened, and are followed by a period of several minutes in which he is partially unaware and is unable to talk. These occur about twice a year. Not on anticonvulsants. An EEG showed a mild generalised abnormality with some paroxysmal features in both tempero-occipital regions, the right more than the left.

(j) *Female*—11 years (case 31). Left hemiplegia. Two major fits at 18 months and 4½ years. Since 4½ years also had other attacks in which she looks vacant and distracted, complains of headache, keeps touching her neck, goes pale, loses touch with her surroundings for about 10 minutes; usually cries afterwards. On regular phenobarbitone.

(k) *Female*—15 years (case 58). Galactosaemia. Fits started 18 months ago. In the fit she gulps, does not speak, appears dazed and either stands still or walks about not knowing what she is doing for 1 to 15 minutes. On regular phenobarbitone and phenytoin sodium. Had 6 to 8 attacks in last year.

Myoclonic Fits

(l) *Female*—13 years. Major fits began at 3 years; 3 fits in last year. Premature birth. Feeding difficulties and episodes of jerking in infancy. Delayed motor milestones. Age 5 years began to have, in addition, a different sort of attack in which she would jerk suddenly and violently (often falling off a chair) and go blank momentarily. These attacks occur several times per day. Age 8 years one left-sided Jacksonian attack. More recently began to have blank spells lasting only a few seconds which are sometimes accompanied by a slight jerk at the outset. These start and end suddenly and are not accompanied by falling. The EEG showed paroxysmal disturbance sometimes confined to the right side. Taking primidone, phenytoin sodium and troxidone.

(m) *Female*—9 years. Major fits since 5 years; fits now about twice a year. A few months after onset of major fits began also to have attacks in which her head jerks violently and her left arm shoots out, her eyes roll upwards and she loses contact with her surroundings for a few moments. Until last few months these attacks occurred nearly daily. Also true petit mal attacks. Taking regular phenobarbitone and phenytoin sodium.

(n) *Male*—10 years. Convulsions as a baby. In last 3 years has had about 6 attacks in which he jerks back violently and falls to the ground. Sometimes he loses consciousness and goes limp, but only momentarily. On regular phenobarbitone.

(o) *Male*—6 years (case 59). Cerebral lipoidosis. Fits in which he goes rigid and arches his back. For some months he has been in more or less continuous status with constant myoclonic jerks and partial consciousness. On regular phenobarbitone and ethosuximide.

(p) *Male*—9 years (case 23). Hemiplegia and fits following encephalitis at 3 years. Fits consist of vertical oculogyric crises associated with sudden upward extension of the arms. These still occur very frequently and 2 years ago he was having fits up to 10 times daily with periods of minor status involving fluctuating consciousness, incontinence and unsteadiness. EEGs have shown a gross generalised abnormality maximal in the posterior two thirds of the right hemisphere. On regular phenobarbitone and phenytoin sodium.

'Salaam' Fits and Infantile Spasms

(q) *Female*—7 years. Fits started at 3 months; last fit 3 years ago but still on regular phenobarbitone and phenytoin sodium. Fit begins by child suddenly falling down, folding at the waist with the right arm coming up. This lasts less than a minute and child carries straight on afterwards. Used to occur 2-3 times per day at one time. Attends normal school.

(r) *Female*—9 years (case 91). As an infant, attacks once or twice per day in which her eyes rolled up and her head flexed suddenly and forcibly. These stopped at age 2 years. Age 4-5 years several major fits. At age 8 years an EEG showed irregular slow activity with spikes and sharp waves; sudden noises invoked K complexes. A few months ago began to have blank spells. Child now very hyperkinetic and severely subnormal. On regular phenobarbitone.

Focal Motor Fits

(s) *Male*—9 years. Only 1 fit a year ago. Took regular phenobarbitone for 3 months subsequently. Fit started by boy feeling peculiar, sat down, slumped unconscious for a few moments with some frothing at the mouth. Left hand and forearm weak and limp for 15 to 20 minutes after regaining consciousness.

(t) *Female*—9 years. Since 18 months had attacks which start with headache and then tingling in the tongue followed by twitching of the right side of the mouth and then the right side of the face, right arm and leg; she is unable to talk and is frightened but does not lose consciousness. The whole attack lasts up to 1½ hours and she is weak in her right arm and leg for some 2 hours afterwards. Last attack 2 years ago but still on regular phenobarbitone. An EEG showed high voltage spike and irregular slow wave disturbance with paroxysmal features more marked on the left.

(u) *Male*—13 years. Fits from age 6 years to 8 years and again at 11 years; still on regular phenobarbitone. Fits began with clonic movements of the left hand which spread to the left side of the face. Sometimes his eyes rolled up and his legs folded from beneath him but he never completely lost consciousness for more than a few minutes. Following the attack (which lasted altogether up to 40 minutes) his left hand was generally weak for about 30 minutes. (*Also* case (1)).

Undifferentiated Minor Fits

(v) *Female*—10 years. Fits started at 7 years; now having about 1 fit per year. Fit starts by child falling to ground with jaw clenched but not otherwise stiff. Unconscious for 1 to 5 minutes. On recovery often nauseated and usually sleepy for several hours. Taking regular phenobarbitone.

(w) *Male*—7 years. Since age 5 years had fits in which he falls and partially loses consciousness but does not have convulsions. The attacks last a few minutes. Taking regular phenobarbitone.

(x) *Female*—9 years. Major fits began at 3 years. These are entirely nocturnal. About 6 months after they began she also started to have attacks in which she would feel peculiar and then fall to the ground, remaining unconscious for about 1 minute. Afterwards she remains quiet for about ½ hour. In addition there are episodes in which she complains of headache and nausea in the evening. After sleeping for a while she gets up and wanders around talking irrelevant nonsense; she is unresponsive to the environment. On recovering she is confused and sleepy. It is uncertain whether these are psychomotor fits or non-epileptic somnambulism. Until recently she took phenobarbitone regularly.

(y) *Male*—10 years. In the last year he developed momentary blank spells in which he had a lapse of consciousness but did not fall. In addition has had attacks in which he loses consciousness (for about 1 minute) and falls to the ground. There are no convulsions. On regular phenobarbitone and troxidone.

(z) *Male*—12 years. Fits since age 2 years in which he feels unwell and then loses consciousness and falls. He remains unconscious for about a minute but does not convulse. Two months ago also had one major fit. On regular phenobarbitone. Ventricular septal defect, very small stature and various other congenital anomalies. Articulation defect, hyperreflexia and constructional dyspraxia.

(aa) *Female*—11 years. Since age 2 years has had attacks in which she feels dizzy and falls down unconscious for 4 or 5 minutes. Sometimes vomits afterwards and always feels sleepy for several hours. On one occasion felt stiff down one side. On phenobarbitone which she takes irregularly.

(bb) *Male*—10 years. From 18 months has had attacks in which he falls and loses consciousness for a few minutes but does not convulse. Also had 2 major fits. On regular phenobarbitone.

(cc) *Female*—12 years. Since 3 months of age has had attacks in which she goes stiff, loses awareness for several seconds and occasionally falls but does not convulse. These now occur about once per week but at age 5 years she was sometimes having 30 per day. Also 1 to 4 major fits every day since age 7 years. On phenobarbitone and phenytoin sodium (previously on primidone). Bilateral hemiplegia.

(dd) *Male*—12 years (case 44). Diplegic. Onset of fits age 3 years. In attack falls to the ground and goes limp and pale. When younger he used to lose consciousness but now he is usually just dazed. Always goes to sleep after fit. Last fit 18 months ago. Previously on primidone but now taking phenobarbitone and phenytoin sodium.

(ee) *Male*—10 years (case 51). Bilateral hemiplegia. Major fits since infancy; now has them about once per month. In recent years has also had minor attacks in which he falls and goes limp but does not always lose consciousness and does not have convulsions. On regular phenobarbitone, primidone and troxidone.

(ff) *Female*—7 years (case 70). Fits since age 4 years. Fit begins by her not being able to see properly, feeling nauseated and occasionally vomiting. She then falls to the ground and remains unconscious for 2 to 30 minutes. Afterwards she is drowsy and usually sleeps for several hours. 7 fits in the last year. Not on anticonvulsants.

APPENDIX C

A Manual of Instructions for the Short Form of the Oseretsky Test of Motor Proficiency

From Sloan's 1955 revision of the Oseretsky Test, 12 items were selected which would discriminate in the age range 9-11 years and which required as little equipment as possible. After the items had been piloted on children on the mainland, ambiguities in both the instructions and the scoring systems were removed. During the Isle of Wight Study, examiners were required to collect more details of the child's performance than were absolutely necessary to get a simple raw score. On analysis of this extra information, it was decided that the scoring criteria given by Sloan were still appropriate for this shortened version.

General Instructions

Preferred Limb

In certain of the sub-tests the preferred hand or foot is treated differently from the other. We shall define 'preferred' as that hand or foot which the subject (S) spontaneously uses for the first trial. In all cases, the examiner (E) must record on the test proforma which limb S elected to use.

There is a possibility that E's demonstration may suggest to S which limb to start off with, but it is more likely that S will perform the task in the more natural way without thinking.

Comprehension

This test is primarily one of motor proficiency, not of intelligence. It is therefore important to minimise the influence of verbal comprehension on S's performance of each task. Anything that can be done to assist S in understanding the task is permissible. E must always demonstrate the required performance and he should be appropriately dressed for this purpose. Where S finds difficulty in performing the task, E should go through the motion in pantomime or use more extensive verbal description, to help S to understand the task required. Where S's first attempt at a task is not correct because of obvious lack of understanding, the item is repeated without penalising S's score. For example, in Item 8, S is required to catch a ball in one hand. If S uses both hands, he should be corrected by E. This trial would not count as one of the five for the hand in question.

Test Order

Test items are arranged in approximate order of difficulty and should be administered in the order presented. E must be thoroughly familiar with the test materials, directions and, especially, the scoring criteria and recording sheet.

Fatigue

Every effort should be made to minimise the influence of fatigue. Adequate rest periods should be allowed and, whenever S shows signs of becoming tired, an additional rest should be given.

Safety

E must guard against S's accidentally hurting himself during any of the tests, particularly where S has to stand on one limb or do things with his eyes closed. E should place himself in such a position that he may be able to catch S in the event of a fall. S should not be tested in his stockinged feet.

Encouragement

Throughout all the tests S must be encouraged to give of his best. This is particularly important in dealing with intellectually retarded children, and in those sub-tests in which speed of performance is critical. S should be exhorted to perform as quickly as possible in Items 5, 7, 9, 10, 11 and 12.

Comfort

E must ensure that S is seated comfortably at the table for performing the finer motor co-ordination tasks. To do this an adequate supply of cushions must be available to adjust the height of the child at the table, so that he can write in a natural, comfortable position.

Scoring and Recording

Our detailed scoring and recording procedures for each item of the scale are given with the instructions for administering the scale. Where an item is failed, we require information on the reasons for failure. Examiners who are familiar with other versions of this battery should note the changes in the administration and scoring of the test and be especially vigilant in following the revised criteria.

The scoring criteria for pass and fail have been made as explicit as possible for each item. When E must judge 'body movement' this usually refers to shifting of the feet from their original position on the floor.

1. WALKING BACKWARDS

Equipment: None.
Number of Trials: Two (if necessary).
Directions: S is to walk backwards for two yards, placing one foot directly behind the other, toe to heel. His arms should hang naturally by his side. E should mark the two yard distance on the floor.

E should demonstrate to S and say, 'I want you to walk like this. Remember your toe must touch your heel each step that you take'.

Scoring Criteria: A trial is failed if:

(*a*) S fails to touch toe to heel. (E corrects S on the first trial only.)
(*b*) S deviates more than one foot in either direction laterally.
(*c*) S uses his arms in order to maintain balance.
(*d*) S does not place his feet directly behind each other in a straight line, although he does touch his heel with his toe. Deviations of 30° and more from the straight are penalised.

Time Limit: Untimed
Points:
3: passing on first trial
2: passing on second trial
1: using arms, or placing feet more than 30° off straight line
0: failing completely on both trials

2. CROUCHING ON TIPTOE

Equipment: Stop-watch.
Number of Trials: Two (if necessary).
Directions: S is to stand on tiptoe (*i.e.* on the balls of the feet, or, at least, with heels raised off the ground) in a semi-crouched position with knees flexed approximately 45°—any angle between 30° and clear of the haunches is acceptable—and arms extended horizontally at the sides. Feet are parallel and approximately one foot apart. The eyes should be closed.

E says 'I want to see how steady you are. Let's see if you can balance on your tiptoes with your arms out like this, when your eyes are closed. (E demonstrates.) Remember, you must stay on your toes with your knees bent, keep your arms out straight and your eyes closed. Ready, go!'

Scoring Criteria: The position must be maintained for 10 seconds for a trial to be passed. A trial is failed if:

(*a*) the position is not held for the full 10 seconds. (E should record the length of time that was able to maintain the position.)
(*b*) S falls.
(*c*) S puts weight on heels.

(*d*) S touches floor with hands.
(*e*) S steps out of place.
(*f*) the arms are not kept in an essentially straight, horizontal position. Moving other parts of the body to maintain balance is permitted.

Time Limit: 10 seconds per trial.

Points: 3: passing on first trial
2: passing on second trial
0: failing on both trials

3. STANDING ON ONE FOOT

Equipment: Stop-watch.

Number of Trials: Two (if necessary) for each leg.

Directions: S is to stand motionless on one leg for 10 seconds with the sole of the other foot placed against the supporting leg. The palms of the hands rest on the outside of the thighs. S may be allowed to start with any leg, but E must note which is used. If the first trial is failed, S should repeat the test using the same leg before proceeding on to the other leg. S is not penalised for failing to keep the flexed leg in contact with the supporting one.

E says, 'Let's see how long you can balance on one leg. Place your hands on your thighs like this and stand on one leg.' (E demonstrates). After the requisite number of trials on one leg he says, 'Now let's try it on the other foot'.

Scoring Criteria: S must maintain the position for 10 seconds for a trial to be passed. A trial is failed if:

(*a*) S does not maintain position for 10 seconds. (E should note the time that S was able to satisfy all the conditions.)
(*b*) S steps on the floor with the flexed leg.
(*c*) S removes his hands from his thighs.
(*d*) S stands on tiptoe.

Time Limit: 10 seconds per trial.

Points: The two legs are scored separately as follows:
3: passing on first trial
2: passing on second trial
0: failing on both trails

4. TOUCHING NOSE

Equipment: None.

Number of Trials: One.

Directions: S is to stretch both arms out to the sides horizontally with index fingers extended and then touch the fleshy part of his nose with the last phalanx of each index finger three times alternately. S should be standing with his eyes closed and his head kept still.

E demonstrates, saying, 'Stretch your arms out like this. Now close your eyes. Now touch your nose with one hand, keeping your head still. That's fine. Now touch it with your other hand.'

Scoring Criteria: The trial is considered passed if each hand touches the nose twice in the three attempts. E must record the number of successful attempts for each hand.

Points: 3: passing
0: failing

5. TOUCHING FINGERTIPS

Equipment: Stop-watch.

Number of Trials: Two (if necessary) for each hand.

Directions: S is to touch all the fingertips of one hand in succession with the thumb of the same hand, beginning with the little finger and moving up to the index finger. This is to be done twice in five seconds.

E says, 'Let me see you touch your fingertips with your thumb. Start with your little finger and touch each finger in order like this. Then go back to the little finger and do it again.' E demonstrates

slowly. 'Watch again.' This time E repeats the demonstration quickly. 'Now you try it.' E should note which hand S uses. 'Now let's try it with your other hand.'
Scoring Criteria: A trial is passed if S touches each finger in order within 5 seconds, *i.e.* eight thumb-to-finger connections have to be made within the 5 second period. A trial is failed if:
(*a*) S takes longer than 5 seconds to complete the task successfully. (E should record the time taken.)
(*b*) S touches a finger more than once.
(*c*) S touches two fingers at the same time with the thumb.
(*d*) S skips one or more fingers.

If the first trial is failed, a second trial should be given to the same hand before the other hand is tested.
Time Limit: 5 seconds per trial.
Points: Each hand is scored separately as follows:
3: passing on first trial
2: passing on second trial
0: failing on both trials

6. STANDING HEEL TO TOE

Equipment: Stop-watch.
Number of Trials: Two (if necessary).
Directions: S stands with the preferred foot placed directly before the other foot, with the heel of the preferred foot touching the toe of the other foot. Both feet should be kept in a straight line. Eyes should be kept closed. Arms should hang naturally beside the body with the palms of the hands turned in.

E demonstrates, saying, 'Stand like this with the toe of one foot touching the heel of the other and with your eyes closed, until I tell you to stop.' E must record which foot S elects to place in front.
Scoring Criteria: The position must be maintained for at least 15 seconds for the item to be passed. The item is failed if:
(*a*) S makes any gross bodily movements, such as waving arms or bending trunk, to maintain balance.
(*b*) S opens his eyes.

Time Limit: 15 seconds per trial.
Points:
3: passing on first trial
2: passing on second trial
1: using arms to maintain balance
0: failing on both trials

7. CLOSING AND OPENING THE HANDS ALTERNATELY

Equipment: Stop-watch.
Number of Trials: Three (if necessary).
Directions: S should be standing. He is to extend his arms full length in front of him, with the palms of the hands turned down. He is then to close his right hand, making a fist, and, at a given signal, to open it and close the left hand, continuing in this manner as fast as possible.

E says, 'Stretch your arms out full length like this (E demonstrates) in front of you with your palms turned down. First I want you to close your right hand like this and keep it closed until I say 'Go'. When I say 'Go', you are to open your right hand and close your left. You are to repeat this order like this (E demonstrates) until I say 'Stop', doing it as quickly as you can. Ready, go!'
Scoring Criteria: A trial is passed if S alternately opens and closes his hands for 10 seconds. A trial is failed if:
(*a*) S opens and closes both hands simultaneously.
(*b*) S bends one or both of his elbows.

Time Limit: 10 seconds per trial.
Points:
3: passing on first trial
2: passing on second trial
1: passing on third trial
0: failing on all trials

8. CATCHING A BALL

Equipment: Regulation squash ball.
Number of Trials: Five (if necessary) with each hand.
Directions: E should toss the ball to S with an underhand motion so that when the ball reaches S it is describing a downward curve and S is able to catch the ball in his cupped hand with the palm facing upward. E is to toss the ball toward the hand the subject is to use in making the catch. If E makes a bad toss, the trial is not counted. S stands at a distance of 10 feet from E, the palms of his hands against his thighs. E precedes each toss with the warning statement, 'Here it comes'. Five tosses are made with S using one hand to catch the ball, and then the test is repeated with the other hand. E should note which hand S elects to use on the first trial.

E says, 'Let's see how well you can catch a ball in one hand. Stand here (designates a point 10 feet distant) and keep your hands at your sides like this (E demonstrates) until I toss the ball. Catch the ball in one hand. Are you ready? Here it comes.' E must record which hand S elects to catch the first ball with.
Scoring Criteria: The number of times the ball is caught is recorded for each hand. In the event of S using the wrong hand to catch the ball, E corrects him but does not count the trial. If the ball is caught between the hand and the body, rather than in the hand, the trial is still counted as a catch. A trial is failed if a well-thrown ball is dropped to the ground.
Time Limit: Untimed.
Points: Each hand is scored separately as follows:

3: 4 catches
2: 2-3 catches
1: 1 catch
0: no catches

9. TAPPING

Equipment: Four sheets of plain, quarto paper. Blunt pencil. Stop-watch.
Number of Trials: Two trials for each hand.
Directions: S is seated at a table on which there is a sheet of plain paper. He is to rest his forearm on the table and take the blunt pencil in his hand. At a given signal, he is to tap the paper with the pencil as quickly as he can, trying not to hit the same spot more than once. Dots may be made anywhere on the paper. Only the hand may be moved. Gross movements of the arms are not permissible, *i.e.*, the arm may not be lifted from the table.

E says, 'I want to see how many dots you can make on this paper with this pencil. You may move your hand, but you may not move your arm from the table. You can make dots anywhere on the paper, but be careful not to tap twice in the same place. (E demonstrates what is required on a scrap piece of paper.) Ready, go.'

Two trials are given consecutively for each hand, with a one minute rest before the other hand is used. A fresh sheet of paper is to be provided each time, and E must note on each sheet which hand and which trial it was used for. S may start with either hand, but E must record which hand is used.
Scoring Criteria: S's score is the average number of dots he makes during the two 15 second periods.
Time Limit: 15 seconds per trial.

Points:	*Preferred hand*	*Other hand*
	(Averaged over 2 trials)	(Averaged over 2 trials)
	3: 80 or more dots	3: 70 or more dots
	2: 70 to 79 dots	2: 60 to 69 dots
	1: 60 to 69 dots	1: 50 to 59 dots
	0: 0 to 59 dots	0: 0 to 49 dots

10. SORTING MATCHSTICKS

Equipment: Two plastic boxes. Forty matchsticks. Stop-watch.
Number of Trials: One trial with each hand.

Directions: S is seated at the table with the two boxes in front of him about 18 inches apart. The 40 matches are placed in the box near S's preferred hand. S is to pick up one match at a time from this box and transfer it to the other box as quickly as he can. Then, with the other hand he is to transfer all the matches back again. S is not to rise from the chair, nor pick up more than one match at a time.

E says, 'Here is a box of matches. I want you to pick up the matchsticks, one at a time, from this box and place them into the other box like this. (E demonstrates.) Do not get up from your chair or pick up more than one match at a time.' E must ask S which hand he wishes to start with and record this choice on the proforma. The matches are placed in the box in front of the chosen hand.

Scoring Criteria: E records the time taken to complete the task. Picking up more than one match at a time and throwing matches constitute errors. E must record the number of such errors made; 5 seconds are added to the time score for each error committed.

Time Limit: None. E records the time taken to complete the task.

Points: The two hands are scored separately as follows:

Preferred hand

Male	*Female*
3: 0 to 44 secs	3: 0 to 47 secs
2: 45 to 54 secs	2: 48 to 63 secs
1: 55 to 69 secs	1: 64 to 87 secs
0: 70 or more secs	0: 88 or more secs

Other hand

3: 0 to 49 secs
2: 50 to 59 secs
1: 60 to 79 secs
0: 80 or more secs

11. DRAWING LINES

Equipment: Pencil. Sheet of lined, white, quarto paper (the lines should be 3/8 of an inch apart). Stop-watch.

Number of Trials: Two trials with each hand.

Directions: S should be seated with his forearm resting on the table, holding the pencil in a writing position. He is to draw perpendicular lines between the ruled lines, touching these lines, but not over-running them by more than 1/8 of an inch. S is allowed 15 seconds for his preferred hand and 20 seconds for his other hand. E must note which is the preferred hand.

E says, 'I want you to draw as many lines as you can between these two lines. I want your line to touch these two lines, but not to run over, like this. (E demonstrates, drawing about a dozen lines as quickly as possible.) Do you understand? Ready, go!'

S is given two trials using the hand that he started with before being given the two trials using his other hand.

Scoring Criteria: The score for each trial is the number of lines correctly drawn during the time limit. A line is not counted if it over-runs or is short of the horizontal lines on the paper by more than 1/8 of an inch. E should identify on the paper each group of lines. S should use a new pair of lines for each of the four trials. E then counts the number of correctly formed lines for each trial and enters this in the record sheet. The final score for each hand is the average number of lines drawn correctly during the two trials.

Time Limit: 15 seconds per trial using the preferred hand.
20 seconds per trial using the other hand.

Points: Each hand is scored separately as follows (averaged over 2 trials):

3: 30 lines and over
2: 20 to 29 lines
1: 10 to 19 lines
0: 0 to 9 lines

12. PUTTING COINS IN A BOX

Equipment: Plastic box. Twenty halfpennies.* Stop-watch.
Number of Trials: One trial with each hand.
Directions: S is seated at the table. The box is placed directly in front of him within his reach. The coins are placed in two rows of ten, with two inches between the rows and between the top row and the box. The coins should be approximately one fourth inch apart. S is to pick up the coins in one hand, one at a time, and place them in the box, as quickly as he can. S may not slide the coins to the edge of the table to pick them up, but must pick them off the table where they lie.

E says, 'Let's see you put these halfpennies into the box as fast as you can. Use only one hand and put in only one halfpenny at a time, like this. (E demonstrates with one or two coins, placing them in quickly.) Put them in the box, do not throw them in.' S may start with either hand. E must note on the proforma which is the 'preferred' hand.
Scoring Criteria: E notes the number of coins correctly placed in 15 seconds, and also records the time taken to place all the coins in the box.
Time Limit: The time taken to complete the task is noted, as is the number of coins placed within 15 seconds.
Points: Each hand is scored separately as follows:

No. of coins placed in 15 *seconds*

3: 17 to 20 coins
2: 14 to 16 coins
1: 11 to 13 coins
0: 0 to 10 coins

*This test was standardised before halfpennies were withdrawn from British currency. Shilling pieces (*i.e.* 5p) might now be preferable.

APPENDIX D

Instructions and Scoring Criteria for the Motor Impersistence Test

1. **Keeping Eyes Closed**

The subject (S) is instructed to close his eyes and keep them closed. Two 20-second trials are given. The examiner (E) records the number of seconds during each trial over which the performance is sustained. A perfect score is 40. Any child scoring less than 40 is deemed impersistent on this task.

2. **Protruding Tongue** (S blindfolded)

S is blindfolded and told to stick out his tongue and keep it out. Two 20-second trials are given, and the total score is the length of time the tongue remains out. Any child scoring less than 40 is deemed impersistent on this task.

3. **Protruding Tongue** (eyes open)

The same procedure as for Task 2 is followed, except that S is not blindfolded. Any child scoring less than 40 is deemed impersistent on this task.

4. **Fixation of Gaze in Lateral Visual Fields**

E and S are seated directly opposite each other in two chairs, with their knees almost touching. With his head fixed in the mid-line position, S is instructed to look at E's finger and to keep looking at it. E extends his index finger vertically at an angle of approximately 45° in the horizontal plane of S's right visual field for 20 seconds. After one trial, the procedure is repeated in S's left visual field. Each time S looks away from the finger, a point is scored in each trial. The total score is the number of times S looks away during both trials. A perfect score is therefore zero. Any child scoring three or more was deemed impersistent on this task.

5. **Keeping Mouth Open**

S is instructed to open his mouth and keep it open. Two 20-second trials are given, and the total score is determined as in Tasks 1, 2 and 3, any child scoring less than 40 being rated impersistent.

6. **Fixation of E's Nose during Confrontation Testing of Visual Fields**

E and S are seated as for Task 4. S is instructed to look at E's nose and to keep looking at it. E gradually brings a finger around the side of S's face, from a point in line with S's ears, until the finger reaches a point at a 45° angle in the horizontal plane of S's right or left visual field. S is told to say when he first sees the finger out of the corner of his eye. Each time S looks away from E's nose, a point is scored, and he is reminded to keep looking at the nose. Two trials of 20 seconds each are given for each visual field, tested alternately. The total score is the number of points scored on all four trials; a score of zero indicates perfect performance. Any child scoring 13 or more is deemed impersistent on this task.

7. **Saying 'Aah'**

E says, 'Take a deep breath and say 'aah', holding it for as long as you can, like this.' E then demonstrates to S, making sure that S understands that he must not exhale before saying 'aah.' Two trials are given. The total score is the sum in seconds of the duration of the responses on both trials. Any score of less than 15 for ten-year-old children, and 13 for nine-year-old children is rated as an impersistent score.

Using these cut-off scores, a child's performance on each task is now characterised as impersistent or not. If the child gets two or more impersistent scores then he is deemed to be pathologically impersistent.

APPENDIX E

Child Health Form (Parents)*

Parents were asked to answer the 23 questions summarised below by putting a cross or number, as appropriate, in the boxes after each question and by writing in extra information when necessary. Most of the questions referred to the school year beginning 1st September 1964.

The first three questions enquired about contact with doctors and other medical facilities (*i.e.* hospital Casualty, Out-patient or In-patient Departments), requesting information about number of visits and reasons in each case.

Question 4 asked whether the child's speech was 'entirely normal', 'not quite distinct or clear but easily understandable', 'understandable with some difficulty', 'understandable with considerable difficulty' or 'hardly understandable at all'.

Questions 5 to 10 enquired about the presence or occurrence of skin rash or spots, severe headaches, attacks of wheezing, sugar diabetes, fits (*i.e.* a spell, convulsion or any other attack that a doctor has called a fit) and weakness or paralysis of the arms or legs. The first three of these items referred to the school year since 1st September 1964. Where the conditions were present, supplementary questions sought out further detailed information, *e.g.*, whether the spots were embarrassing and required bandages or ointments, whether headaches were accompanied by vomiting, whether injections were required for wheezing or diabetes. Parents were asked to give a description of any fits, turns, wasting or paralysis and to state the frequency of occurrence.

The next four questions (11 to 14) dealt with medication and possible limitations to the child's activities, *i.e.* regular medication for periods over two weeks, restriction of physical activities, special diet or any other extra care such as taking to the toilet, getting up at night, wheelchair, *etc.*

Questions 15 to 19 comprised one question on whether, in the parents' opinion, the child was having the right kind of schooling, and four questions on his general health, *i.e.* whether the child was 'bounding with energy', had 'just normal amount of energy', was 'tired, sluggish or lacking in energy' or was '*very* sluggish, tired or lacking in energy'; whether he/she had any difficulty with hearing; whether there were any other medical or health problems present such as heart trouble, bladder trouble including bed-wetting, or difficulties in seeing even when wearing spectacles; and whether there were any other problems in the care of the child which had not been mentioned in answering the previous questions.

The last four questions (20 to 23) concerned family employment and housing. Parents were asked to state the usual job of the head of the household or usual job before retirement, whether paid weekly, monthly or self-employed, how much the head of the household had been off work since 1st September 1964 and for what reasons, whether anybody else living at home had had problems with his/her health. In addition, they were asked how many rooms there were in the house that were used by the family, and how many people there were in the household.

Finally, space was left for any other comments the parents wished to make about medical conditions or health problems in the family.

*The Parental and Teacher's Child Health Forms and Child Scales A and B are reproduced in full in *Education, Health and Behaviour* (Rutter *et al.* 1970).

APPENDIX F

Child Health Form (Teachers)

Teachers were asked to answer the 22 questions summarised below by putting a cross or number' as appropriate, in the boxes after each question, giving approximate numbers in cases of uncertainty' Questions referred to the school year beginning 1st September 1964.

The first three questions enquired about the amount of schooling missed for any reason during the school year, whether the child had had to be sent home for any medical reason and whether the child had been admitted to hospital. Teachers were asked to specify reasons if known.

Questions 4 to 9 dealt with special arrangements for the child's care at school, *i.e.* did the school staff have to supervise medical dressings or the taking of tablets or medicine (if so, how often and why); were there any school activities in which the child was not allowed to take part and by whose authority; did the child have a special diet for meals at school or have to go home to lunch because of a special diet; were special arrangements necessary for transport to and from school; and were any other special arrangements necessary at school such as help with feeding or toileting, provision for wheelchair?

Questions 10 to 20 enquired about fits, diabetes, asthma, skin conditions, speech, severe headaches, weakness or paralysis, energy, hearing, sight and co-ordination. Whenever a condition was present or there was some abnormality or difficulty, supplementary information was requested including details of frequency of occurrence where appropriate and whether the child had to be sent home from school. Question 20 asked whether there were any other problems in the health or education of the child.

The last two questions dealt with schooling, *i.e.* what kind of school and class the child was in, whether he was as well placed as possible and if not, in what sort of school and class he would be better placed.

APPENDIX G Child Scale A (Parents)

The questionnaire asks about various kinds of behaviour that many children show at some time. Parents were asked to cross the answers according to the way their child was at the time of the survey.

Health Problems

Below is a list of minor health problems which most children have at some time. Parents were requested to state whether each happened: (i) never in the last year, (ii) less often than once per month, (iii) at least once per month and (iv) at least once per week, by putting a cross in the appropriate box.

The items were: complains of headaches; has stomach-ache or vomiting; complains of biliousness; wets his/her bed or pants; soils him/herself or loses control of bowels; has temper tantrums (*i.e.* complete loss of temper with shouting, angry movements, etc.); had tears on arrival at school or refused to go into the building; truants from school.

Habits

Parents were required to answer 'No', Yes- mildly/occasionally' or 'Yes—severely/frequently' to the following questions.

1. Does he/she stammer or stutter?
2. Has he/she any difficulty with speech other than stammering or stuttering? If Yes, is the difficulty 'lisping', 'cannot say words properly' or 'other (please describe)'?
3. Does he/she ever steal things? If so, does it involve 'minor pilfering of pens, sweets, toys, small sums of money, etc.', 'stealing of big things' or 'both'? Is it done 'in the home', 'elsewhere' or 'both'? Does he/she do it 'on his/her own', 'with other children or adults', 'both'?
4. Does he/she have any eating difficulty? If so, is it 'faddiness', 'not eating enough', 'eating too much' or 'other (please describe)'?
5. Does he/she have any sleeping difficulty? If so, is it 'getting off to sleep', 'waking during the night', 'waking early in the morning' or 'other (please describe)'?

Behaviour

Below are a series of descriptions of behaviour often shown by children. After each statement, parents were asked to place a cross in a box in one of three columns: 'Doesn't Apply', 'Applies Somewhat' or 'Certainly Applies'.

1. Very restless. Often running about or jumping up and down. Hardly ever still.
2. Squirmy, fidgety child.
3. Often destroys own or others' belongings.
4. Frequently fights with other children.
5. Not much liked by other children.
6. Often worried, worries about many things.
7. Tends to do things on his own—rather solitary.
8. Irritable. Is quick to 'fly off the handle'.
9. Often appears miserable, unhappy, tearful or distressed.
10. Has twitches, mannerisms or tics of the face or body.
11. Frequently sucks thumb or finger.
12. Frequently bites nails or fingers.
13. Is often disobedient.
14. Cannot settle to anything for more than a few moments.
15. Tends to be fearful or afraid of new things or new situations.
16. Fussy or over-particular child.
17. Often tells lies.
18. Bullies other children.

Parents were then asked whether there were any other problems of behaviour.

APPENDIX H

Child Scale B (Teachers)

Below are a series of descriptions of behaviour often shown by children. After each statement, teachers were asked to place a cross in a box in one of three columns: 'Doesn't Apply', 'Applies Somewhat', or 'Certainly Applies'.

This questionnaire includes all the statements listed under *Behaviour* in Appendix G, plus the following 8 items.

19. Truants from school.
20. Tends to be absent from school for trivial reasons.
21. Has stolen things on one or more occasions.
22. Has wet or soiled self at school this year.
23. Often complains of pains or aches.
24. Has had tears on arrival at school *or* has refused to come into the building this year.
25. Has a stutter or stammer.
26. Has other speech difficulty.

Teachers were also asked to state whether there were any other problems of behaviour and whether they knew the child: "Very well', Moderately well", or 'Not very well'.

REFERENCES

Ackerly, S. S. (1964) 'A case of paranatal bilateral frontal lobe defect observed for thirty years.' *in* Warren, J. M., Akert, K. (Eds.). The Frontal Granular Cortex and Behaviour. New York: McGraw-Hill.

Aird, R. B., Yamamoto, T. (1966) 'Behaviour disorders of childhood.' *Electroenceph. clin. Neurophysiol.*, **21,** 148.

Akert K., Orth, O. S., Harlow, H. F., Schiltz, K. A. (1960) 'Learned behaviour of Rhesus monkeys following neonatal bilateral prefrontal lobotomy.' *Science*, **132,** 1944.

Alajouanine, Th., Lhermitte, F. (1965) 'Acquired aphasia in children.' *Brain*, **88,** 653.

Allen, R. M. (1947) 'The test performance of brain injury.' *J. clin. Psychol.*, **3,** 225.

Andersen, B. (1954) 'Cerebral palsy.' *J. Oslo Cy. Hosp.*, **4,** 65.

André-Thomas, S., Chesni, Y., Saint-Anne Dargassies, S. (1960) The Neurological Examination of the Infant. Little Club Clinics in Developmental Medicine No. 1. London: SIMP/Heinemann Medical.

Annett, M., Lee, D., Ounsted, C. (1961) 'Intellectual disabilities in relation to lateralized features in the EEG.' *in* Hemiplegic Cerebral Palsy in Children and Adults. Little Club Clinics in Developmental Medicine No 4. London: SIMP/Heinemann Medical.

Asher, P., Schonell, F. E. (1950) 'A survey of 400 cases of cerebral palsy in childhood.' *Arch. Dis. Childh.*, **25,** 360.

Ashley-Miller, M. (1965) 'Selective school medical inspection.' *Med. Offr.*, **113,** 119.

Bakwin, H. (1949) 'Cerebral damage and behaviour disorders in children.' *J. Pediat.*, **34,** 371.

—— Bakwin, R. M. (1966) Clinical Management of Behaviour Disorders in Children (3rd Edn.) Philadelphia: W. B. Saunders.

Baldwin, W. K. (1958) 'The social position of the educable mentally retarded child in the regular grades of public schools.' *Except. Child*, **25,** 106.

Balf, C. L., Ingram, T. T. S. (1955) 'Problems in the classification of cerebral palsy in childhood.' *Brit. med. J.*, **ii,** 163.

Banas, P. A., Dawis, R. V. (1962) 'Identifying the physically handicapped through survey methods.' *Amer. J. publ. Hlth.*, **52,** 443.

Barclay, J. (1956) 'A survey of cerebral palsy in Otago.' *N.Z. med. J.*, **55,** 199.

Barker, R. G., Wright, B. A., Myerson, L., Gonick, M. R. (1953) 'Adjustment to physical handicap and illness: a survey of the social psychology of physique and disability.' *Soc. Sci. Res. Council Bull.*, No. 55.

Basser, L. S. (1962) 'Hemiplegia of early onset and the faculty of speech with special reference to the effects of hemispherectomy.' *Brain*, **85,** 427.

Bax, M., Mac Keith, R. (Eds.) (1963) Minimal Cerebral Dysfunction. Clinics in Developmental Medicine No. 10. London: SIMP/Heinemann Medical.

Bayley, N. (1968) Infant Scales of Development. New York: Psychological Corporation.

Beach, F. A. (1938) 'The neural basis of innate behaviour. II. Relative effects of partial decortication in adulthood and infancy upon the maternal behaviour of the primiparous rat.' *J. genet. Psychol.*, **53,** 109.

Beck, H., Lam, R. L. (1955) 'The use of the WISC in predicting organicity.' *J. clin. Psychol.*, **11,** 154.

Becker, W. C., Madsen, C. H., Arnold, C. R., Thomas, D. R. (1967) 'The contingent use of teacher attention and praise in reducing classroom behaviour problems.' *J. spec. Educ.*, **1,** 287.

Beintema, D. J. (1968) A Neurological Study of Newborn Infants. Clinics in Developmental Medicine No. 28. London: SIMP/Heinemann Medical.

Belmont, L. (1968) Personal communication.

—— Birch, H. G. (1960) 'The relation of time of life to behavioural consequence in brain damage. I. The performance of brain-injured adults on the marble-board test.' *J. nerv. ment. Dis.*, **131,** 91.

—— —— (1965) 'Lateral dominance, lateral awareness, and reading disability.' *Child Develop.*, **36,** 57.

Bender, L. (1956) Psychopathology of Children with Organic Brain Disorders. Springfield, Ill.: C. C. Thomas.

Bender, M., Fink, M., Green, M. (1951) 'Patterns in perception on simultaneous tests of face and hand.' *Arch. Neurol. Psychiat. (Chic.)*, **66,** 355.

Benjamin, R. M., Thompson, R. F. (1959) 'Differential effects of cortical lesions in infant and adult cats on roughness discrimination.' *Exp. Neurol.*, **1,** 305.

Benson, D. F., Geschwind, N. (1968) 'Cerebral dominance and its disturbances.' *Pediat. Clin. N. Amer.*, **15,** 759.

Benton, A. L. (1962) 'Behavioral indices of brain injury in school children.' *Child Develop.*, **33,** 199.

—— (1964) 'Developmental aphasia and brain damage.' *Cortex*, **1,** 40.

—— Garfield, J. C., Chiorini, J. C. (1964) 'Motor impersistence in mental defectives'. *in* Oster, J. (Ed.) Proceedings of the International Copenhagen Conference on the Scientific Study of Mental Retardation. Copenhagen: Statens & Andssvageforsorg. p. 746.

Berkson, J. (1946) 'Limitations of the application of four-fold table analysis to hospital data.' *Biometrics*, **2,** 264.
Berlin, L. (1955) 'Compulsive eye-opening and associated phenomena.' *Arch. Neurol. Psychiat., (Chic.)*, **73,** 597.
Bijou, S. W. (1968) 'Research on the academic education of the retarded.' *in* Jervis, G. A. (Ed.) Expanding Concepts in Mental Retardation. Springfield, Ill.: C. C. Thomas.
Bingley, T. (1958) 'Mental symptoms in temporal lobe epilepsy and temporal lobe gliomas.' *Acta psychiat. scand.*, **33,** Suppl. 120.
Birch, H. G. (1964) Brain Damage in Children: The Biological and Social Aspects. Baltimore: Williams and Wilkins.
—— Belmont, L. (1960) 'The relation of time of life to behavioural consequence in brain damage: II. The organisation of tactical form experience in brain-injured adults.' *J. nerv. ment. Dis.*, **131,** 489.
—— —— (1964) 'Auditory-visual integration in normal and retarded readers.' *Amer. J. Orthopsychiat.*, **34,** 852.
—— —— (1965*a*) 'Auditory-visual integration in brain-damaged and normal children.' *Develop. Med. Child Neurol.*, **7,** 135.
—— —— (1965*b*) 'Auditory-visual integration, intelligence and reading ability in school children.' *Percept. Mot. Skills*, **20,** 295.
—— Lefford, A. (1963) 'Intersensory development in children.' *Monogr. Soc. Res. Child Develop.*, **28** (5), 1.
—— Belmont, L., Belmont, I., Taft, L. T. (1967) 'Brain damage and intelligence in educable mentally subnormal children.' *J. nerv. ment. Dis.*, **144,** 247.
Blank, M., Bridger, W. H. (1964) 'Cross-modal transfer in nursery school children.' *J. comp. Physiol. Psychol.*, **58,** 277.
—— —— (1967) 'Perceptual abilities and conceptual deficiencies in retarded readers.' *in* Zubin, J., Jervis, G. A. (Eds.) Psychopathology of Mental Development. New York: Grune and Stratton.
Bond, E. P., Partridge, C. E. (1926) 'Post-encephalitic behaviour disorders in boys and their management in a hospital.' *Amer. J. Psychiat.*, **6,** 25.
Bower, B. D. (1969) 'Epilepsy in childhood.' *Brit. J. hosp. Med.*, **2,** 454.
Bower, E. M. (1960) Early Identification of Emotionally Handicapped Children. Springfield, Ill.: C. C. Thomas.
Bradley, C. (1937) 'The behaviour of children receiving benzedrine.' *Amer. J. Psychiat.*, **94,** 577.
—— (1951) 'Behaviour disturbances in epileptic children.' *J. Amer. med. Ass.*, **146,** 436.
—— (1955) 'Organic factors in the psychopathology of childhood.' *in* Hoch, P. H., Zubin, J. (Eds.) Psychopathology of Childhood. New York: Grune & Stratton.
Bradway, K. P. (1937) 'Birth lesions in identical twins.' *Amer. J. Orthopsychiat.*, **7,** 194.
Brain, W. R. (1955) Diseases of The Nervous System (5th Ed.). London: Oxford University Press.
Brandt, S., Kristensen, K. H., Plum, P. (1964) 'A lowered incidence of infantile cerebral palsy?' *Develop. Med. Child Neurol.*, **6,** 536.
Brante, G. (1949) 'Studies on lipids in the nervous system with special reference to quantitative chemical determination and topical distribution.' *Acta. physiol. scand.*, **18,** Suppl. 633.
Brenner, M. W., Gillman, S. (1966) 'Visuomotor ability in school children—a survey.' *Develop. Med. Child Neurol.*, **8,** 686.
—— —— Zangwill, O. L., Farrell, M. (1967) 'Visuomotor disability in school children.' *Brit. med. J.*, **4,** 259.
Brewis, M., Poskanzer, D. C., Rolland, C., Miller, H. (1966) 'Neurological disease in an English City.' *Acta. neurol. scand.*, Suppl. 24 Vol. 42, 1.
Bridge, E. M. (1949) Epilepsy and Convulsive Disorders in Children. New York: Mcgraw-Hill.
British Council for the Welfare of Spastics (1948) 'The incidence of cerebral palsy.' (Unpublished report).
British Medical Journal (1962) Leading Article 'Clumsy Children.' *Brit. med. J.*, **ii,** 1665.
Brodman, K., Eerdmann, A. J., Lorge, I., Wolff, H. G., Broadbent, T. H. (1949) 'The Cornell Medical Index—an adjunt to medical interview.' *J. Amer. med. Ass.*, **140,** 530.
—— —— —— Gershenson, C. P., Wolff, H. G., Broadbent, T. H. (1952) 'The Cornell Medical Index Health Questionnaire. IV. The recognition of emotional disturbances in a general hospital.' *J. clin. Psychol.*, **8,** 289.
Brown, G. W., Bone, M., Dalison, B., Wing, J. K. (1966) Schizophrenia and Social Care. Maudsley Monograph No. 17. London: Oxford University Press.
Butler, N. R., Bonham, D. C. (1963) Perinatal Mortality. Edinburgh: E. & S. Livingstone.
Burt, C. (1959) 'The accomplishment quotient: a reply.' *Brit. J. educ. Psychol.*, **29,** 259.
Byers, R. K., Lord, E. E. (1943) 'Late effects of lead poisoning on mental development.' *Amer. J. Dis. Childh.*, **66,** 471.
Caldwell, B. M., Guze, S. B. (1960) 'A study of the adjustment of parents and siblings of institutionalised and non-institutionalised retarded children.' *Amer. J. ment. Defic.*, **64,** 845.
Carey, A. (1967) 'The Hawthorne studies: a radical criticism.' *Amer. sociol. Rev.* **32,** 403.
Carter, C. (1958) 'A life-table for mongols with the causes of death.' *J. ment. Def. Res.*, **2,** 64.

Chase, H. C. (1967) 'Perinatal and infant mortality in the United States and six West European countries.' *Amer. J. publ. Hlth.*, **57,** 1735.
Chaudhry, M. R., Pond, D. A. (1961) 'Mental deterioration in epileptic children.' *J. Neurol. Neurosurg. Psychiat.*, **24,** 213.
Clausen, J. A. (1966) 'Family structure, socialisation and personality.' *in* Hoffman, L. W., Hoffman, H. L. (Eds.) Review of Child Development Research. Vol. 2. New York: Russell Sage Foundation.
Clements, S. D., Peters, J. E. (1962) 'Minimal brain dysfunction in the school age child.' *Arch. gen. Psychiat.*, **6,** 185.
Cockburn, J. M. (1961) 'Psychological aspects.' *in* Henderson, J. L. (Ed.) Cerebral Palsy in Childhood and Adolescence. Edinburgh: E. & S. Livingstone. p. 281.
Cohen, H. J., Taft, L. T. Mahadeviah, M. S., Birch, H. G. (1967) 'Developmental changes in overflow in normal and aberrantly functioning children.' *J. Pediat.*, **71,** 39.
—— Molnar, G. E., Taft, L. T. (1968) 'The genetic relationship of progressive muscular dystrophy (Duchenne type) and mental retardation.' *Develop. Med. Child Neurol.*, **10,** 754.
Cohen, H. M. (1953) *in* Ministry of Health Memorandum No. 26. Cited by Henderson, J. L. (1961).
—— (1954) Personal communication. Cited by Ingram (1955).
Cohen, J. (1959) 'The factorial structure of the WISC at ages 7.6, 10.6, and 13.6.' *J. consult. Psychol.*, **23,** 285.
College of General Practitioners Research Committee (1960) 'A survey of the epilepsies in general practice.' *Brit. med. J.* **ii,** 416.
Combs, R. H., Harper, J. L. (1967) 'Effects of labels on attitudes of educators towards handicapped children.' *Except. Child*, **33,** 399.
Committee on Child Psychiatry (1966) Psychopathological Disorders in Childhood: Theoretical Considerations and a Proposed Classification. New York: Group for the Advancement of Psychiatry.
Committee on Training in Clinical Psychology (1947) 'Recommended graduate training program in clinical psychology.' *Amer. Psychol.*, **2,** 539.
Conel, J. L. (1939-63) The Postnatal Development of the Human Cerebral Cortex. Vols. I-VI. Cambridge, Mass.: Harvard University Press.
—— (1952) 'Histologic development of the cerebral cortex.' *in* The Biology of Mental Health and Disease. Proceedings of Twenty-seventh Annual Conference of the Milbank Memorial Fund. New York: Hoeber.
Connolly, K. (1968) 'The application of operant conditioning to the measurement and development of motor skill in children,' *Develop. Med. Child Neurol.*, **10,** 697.
Cooper, J. E. (1965) 'Epilepsy in a longitudinal survey of 5,000 children.' *Brit. med. J.*, **i,** 1020.
Costeff, H. (1965) 'Convulsions in childhood: their natural history and indications for treatment.' *New Eng. J. Med.*, **273,** 1410.
County Medical Officer of Health (1963) Annual Report for the Isle of Wight, 1962. Isle of Wight: County Hall.
County Medical Officer of Health (1969) Annual Report for the Isle of Wight, 1968. Isle of Wight: County Hall.
Courville, C. B. (1958) 'Structural changes in the brain in cerebral palsy.' *in* Illingworth, R. S. (Ed.) Recent Advances in Cerebral Palsy. London: J. & A. Churchill.
Craig, M. M., Glick, S. J. (1965) A Manual of Procedures for Application of the Glueck Prediction Table. London: University of London Press.
Crane, A. R. (1959) 'A historical and critical account of the accomplishment quotient idea.' *Brit. J. educ. Psychol.*, **29,** 252.
Critchley, M. (1964) Developmental Dyslexia. London: Heinemann.
Crome, L. (1960) 'The brain and mental retardation.' *Brit. med. J.*, **1,** 897.
Cronbach, L. J. (1949) 'Statistical methods applied to Rorschach score: a review.' *Psychol. Bull*, **46,** 393.
Cruickshank, W. M., Bice, H. V. (1955) 'Personality characteristics.' *in* Cruickshank, W. M., Raus, G. M. (Eds.) Cerebral Palsy: its Individual and Community Problems. Syracuse: Syracuse University Press.
—— Raus, G. M. (Eds.) (1955) Cerebral Palsy: Its Individual and Community Problems. Syracuse: Syracuse University Press.
Culpan, R. H., Davies, B. M., Oppenheim, A. N. (1960) 'Incidence of psychiatric illness among hospital out-patients: an application of the Cornell Medical Index.' *Brit. med. J.*, **i,** 855.
Cummings, S. T., Bayly, H. C., Rie, H. E. (1966) 'Effects of the child's deficiency on the mother: a study of mothers of mentally retarded, chronically ill and nuerotic children.' *Amer. J. Orthopsychiat.*, **36,** 595.
Curran, A. P., McSwan, E., Jefferson, E., Baker, P. (1964) Handicapped Children and Their Families. Dunfermline: Carnegie U.K. Trust.
Davies-Eysenck, M. (1966) Paper presented at Day Conference for Medical Officers, London. Nov. Unpublished paper.

D'Avignon, M. (1963) 'Acquired cerebral palsy: history, symptoms, treatment.' *Develop. Med. Child Neurol.*, **5,** 626.
de Haas, A. M. L. (1962) 'Social aspects of epilepsy in childhood.' *Epilepsia*, **3,** 44.
Denhoff, E. (1955) 'Cerebral palsy: medical aspects.' *in* Cruickshank, W. M., Raus, G. M. (Eds.) Cerebral Palsy: Its Individual and Community Problems. Syracuse: Syracuse University Press.
—— Robinault, I. P. (1960) Cerebral Palsy and Related Disorders. New York: McGraw-Hill.
Department of Education and Science (1964) 'Slow learners at school.' Educational Pamphlet No. 46. London: H.M.S.O.
Dobbing, J. (1968) 'Vulnerable periods in developing brain.' *in* Davison, A. N., Dobbing, J. (Eds.) Applied Neurochemistry. Oxford: Blackwell.
Douglas, A. A. (1961) 'Ophthalmological aspects.' *in* Henderson, J. L. (Ed.) Cerebral Palsy in Childhood and Adolescence. Edinburgh: E. & S. Livingstone. p. 197.
Douglas, J. W. B., Ross, J. M., Cooper, J. E. (1967) 'The relationship between handedness, attainment and adjustment in a national sample of school children.' *Educ. Res.*, **9,** 223.
Drillien, C. M. (1964) The Growth and Development of the Prematurely Born Infant. Edinburgh: E. & S. Livingstone.
—— Ingram, T. T. S., Russell, E. M. (1962) 'Comparative aetiological studies of congenital diplegia in Scotland.' *Arch. Dis. Childh.*, **37,** 282.
Dunn, L. M. (1965) Peabody Picture Vocabulary Test: An expanded manual. Minneapolis: American Guidance Service.
Dunsdon, M. I. (1952) The Educability of Cerebral Palsied Children. London: National Foundation for Educational Research.
Ebaugh, F. G. (1923) 'Neuropsychiatric sequelae of acute epidemic encephalitis in children.' *Amer. J. Dis. Child.*, **25,** 89.
Eckstein, H. B. (1968) 'Myelomeningocele, basic considerations.' *Hosp. Med.*, **2,** 896.
Edwards, J. H. (1958) 'Congenital malformations of the central nervous system in Scotland.' *Brit. J. prev. soc. Med.*, **12,** 115.
Edwards, W. R. (1968) 'G.P. obstetric beds.' *Brit. med. J.*, **3,** 315.
Egan, D. F., Illingworth, R. S., Mac Keith, R. C. (1969) Developmental Screening 0-5 Years. Clinics in Developmental Medicine No. 30. London: SIMP/Heinemann Medical.
Eisenberg, L. (1966) 'The management of the hyperkinetic child.' *Develop. Med. Child Neurol.*, **8,** 593.
Ellingson, R. (1954) 'The incidence of EEG abnormality among patients with mental disorders of apparently non-organic origin: a critical review.' *Amer. J. Psychiat.*, **111,** 263.
Elser, R. P. (1959) 'The social position of hearing-handicapped children in the regular grades.' *Except. Child*, **25,** 305.
Ernhart, C. B., Graham, F. K., Eichman, P. L., Marshall, J. M., Thurston, D. (1963) 'Brain injury in the preschool child: some developmental considerations. II. Comparison of brain-injured and normal children.' *Psychol. Monogr.*, **77,** No. 11.
Eysenck, H. J. (1968) 'The contribution of clinical psychology to psychiatry.' *in* Howells, J. G. (Ed.) Modern Perspectives in World Psychiatry. Edinburgh: Oliver and Boyd.
Farber, B. (1959) 'Effects of a severely mentally retarded child on family integration.' *Monogr. Soc. Res. Child. Dev.*, **24,** (2).
Falconer, M. A., Serafetinides, E. A. (1963) 'A follow-up study of surgery in temporal lobe epilepsy.' *J. Neurol. Neurosurg. Psychiat.*, **26,** 154.
Falkner, F. (1966) (Ed.) Human Development. Philadelphia: W. B. Saunders.
Field, J. G. (1960) 'Two types of tables for use with Wechsler's intelligence scales.' *J. clin. Psychol.*, **16,** 3.
Finley, K. H. (1958) 'Postencephalitic manifestations of viral encephalitides.' *in* Fields, W. S., Blattner, R. J. (Eds.) Viral Encephalitis. Springfield, Ill.: C. C. Thomas.
Fisch, L. (1957) 'Hearing impairment and cerebral palsy.' *Speech*, **21,** 43.
Fisher, M. (1956) 'Left hemiplegia and motor impersistence.' *J. nerv. ment. Dis.*, **123,** 201.
Flory, C. D. (1935) 'Sex differences in skeletal development.' *Child Develop.*, **6,** 205.
Floyer, E. B. (1955) A Psychological Study of a City's Cerebral Palsied Children. London: British Council for the Welfare of Spastics.
Fog, E., Fog, M. (1963) 'Cerebral inhibition examined by associated movements.' *in* Bax, M., Mac Keith, R. (Eds.) Minimal Cerebral Dysfunction. Clinics in Developmental Medicine No. 10. London: SIMP/Heinemann Medical.
Folch-Pi, J. (1952) 'Chemical constituents of brain during development and in maturity.' *in* The Biology of Mental Health and Disease. Proceedings of the Twenty-seventh Annual Conference of the Milbank Memorial Fund. New York: Hoeber.
—— (1955) 'Composition of the brain in relation to maturation.' *in* Waelsch, H., (Ed.) Biochemistry of the Developing Nervous System. New York: Academic Press.
Foley, J. (1968) 'Deterioration in the EEG in children with cerebral palsy.' *Develop. Med. Child. Neurol.*, **10,** 287.
Force, D. G. (1956) 'Social status of physically handicapped children.' *Except. Child*, **23;** 104, 132.
Ford, F. R. (1960) Diseases of the Nervous System in Infancy, Childhood and Adolescence (4th ed.). Springfield, Ill.: C. C. Thomas.

Forrester, R. M. (1967) 'Motor handicap in children: a study of a population in 1965.' *Develop. Med. Child Neurol.*, **9,** 22.
Fransella, F., Gerver, D. (1965) 'Multiple regression equations for predicting reading age from chronological age and WISC verbal I.Q.' *Brit. J. educ. Psychol.*, **35,** 86.
Freud, A. (1945) 'Indications for child analysis.' *Psychoanal. Stud. Child*, **1,** 127.
—— (1966) Normality and Pathology in Childhood. London: Hogarth Press.
Frostig, M., Lefever, D. W., Whittlesey, J. (1961) 'A developmental test of visual perception for evaluating normal and neurologically handicapped children.' *Percept. mot. Skills*, **12,** 383.
—— —— —— (1964) Developmental Test of Visual Perception. Palo Alto, Calif.: Consulting Psychologists Press.
Fulton, J. F., Keller, A. D. (1932) The Sign of Babinski: a Study of the Evolution of Cortical Dominance in Primates. Springfield, Ill.: C. C. Thomas.
Gallagher, J. J. (1957) 'A comparison of brain injured and non-brain-injured mentally retarded children on several psychological variables.' *Mon. Soc. Res. Child Develop.*, **22,** (2).
Gardner, L. (1961) 'Some educational and psychological problems associated with hemiplegia.' *in* Hemiplegic Cerebral Palsy in Children and Adults. Little Club Clinics in Developmental Medicine, No. 4. London: SIMP/Heinemann Medical.
Garfield, J. C. (1964) 'Motor impersistence in normal and brain damaged children.' *Neurology (Minneap.)*, **14,** 623.
—— Benton, A. L., MacQueen, J. C. (1966) 'Motor impersistence in brain damaged and cultural-familial defectives.' *J. nerv. ment. Dis.*, **142,** 434.
Garrard, S. D., Richmond, J. B. (1957) 'Psychological aspects of the management of children with defects or damage of the central nervous system.' *Pediat. Clin. N. Amer.* **4,** 1033.
Gelfand, D. M., Hartmann, D. P. (1968) 'Behaviour therapy with children: a review and evaluation of research methodology.' *Psychol. Bull.*, **3,** 204.
Gesell, A. L., Amatruda, C. S. (1947) Developmental Diagnosis: Normal and Abnormal Child Development. New York: Hoeber.
Gibbens, T. C. N., Pond, D. A., Stafford-Clark, D. (1959) 'A follow-up study of criminal psychopaths.' *J. ment. Sci.*, **105,** 108.
Gibberd, F. B. (1966*a*) 'The clinical features of petit mal.' *Acta Neurol. Scand.*, **42,** 176.
—— (1966*b*) 'The prognosis of petit mal.' *Brain*, **89,** 531.
Gibbs, E. L., Gillen, H. W., Gibbs, F. A. (1954) 'Disappearance and migration of epileptic foci in childhood.' *Amer. J. Dis. Child.*, **88,** 596.
Gibbs, F. A. (1951) 'Ictal and non-ictal psychiatric disorders in temporal lobe epilepsy.' *J. nerv. ment. Dis.*, **113,** 522.
—— Knott, J. R. (1949) 'Growth of the electrical activity of the cortex.' *Electroenceph. clin. Neurophysiol.*, **1,** 223.
—— Gibbs, E. L., Lennox, W. C. (1937) 'Epilepsy: a paroxysmal cerebral dysrythmia.' *Brain*, **60,** 377.
Gibbs, N. (1958) 'Psychological aspects of cerebral palsy.' *in* Illingworth, R. S. (Ed.) Recent Advances in Cerebral Palsy. London: J. and A. Churchill. p. 108.
Gibson, H. B., Hanson, R., West, D. J. (1967) 'A questionnaire measure of neuroticism using a shortened scale derived from the Cornell Medical Index.' *Brit. J. soc. clin. Psychol.*, **6,** 129.
Glaser, G. H., Dixon, M. S. (1956) 'Psychomotor seizures in childhood: a clinical study.' *Neurology (Minneap.)*, **6,** 646.
—— Golub, L. M. (1955) 'The electroencephalogram of psychomotor seizures in childhood.' *Electroenceph. clin. Neurophysiol.*, **7,** 329.
Goldstein, K. (1940) Human Nature in the Light of Psychopathology. Cambridge, Mass.: Harvard University Press.
Goodman, N., Tizard, J. (1962) 'Prevalence of imbecility and idiocy among children.' *Brit. med. J.* **5723,** 216.
Goodman, N., Richardson, S. A., Dornbusch, S. M., Hastort, A. H. (1963) 'Variant reactions to physical disabilities.' *Amer. sociol. Rev.*, **28,** 429.
Gordon, N. (1958) 'The minor epilepsies of childhood.' *Postgrad. med. J.*, **34,** 474.
—— (1965) 'The natural history of petit mal epilepsy.' *Develop. Med. Child Neurol.*, **7,** 537.
—— (1968) 'Folic acid deficiency from anticonvulsant therapy.' *Develop. Med. Child Neurol.*, **10,** 497.
—— Taylor I. G. (1964) 'The assessment of children with difficulties of communication.' *Brain*, **87,** 121.
Grady, P. A. E., Daniels, J. C. (1964) 'A survey of the incidence of speech defect in children.' University of Nottingham Institute of Education, Educational Papers No. 1. Nottingham: University of Nottingham.
Graham, F. K., Berman, P. W. (1961) 'Current status of behavior tests for brain damage in infants and pre-school children.' *Amer. J. Orthopsychiat.*, **31,** 713.
Graham, P., Rutter, M. (1968) 'The reliability and validity of the psychiatric assessment of the child. II. Interview with the parent.' *Brit. J. Psychiat.*, **114,** 581.
Grant, Q. A. F. R. (1958) Age and Sex Trends in the Symptomatology of Disturbed Children. Unpublished D.P.M. Dissertation, University of London.

Greulich, W. W., Crismon, C. S., Turner, M. L. (1953) 'The physical growth and development of children who survived the atomic bombing of Hiroshima or Nagasaki.' *J. Pediat.*, **43**, 121.
Griffith, H., Davidson, M. (1966) 'Long-term changes in intellect and behaviour after hemispherectomy.' *J. Neurol. Neurosurg. Psychiat.*, **29**, 571.
Griffiths, M. I., Barrett, N. M. (1967) 'Cerebral palsy in Birmingham.' *Develop. Med. Child Neurol.*, **9**, 33.
Griffiths, R. (1954) The Abilities of Babies. London: University of London Press.
Gronlund, N. E. (1959) Sociometry in the Classroom. New York: Harper & Row.
Gruenberg, E. M. (1966) 'Epidemiology of mental illness.' *Int. J. Psychiat.*, **2**, 78.
Grünberg, F., Pond, D. A. (1957) 'Conduct disorders in epileptic children.' *J. Neurol. Neurosurg. Psychiat.*, **20**, 65.
Gubbay, S. S., Ellis, E., Walton, J. N., Court, S. D. M. (1965) 'Clumsy children: a study of apraxic and agnosic defects in 21 children.' *Brain*, **88**, 295.
Gudmundsson, G. (1966) 'Epilepsy in Iceland: a clinical and epidemiological investigation.' *Acta. Neurol. scand.*, **43**, Suppl. 25.
Gudmundsson, K. R. (1967) 'Cerebral palsy in Iceland.' *Acta neurol. scand.*, Suppl. 34.
Guttman, E. (1942) 'Aphasia in children.' *Brain*, **65**, 205.
Halstead, H. (1957) 'Abilities and behaviour of epileptic children.' *J. ment. Sci.*, **103**, 28.
Hamilton, M., Pond, D. A., Ryle, A. (1962) 'Relation of C.M.I. responses to some social and psychological factors.' *J. psychosom. Res.*, **6**, 157.
Hansen, E. (1960) 'Cerebral palsy in Denmark.' *Acta psychiat. neurol. scand.*, Suppl. 146.
Harlow, H. F., Akert, K., Schiltz, K. A. (1964) 'The effects of bilateral prefrontal lesions on learned behaviour of neonatal infant and preadolescent monkeys.' *in* Warren, J. M., Akert, K. (Eds.) The Frontal Granular Cortex and Behaviour. New York: McGraw-Hill.
—— Blomquist, A. J., Thompson, C. I., Schiltz, K. A., Harlow, M. K. (1968) 'Effects of induction age and size of frontal lobe lesions on learning in Rhesus monkeys.' *in* Isaacson, R. L. (Ed.) The Neuropsychology of Development. New York: Wiley.
Harper, J. R. (1968) 'True myoclonic epilepsy in childhood.' *Arch. Dis. Childh.*, **43**, 28.
Harrington, J. A., Letemendia, F. J. J. (1958) 'Persistent psychiatric disorders after head injuries in children.' *J. ment. Sci.*, **104**, 1205.
Harvald, B. (1954) Heredity in Epilepsy. Copenhagen: Munksgaard.
Hatton, D. A. (1966) 'The child with minimal cerebral dysfunction.' *Develop. Med. Child Neurol.*, **8**, 71.
Hebb, D. O. (1942) 'The effect of early and late brain injury upon test scores, and the nature of normal adult intelligence.' *Proc. Amer. phil. Soc.*, **85**, 275.
Hecaen, H. (1962) 'Clinical symptomatology in right and left hemispheric lesions.' *in* Mountcastle, V. B. (Ed.) Interhemispheric Relations and Cerebral Dominance. Baltimore: Johns Hopkins.
Hefferline, R. F. (1958) 'The role of proprioception in the control of behavior.' *Trans. N.Y. Acad. Sci.*, **20**, 739.
Hellebrandt, F. A., Waterland, J. C. (1962) 'Expansion of motor patterning under exercise stress.' *Amer. J. phys. Med.*, **41**, 56.
Henderson, J. L. (Ed.) (1961) Cerebral Palsy in Childhood and Adolescence: a Medical, Psychological and Social Study. Edinburgh: E. & S. Livingstone.
Henderson, P. (1953) 'Epilepsy in school children.' *Brit. J. prev. soc. Med.*, **7**, 9.
Herbert, M. (1964) 'The concept and testing of brain damage in children: a review.' *J. Child. Psychol. Psychiat.*, **5**, 197.
Herlitz, G., Redin, B. (1955) 'The prevalence of cerebral palsy.' *Acta paediat. scand.*, **44**, 146.
Hersov, L. A. (1963) 'Emotional factors in cerebral palsy.' *Develop. Med. Child Neurol.*, **5**, 504.
Hertzig, M. E., Bortner, M., Birch, H. G. (1969) 'Neurologic findings in children educationally designated as 'brain-damaged'.' *Amer. J. Orthopsychiat.*, **39**, 437.
Hewett, S., Newson, J., Newson, E. (1970) The Family and the Handicapped Child: A Study of Cerebral Palsied Children in their Homes. London: Allen & Unwin.
Hill, D., Falconer, M. A., Pampiglione, G., Liddell, D. W. (1953) 'Discussion on the surgery of temporal lobe epilepsy: the clinical study and selection of patients.' *Proc. roy. Soc. Med.*, **46**, 965.
Hill, R. (1949) Families Under Stress: Adjustment to the Crisis of War, Separation and Reunion. New York: Harper.
Hjern, B., Nylander, I. (1962) 'Late prognosis of severe head injuries in childhood.' *Arch. Dis. Childh.*, **37**, 113.
Holden, R. H., Solomons, G. (1962) 'Relations between pediatric, psychological and neurological examinations during the first year of life.' *Child Develop.*, **33**, 719.
Holoran, I. M. (1952) 'The incidence and prognosis of cerebral palsy: an interim report.' *Brit. med. J.*, **i**, 214.
Holowach, J., Thurston, D. L., O'Leary, J. L. (1962) 'Petit mal epilepsy.' *Pediatrics*, **30**, 893.
Holroyd, J., Wright, F. (1965) 'Neurological implications of WISC verbal-performance discrepancies in a psychiatric setting.' *J. consult. Psychol.*, **29**, 206.
Holt, K. S. (1961) 'The plantar response in infants and children.' *Cerebral Palsy Bull.*, **3**, 449.

Hopkins, K. D. (1964) 'An empirical analysis of the efficacy of the WISC in the diagnosis of organicity in children of normal intelligence.' *J. genet. Psychol.*, **105**, 163.
Horne, B. M., Justiss, W. A. (1967) 'Clinical indicators of brain damage in mentally retarded children.' *J. clin. Psychol.*, **23**, 464.
Hutt, S. J. (1967) 'Epilepsy and education' *in* What is Special Education? *Proc. First Int. Conf. Ass. Spec. Educ.* 25th-28th July 1966. London: Association for Special Education.
—— Hutt, C. (1964) 'Hyperactivity in a group of epileptic (and some non-epileptic) brain damaged children.' *Epilepsia*, **5**, 334.
—— Jackson, P. M., Belsham, A., Higgins, G. (1968) 'Perceptual motor behaviour in relation to blood phenobarbitone level: a preliminary report.' *Develop. Med. Child Neurol.*, **10**, 626.
Illingworth, R. S. (Ed.) (1958) Recent Advances in Cerebral Palsy. London: J. & A. Churchill.
—— (1961) An Introduction to Developmental Assessment in the First Year. Little Club Clinics No. 3. London: SIMP/Heinemann Medical.
—— Woods, G. E., Gordon, R. R., Roberts, L. (1961) 'Social status of the parents of cerebral palsied children.' *Cerebral Palsy Bull.*, **3**, 157.
Ingram, T. T. S. (1955) 'A study of cerebral palsy in the childhood population of Edinburgh.' *Arch. Dis. Childh.*, **30**, 85.
—— (1956) 'A characteristic form of overactive behaviour in brain-damaged children.' *J. ment. Sci.*, **102**, 550.
—— (1959*a*) 'A description and classification of the common disorders of speech in children.' *Arch. Dis. Childh.*, **30**, 444.
—— (1959*b*) 'Specific developmental disorders of speech in childhood.' *Brain*, **82**, 450.
—— (1963*a*) 'The association of speech retardation and educational difficulties.' *Proc. roy. Soc. Med.*, **56**, 199.
—— (1963*b*) 'Chronic brain syndromes in childhood other than cerebral palsy, epilepsy and mental defect.' *in* Bax, M., Mac Keith, R. (Eds.) Minimal Cerebral Dysfunction. Clinics in Developmental Medicine No. 10. London: SIMP/Heinemann Medical.
—— (1963*c*) Report of the Dysphasia Subcommittee of the Scottish Paediatric Society. Unpublished report.
—— (1964) Paediatric Aspects of Cerebral Palsy. Edinburgh: E. & S. Livingstone.
—— (1968) 'Speech disorders in childhood.' *Pediat. Clin. N. Amer.*, **15**, 611.
—— (1970) Edinburgh Tests of Phonetic Maturation. Edinburgh: Edinburgh University Press.
—— Barn, J. (1960) 'A description and classification of common speech disorders associated with cerebral palsy.' *Cerebr. Palsy Bull.*, **3**, 57.
—— Russell, E. M. (1961) 'The reproductive histories of mothers of patients suffering from congenital diplegia.' *Arch. Dis. Childh.*, **36**, 34.
Isaacson, R. L., Nonneman, A. J., Schmaltz, L. W. (1968) 'Behavioural and anatomical sequelae of the infant limbic system.' *in* Isaacson, R. L. (Ed.) The Neuropsychology of Development. New York: Wiley.
Jackson, H. (1878) 'Remarks on non protrusion of the tongue in some cases of aphasia.' *Lancet*, **1**, 716.
Jackson, S. (1966) Special Education in England and Wales. London: Oxford University Press.
Jacobs, J. F., Pierce, M. L. (1968) 'The social position of retardates with brain-damage-associated characteristics.' *Except. Child*, **34**, 677.
Jaeger, R. (1953) 'Congenital spinal meningocele.' *J. Amer. med. Ass.*, **153**, 792.
James, I. P. (1960) 'Temporal lobectomy for psychomotor epilepsy.' *J. ment. Sci.*, **106**, 543.
Jenkins, R. L. (1935) 'Dissimilar identical twins: results of brain injury at birth.' *Amer. J. Orthopsychiat.*, **5**, 39.
Jensen, A. R. (1964) 'The Rorschach technique: a re-evaluation.' *Acta psychol.*, **22**, 60.
Jones, R. L., Gottfried, N. W., Owens, A. (1966) 'The social distance of the exceptional: a study at the high school level.' *Except. Child*, **32**, 551.
Jones, S. (1962) 'The Wechsler Intelligence Scale for Children applied to a sample of London primary school children.' *Brit. J. Educ. Psychol.*, **32**, 119.
Jordan, T. E. (1962) 'Research on the handicapped child and the family.' *Merrill Palmer Quart. Behav. Develop.*, **8**, 243.
Joynt, R. J., Benton, A. L., Fogel, M. L. (1962) 'Behavioural and pathological correlates of motor impersistence.' *Neurology (Minneap.)*, **12**, 876.
Kahn, E., Cohen, L. H. (1934) 'Organic drivenness: a brain stem syndrome and an experience.' *New Eng. J. Med.*, **210**, 748.
Kaplan, F. (1969) 'Siblings of the retarded.' *in* Sarason, S. B., Doris, J. (Eds.) Psychological Problems in Mental Deficiency. New York: Harper and Row.
Keating, L. E. (1961) 'Epilepsy and behaviour disorder in school children.' *J. ment. Sci.*, **107**, 161.
Kennard, M. A. (1936) 'Age and other factors in motor recovery from precentral lesions in monkeys.' *Amer. J. Physiol.*, **115**, 138.
—— (1938) 'Reorganisation of motor function in the cerebral cortex of monkeys deprived of motor and premotor areas in infancy.' *J. Neurophysiol.*, **1**, 477.

—— (1942) 'Cortical reorganisation of motor function: studies on series of monkeys of various ages from infancy to maturity.' *Arch. Neurol. Psychiat.*, **48,** 227.
——(1960) 'Value of equivocal signs in neurologic diagnosis.' *Neurology* (*Minneap*)., **10,** 753.
Kling, A., Tucker, T. J. (1968) 'Sparing of function following localised brain lesions in neonatal monkeys. *in* Isaacson, R. L. (Ed.) The Neuropsychology of Development. New York: Wiley.
Klonoff, H., Robinson, G. C., Thompson, G. (1969) 'Acute and chronic brain syndromes in children.' *Develop. Med. Child Neurol.*, **11,** 198.
Knights, R. M., Tymchuk, A. J. (1968) 'An evaluation of the Halstead-Reitan category tests for children.' *Cortex*, **4,** 403.
Knobel, M., Wolman, M. B., Mason, E. (1959) 'Hyperkinesis and organicity in children.' *Arch. gen. Psychiat.*, **1,** 310.
Knobloch, H., Pasamanick, B. (1962) 'The developmental behavioural approach to the neurologic examination in infancy.' *Child Develop.*, **33,** 181.
—— —— (1966) 'Prospective studies on the epidemiology of reproductive casualty: methods, findings and some implications.' *Merrill Palmer Quart. Behav. Develop.*, **12,** 27.
—— —— (1967) 'Prediction from the assessment of neuromotor and intellectual status in infancy.' *in* Zubin, J., Jervis, C. A. (Eds.) Psychopathology of Mental Development. London: Grune & Stratton.
Kurland, L. T. (1958) 'Descriptive epidemiology of selected neurologic and myopathic disorders with particular reference to a survey in Rochester, Minnesota.' *J. chron. Dis.*, **8,** 378.
—— (1959) 'The incidence and prevalence of convulsive disorders in a small urban community.' *Epilepsia*, **1,** 143.
Kushlick, A. (1961) 'Subnormality in Salford.' *in* Susser, M. W., Kushlick, A. A Report on the Mental Health Services of Salford for the Year 1960. Salford Health Dept.
—— (1964) 'The prevalance of recognised mental subnormality of I.Q. under 50 among children in the South of England.' Proceedings of the International Conference on the Scientific Study of Mental Retardation, Copenhagen. Copenhagen: Statens & Andssvageforsorg. p. 550.
—— (1965) 'Community services for the mentally subnormal: a plan for experimental evaluation.' *Proc. roy. Soc. Med.*, **58,** 374.
Kuzma, J. W., Tourtellotte, W. W., Remington, R. D. (1965) 'Quantitative clinical neurological testing. II. Some statistical considerations of a battery of tests.' *J. chron. Dis.*, **18,** 303.
Landau, W. M., Goldstein, R., Kleffner, F. R. (1960) 'Congenital aphasia: a clinicopathologic study.' *Neurology* (*Minneap.*), **10,** 915.
Lapouse, R. (1965) 'The relationship of behaviour to adjustment in a representative sample of children.' *Amer. J. publ. Hlth.*, **55,** 1130.
Lassner, R. (1948) 'Annotated bibliography on the Oseretsky tests of motor proficiency.' *J. consult. Psychol.*, **12,** 37.
Laufer, M. W., Denhoff, E., Solomons, G. (1957) 'Hyperkinetic impulse disorder in children's behaviour problems.' *Psychosom. Med.*, **19,** 38.
Laurence, K. M., Carter, C. O., David, P. A. (1967) 'Major central nervous system malformations in South Wales. I. Incidence, local variations and geographical factors.' *Brit. J. prev. Soc. Med.*, **22,** 146.
Lawson, D., Metcalfe, M., Pampiglione, G. (1965) 'Meningitis in childhood.' *Brit. med. J.*, **i,** 557.
Lee, J. A. H. (1958) 'The effectiveness of routine examination of school children.' *Brit. med. J.*, **i,** 573.
Lees, F., Liversedge, L. A. (1962) 'The prognosis of petit mal and minor epilepsy.' *Lancet*, **ii,** 797.
Leeson, J. (1965) 'Evaluation of a questionnaire to parents as a method of screening school children.' *Med. Offr.*, **113,** 313.
Leff, R. (1968) 'Behavior modification and the psychoses of childhood.' *Psychol. Bull.*, **369,** 396.
Lenneberg, E. H. (1967) Biological Foundations of Language. New York: Wiley.
Lewandowsky, M. von (1907) 'Uber Apraxie des Lidschlusses.' *Neurol. Zbl.*, **26,** 720
Levy, P. M. (1962) 'Ability and attainment: a new psychometric formulation of the concept of educational retardation.' *Brit. J. statist. Psychol.*, **15,** 137.
Lewis, E. O. (1929) Report of the mental deficiency committee, Part IV. Report of an investigation into the incidence of mental deficiency in 6 areas, 1925-1927. London: H.M.S.O.
Lewis, M. M. (1963) Language, Thought and Personality in Infancy and Childhood. London: Harrap.
Lindsay, J. M. M. (1966) 'Biological factors in temporal lobe epilepsy.' Ph.D. Thesis, Belfast (cited in Hutt, S. J., 'Epilepsy and education' *in* What is Special Education?). London: Association for Special Education.
Lishman, W. A. (1968) 'Brain damage in relation to psychiatric disability after head injury.' *Brit. J. Psychiat.*, **114,** 373.
Littell, W. M. (1960) 'Wechsler Intelligence Scale for Children: review of a decade of research.' *Psychol. Bull.*, **57,** 132.
Lockyer, L., Rutter, M. (1970) 'A five to fifteen year follow-up study of infantile psychosis. IV. Patterns of cognitive ability.' *Brit. J. soc. clin. Psychol.* (in press)
Lorber, J. (1961) 'Long-term follow-up of 100 children who recovered from tuberculous meningitis.' *Pediatrics*, **28,** 778.

Lucas, A. R., Rodin, E. A., Simson, C. B. (1965) 'Neurological assessment of children with early school problems.' *Develop. Med. Child Neurol.*, **7,** 145.
Luria, A. R. (1957) 'The role of language in the formation of temporary connections.' *in* Simon, B. (Ed.) Psychology in the Soviet Union. London: Routledge and Kegan Paul.
Luria, A. R. (1966) Higher Cortical Functions in Man. London: Tavistock Publications.
—— Yudovich, F. I. (1959) Speech and the Development of Mental Processes in the Child. London: Staples Press.
Luszki, W. A. (1965) 'Hearing loss and intelligence among retardates.' *Amer. J. ment. Defic.* **70,** 93.
Macfarlane, J. W., Allen, L., Honzik, M. P. (1954) 'A developmental study of the behaviour problems of normal children between 21 months and 14 years.' Berkeley: University of California Press.
MacGregor, M., Pirrie, D., Shaddick, C. W. (1957) 'Cerebral palsy in the county of London.' *Med. Offr.*, **98,** 367.
Mac Keith, R. C. (1963) 'Defining the concept of 'minimal brain damage.' *in* Bax, M., Mac Keith, R. (Eds.) Minimal Cerebral Dysfunction. Clinics in Developmental Medicine No. 10. London: SIMP/Heinemann Medical.
—— Mackenzie, I. C. K., Polani, P. E. (1959) 'The Little Club Memorandum on terminology and classification of cerebral palsy.' *Cerebral Palsy Bull.*, **1,** (5), 27.
Madonick, M. J. (1960) 'Statistical control studies in neurology: relationship between frequencies of reflexes in a group of 2500 non-neurologic patients. Babinski, Hoffman, Rossolimo, Oppenheim, Gordon signs and absent cutaneous abdominal reflexes.' *J. nerv. ment. Dis.*, **131,** 547.
Malmquist, E. (1958) 'Factors related to reading disability in the first grade of the elementary school.' Acta Universitatis Stockholmiensis. Stockholm: Alinquist & Wiksell.
Margerison, J. H., Corsellis, J. A. N. (1966) 'Epilepsy and the temporal lobes: a clinical, electroencephalographic and neuropathological study of the brain in epilepsy, with particular reference to the temporal lobes.' *Brain*, **89,** 499.
—— Liddell, D. W. (1961) 'The incidence of temporal lobe epilepsy among a hospital population of long-stay female epileptics. *J. ment. Sci.*, **107,** 909.
Marshall, W. A. (1968) Development of the Brain. Edinburgh: Oliver & Boyd.
Marstrander, J. (1968) 'A longitudinal study of mental and motor development in children with a birth weight of less than 2,000 grams: the prognostic value of neurological signs in infancy.' *J. Oslo. Cy. Hosp.*, **18,** 61.
Mason, A. W. (1967) 'Specific (developmental) dyslexia.' *Develop. Med. Child Neurol.*, **9,** 183.
Maxwell, A. E. (1959) 'A factoral analysis of the Wechsler Intelligence Scale for Children.' *Brit. J. educ. Psychol.*, **29,** 237.
—— (1962) Personal communication.
McCance, C., Watt, J. A., Hall, D. J. (1968) 'An evaluation of the reliability and validity of the plantar response in a psychogeriatric population.' *J. Chron. Dis.*, **21,** 369.
McCarthy, J. J., Kirk, S. A. (1961) Illinois Test of Psycholinguistic Abilities: experimental edition. Urbana, Ill.: University of Illinois Press.
McCord, W., McCord, J., Zola, I. K. (1959) Origins of Crime. New York: Columbia University Press.
McDonald, A. D. (1963) 'Cerebral palsy in children of very low birth weight.' *Arch. Dis. Childh.*, **38,** 579.
McFie, J. (1961*a*) 'The effects of hemispherectomy on intellectual functioning in cases of infantile hemiplegia.' *J. Neurol. Neurosurg. Psychiat.*, **24,** 240.
—— (1961*b*) 'Intellectual impairment in children with localised post-infantile cerebral lesions.' *J. Neurol. Neurosurg. Psychiat.*, **24,** 361.
—— (1963) 'An introduction to the problem of 'minimal brain damage'.' *in* Bax, M., Mac Keith, R. (Eds.) Minimal Cerebral Dysfunction. Clinics in Developmental Medicine No. 10. London: SIMP/Heinemann Medical.
McGreal, D. A. (1966) 'A survey of cerebral palsy in Windsor and Essex County, Ontario.' *Canad. med. Ass. J.*, **95,** 1237.
Meade, T. W., Gardner, M. J. (1968) 'Observer variability in cardiology.' *Proc. Roy. Soc. Med.*, **61,** 451.
Menyuk, P. (1964) 'Comparison of grammar of children with functionally deviant and normal speech.' *J. speech hearing Res.*, **7,** 109.
Meyer, E., Byers, R. K. (1952) 'Measles encephalitis: a follow-up study of sixteen patients.' *Amer. J. Dis. Child.*, **84,** 543.
Meyer, V. (1957) 'Critique of psychological approaches to brain damage.' *J. ment. Sci.*, **103,** 80.
Miles, T. R. (1967) 'In defence of the concept of dyslexia.' *in* Downing, J., Brown, A. L. (Eds.) The Second International Reading Symposium. London: Cassell.
Miller, B. (1964) 'Some effects of frontal lobectomy in man.' *in* Warren, J. M., Akert, K. (Eds.) The Frontal Granular Cortex and Behaviour. New York: McGraw-Hill.
Miller, F. J. W., Court, S. D. M., Walton, W. S., Knox, E. G. (1960) Growing Up in Newcastle-on-Tyne. London: Oxford University Press.
Miller, J. D., Ross, C. (1968) 'Encephalitis, a four-year survey.' *Lancet*, **i,** 1121.

Milner, B. (1962) 'Laterality effects in audition.' *in* Mountcastle, V. B. (Ed.) Interhemispheric Relations and Cerebral Dominance. Baltimore: Johns Hopkins Press.
Ministry of Education (1955) Report of the Committee on Maladjusted Children. London: H.M.S.O.
—— (1962) The Health of the School Child, 1960-61: Chapter 10 'Children with Epilepsy'. London: H.M.S.O.
—— (1963) A Report on a Survey of Deaf Children who have been Transferred from Special Schools or Units to Ordinary Schools. London: H.M.S.O.
Minkowski, A. (Ed.) (1967) Regional Development of The Brain in Early Life. Oxford: Blackwell.
Mitchell, R. G. (1961) 'The definition and classification of cerebral palsy.' *in* Henderson, J. L. (Ed.) Cerebral Palsy in Childhood and Adolescence. Edinburgh: E. & S. Livingstone.
Morley, M. E. (1965) The Development and Disorders of Speech in Childhood. Edinburgh: E. & S. Livingstone.
—— Court, D., Miller, H., Garside, R. F. (1955) 'Delayed speech and developmental aphasia.' *Brit. med. J.*, **ii,** 463.
Morrell, F. (1956) 'Interseizure disturbances in focal epilepsy.' *Neurology* (*Minneap.*), **6,** 327.
Mowat, J. (1961) 'Ear, nose and throat disorders: deafness.' *in* Henderson, J. L. (Ed.) Cerebral Palsy in Childhood and Adolescence. Edinburgh: E. & S. Livingstone. p. 242.
Munro, D. (1961) 'Dental features.' *in* Henderson, J. L. (Ed.) Cerebral Palsy in Childhood and Adolescence. Edinburgh: E. & S. Livingstone. p. 254.
Myklebust, H. R. (1960) The Psychology of Deafness. London: Grune and Stratton.
Napier, J. A. (1962) 'Field methods and response rates in the Tecumseh community health study.' *Amer. J. publ. Hlth.*, **52,** 208.
Nathan, P. W., Smith, M.C. (1955) 'The Babinski response: a review and new observations.' *J. Neurol. Neurosurg. Psychiat.*, **18,** 250.
Neale, M. D. (1958) Neale Analysis of Reading Ability Manual. London: Macmillan.
Nelson, K. B. (1968) 'The continuum of reproductive casualty.' *in* Mac Keith, R., Bax, M. (Eds.) Studies in Infancy. Clinics in Developmental Medicine. No. 27. London: SIMP/Heinemann Medical.
Netley, C., Rachman, S., Turner, R. K. (1965) 'The effect of practice on performance in a reading attainment test.' *Brit. J. educ. Psychol.*, **35,** 1.
Newman, J. R., Loos, F. M. (1955) 'Differences between verbal and performance IQs with mentally defective children on the WISC.' *J. consult. Psychol.*, **19,** 16.
Newson, J., Newson, E. (1968) Four Years Old in an Urban Community. London: Allen & Unwin.
Nielsen, H. H. (1966) A Psychological Study of Cerebral Palsied Children. Copenhagen: Munksgaard.
Norman, R. M. (1945) 'Thalamic degeneration following bilateral premotor frontal lobe atrophy of the Strümpell type.' *J. Neurol. Neurosurg. Psychiat.*, **8,** 52.
Norris, H. (1960) 'The WISC and diagnosis of brain damage.' University of London Dissertation (unpublished).
Nuffield, E. J. A. (1961) 'Neurophysiology and behaviour disorders in epileptic children.' *J. ment. Sci.*, **107,** 438.
Nyhan, W. L., Richardson, F. (1963) 'Complications of meningitis.' *Ann.. rev. Med.*, **14,** 243.
O'Connor, N. (1956) 'The evidence for the permanently disturbing effects of mother-child separation.' *Acta psychol.*, **12,** 174.
—— (1968) 'Children in restricted environments.' *in* Newton, G., Levine, S. (Eds.) Early Experience and Behaviour. Springfield, Ill.: C. C. Thomas.
—— Hermelin, B. (1963) Speech and Thought in Severe Subnormality. London: Pergamon.
Ogden, D. A. (1959) 'Use of surgical rehabilitation in young delinquents.' *Brit. Med. J.*, **i,** 432.
Oldfield, R. C., Williams, M. (1961) 'Cerebral trauma in infancy and intellectual defect.' *J. Neurol. Neurosurg. Psychiat.*, **24,** 32.
Oldham, P. D. (1968) 'Observer error in medicine. Observer error—a potential asset.' *Proc. Roy. Soc. Med.*, **61,** 447.
Orlansky, H. (1949) 'Infant care and personality.' *Psychol. Bull.* **46,** 1.
Oseretsky, N. (1931) 'Psychomotorik Methoden zur untersuchung der Motorik.' *Z. angewandt. Psychol.*, **17,** 1. (Unpublished translation, Lang, E., (1949), quoted by Sloan, 1955).
Oswin, M. (1967) Behaviour Problems Among Children with Cerebral Palsy. Bristol: Wright.
Ounsted, C. (1955) 'The hyperkinetic syndrome in epileptic children.' *Lancet*, **ii,** 303.
—— (1968) 'Attention, intelligence and seizures of the immature brain.' Third Shorvon Memorial Lecture (unpublished).
—— (1970) 'A biological approach to autistic and hyperkinetic syndromes.' *in* Apley, J. (Ed.) Modern Trends in Paediatrics. London: Butterworths.
—— Lindsay, J., Norman, R. (1966) Biological Factors in Temporal Lobe Epilepsy. Clinics in Developmental Medicine. No. 22. London: SIMP/Heinemann Medical.
Paine, R. S. (1962) 'Minimal chronic brain syndromes in children.' *Develop. Med. Child. Neurol.*, **4,** 21.
—— (1968) 'Syndromes of "minimal cerebral damage".' *Pediat. Clin. N. Amer.*, **15,** 779.
—— Oppé, T. E. (1966) Neurological Examination of Children. Clinics in Developmental Medicine No. 20/21. London: SIMP/Heinemann Medical.

—— Werry, J. S., Quay, H. C. (1968) 'A study of 'minimal cerebral dysfunction'.' *Develop. Med. Child Neurol.*, **10**, 505.
Pasamanick B., Knobloch, H. (1961) 'Epidemiologic studies on the complications of pregnancy and the birth process,' *in* Caplan, G. (Ed.) Prevention of Mental Disorders in Children. New York: Basic Books.
—— ——(1966) 'Retrospective studies on the epidemiology of reproductive casualty: old and new.' *Merrill Palmer Quart. Behav. Develop.*, **12**, 7.
Patterson, C. H. (1953) The Wechsler-Bellevue Scales—a Guide for Counsellors. Springfield, Ill.: C. C. Thomas.
Payne, R. W. (1955) 'L'utilité du test de Rorschach en psychologie clinique.' *Rev. Psychol. appl.*, **5**, 255.
Peiper, A. (1963) Cerebral Function in Infancy and Childhood. London: Pitman.
Penrose, L. S. (1963) The Biology of Mental Defect. (3rd Edn.) London: Sidgwick & Jackson.
—— Smith, C. F. (1966). Down's Anomaly. London: J. & A. Churchill.
Perlstein, M. A. (1952) 'Infantile cerebral palsy; classification and clinical correlations.' *J. Amer. med. Ass.*, **149**, 30.
—— Barnett, H. E. (1952) 'Nature and recognition of cerebral palsy in infancy.' *J. Amer. med. Ass.*, **148**, 1389.
Peterman, M. G. (1946) 'Convulsions in childhood; twenty year study of 2,500 cases.' *Amer. J. Dis. Child.*, **72**, 399.
Phelps, W. M. (1941) 'The rehabilitation of cerebral palsy.' *Sth. Med. J.*, **34**, 770.
—— (1949) 'Description and differentiation of types of cerebral palsy.' *Nerv. Child*, **8**, 107.
Pickles, D. C. (1966) 'The Wechsler Performance Scale and its relationship to speech and educational response in deaf slow-learning children.' *Teacher of the Deaf*, 382.
Piercy, M. F. (1964) 'The effects of cerebral lesions on intellectual function: a review of recent research trends.' *Brit. J. Psychiat.*, **110**, 310.
Pineas, H. (1924) 'Hirnbedfunde bei Apraxie.' *Zbl. f. d. ges. Neurol. Psychiat.*, **35**, 446.
Pinneau, S. R. (1955) 'The infantile disorders of hospitalism and anaclitic depression.' *Psychol. Bull.*, **52**, 429.
Pond, D. A. (1951) 'L'electroencephalographie en psychiatrie infantile.' Psychiatrie Sociale de l'Enfant. Centre Internationale de l'Enfance, Travaux et Documents, II. Paris: Centre Internationale de l'Enfance.
—— (1960) 'Is there a syndrome of 'brain damage' in children?' *Cerebral Palsy Bull.*, **2**, 296.
—— (1961) 'Psychiatric aspects of epileptic and brain-damaged children'. *Brit. med. J.*, **ii**, 1378, 1454.
—— (1963) 'The EEG in paediatrics.' *in* Hill, J. D. N., Parr, G. (Eds.) Electroencephalography: A Symposium on its Various Aspects (2nd Ed.). London: MacDonald.
—— Bidwell, B. H. (1960) 'A survey of epilepsy in fourteen general practices. II. Social and psychological aspects.' *Epilepsia*, **1**, 285.
—— Burden, G. S. (1963) 'Review of the social and medical services for the epileptic patient in England and Wales.' *Epilepsia*, **4**, 77.
—— Landucci, L. (1954) 'L'elettroencefalografia in psichiatria infantile.' *Minerva Med.*, **1**, 188.
—— Bidwell, B. H., Stein, L. (1960) 'A survey of epilepsy in fourteen general practices. I. Demographic and medical data.' *Psychiat. Neurol. Neurochir.* (*Amst.*), **63**, 217.
Prechtl, H. F. R. (1965) 'Neurologische afwigkingen na pre-en paranatale hypoxie.' *Ned. Tid. Geneesk.*, **109**, 1991.
—— (1967) 'Neurologic sequelae of prenatal and perinatal complications.' *Brit. med. J.*, **iv**, 763.
—— Beintema, D. J. (1964) Neurological Examination of the Full Term Newborn Infant. Clinics in Developmental Medicine No. 12. London: SIMP/Heinemann Medical.
Preston, M. I. (1945) 'Late behavioural aspects found in cases of prenatal, natal and postnatal anoxia.' *J. Pediat.*, **26**, 353.
Price, J. C. (1950) 'The epileptic child in school.' *Ohio State J. Med.*, **46**, 794.
Pringle, M. L. K. (1964) The Emotional and Social Adjustment of Physically Handicapped Children. London: National Foundation for Educational Research.
Ravenette, A. T. (1961) 'Vocabulary level and reading attainment; an empirical approach to the assessment of reading retardation.' *Brit. J. educ. Psychol.*, **31**, 96.
Rawnsley, K. (1966) 'Congruence of independent measures of psychiatric morbidity.' *J. psychosom. Res.*, **10**, 84.
Registrar-General (1964) Statistical Review of England and Wales for the Year 1962. Part I. Tables, Medical. London: H.M.S.O.
Reitan, R. M. (1967) 'Psychological assessment of deficits associated with brain lesions in subjects with normal and subnormal intelligence.' *in* Khanna, J. L. (Ed.) Brain Damage and Mental Retardation: a Psychological Evaluation. Springfield Ill.: C. C. Thomas.
—— Heineman, C. E. (1968) 'Interactions of neurological deficits and emotional disturbance in children with learning disorders: methods for differential diagnosis.' *in* Hellmuth, J. (Ed.) Learning Disorders. Vol. 3. Seattle: Special Child Publications.
Renfrew, C. (1966) Articulation Attainment Test. Abingdon: Abbey Press.
Reuben, R. N., Bakwin, H. (1968) 'Developmental clumsiness.' *Pediat. Clin. N. Amer.*, **15**, 601.

Reynell, J. (1970) Language Scales. Slough, Bucks.: National Foundation for Educational Research.
Reynolds, E. H. (1968) 'Mental effects of anticonvulsants and folic acid metabolism.' *Brain*, **91,** 197.
Richardson, S. A., Royce, J. (1968) 'Race and physical handicap in children's preference for other children.' *Child Develop.* **39,** 467.
—— Goodman, N., Hastorf, A. H., Dornbusch, S. (1961) 'Cultural uniformity in reaction to physical disabilities.' *Amer. Sociol. Rev.*, **26,** 241.
Riesen, A. (1965) 'Effects of early deprivation of photic stimulation.' *in* Osler, S. F , Cooke, R. E., (Eds.) The Biosocial Basis of Mental Retardation. Baltimore: Johns Hopkins.
Robins, L. N. (1966) Deviant Children Grown Up. Baltimore: Williams and Wilkins.
—— (1970) 'Social correlates of psychiatric illness: can we tell causes from consequences?' *Ass. Res. nerv. ment. Dis. Proc.* (in press).
Rodin, E., Lucas, A., Simpson, C. (1963) 'A study of behaviour disorders in children by means of general purpose computers.' *in* Enslein, K. (Ed.) Data Acquisition and Processing in Biology and Medicine, Vol. 3. London: Pergamon. p. 115.
Roethlisberger, F. J., Dickson, W. (1939) Management and the Worker. Cambridge Mass.: Harvard University Press.
Rogers, C. R. (1942) 'The criteria used in a study of mental health problems.' *Educ. Res. Bull.*, **21,** 29.
Rogers, M. E., Lilienfeld, A. M., Pasamanick, B. (1955) 'Prenatal and paranatal factors in the development of childhood behaviour disorders.' *Acta psychiat. neurol. scand.*, Suppl. 102.
Rose, A. W., Peace, L., McBride, M. (1955) 'On changing social concepts of epilepsy.' *Epilepsia*, **4,** 99.
Rosenblith, J. F. (1966) 'Prognostic value of neonatal assessment.' *Child Develop.*, **37,** 623.
Rosenzweig, M. R., Bennett, E. L., Diamond, M. C. (1967) 'Effects of differential environments on brain anatomy and brain chemistry.' *in* Zubin, J., Jervis, G. A. (Eds.) Psychopathology of Mental Development. New York: Grune and Stratton.
Russell, W. R. (1948) 'Functions of the frontal lobes.' *Lancet*, **i,** 356.
—— (1959) Brain, Memory and Learning. Oxford: Clarendon Press.
Rutter, M. (1965) 'Classification and categorisation in child psychiatry.' *J. Child Psychol. Psychiat.* **6,** 71.
—— (1966) Children of Sick Parents: An Environmental and Psychiatric Study. Maudsley Monograph No. 16. London: Oxford University Press.
—— (1967*a*) 'Psychotic disorders in early childhood.' *in* Coppen, A., Walk, A. (Eds.) Recent Developments in Schizophrenia. London: Royal Medico-psychological Association.
—— (1967*b*) 'Children's behaviour questionnaire for completion by teachers. Preliminary findings.' *J. Child Psychol. Psychiat.*, **8,** 1.
—— (1967*c*) 'Brain-damaged children.' *New Educ.*, **3,** 10.
—— (1968) 'Lésion cérébrale organique, hyperkinésie et retard mental.' *Psychiat. Enfant*, **11,** 475.
—— (1969*a*) 'The description and classification of infantile autism.' *in* Proceedings of the Indiana University Colloquium on Infantile Autism. (in press.)
—— (1969*b*) The education of autistic children. *in* Proceedings of the First Australian Conference on the Autistic Child, Adelaide, 1967.
—— (1970) 'Sex differences in children's responses to family stress.' *in* Anthony, E. J., Koupernik, C. (Eds.) International Year Book of Child Psychiatry, Vol. I. The child in his family. New York: Wiley.
—— Graham, P. (1966) 'Psychiatric disorder in 10 and 11 year old children.' *Proc. roy. Soc. Med.*, **59,** 382.
—— —— (1968) 'The reliability and validity of the psychiatric assessment of the child. I. Interview with the child.' *Brit. J. Psychiat.*, **114,** 563.
—— —— Birch, H. (1966) 'Inter-relations between the choreiform syndrome, reading disability and psychiatric disorder in children of 8-11 years.' *Develop. Med. Child Neurol.*, **8,** 149.
—— Greenfield, D., Lockyer, L. (1967*a*) 'A 5-15 year follow-up study of infantile psychosis. II. Social and behavioural outcome.' *Brit. J. Psychiat.*, **113,** 1183.
—— Yule, W., Tizard, J., Graham, P. (1967*b*) 'Severe reading retardation: its relationship to maladjustment, epilepsy and neurological disorders.' *in* What is Special Education? Proceedings of the First International Conference of the Association for Special Education. London: Association for Special Education.
—— Tizard, J., Whitmore, K. (Eds.) (1970) Education, Health and Behaviour. London: Longmans, Green.
Sainsbury, P., Grad, J. (1966) 'Evaluating the community psychiatric service in Chichester.' *Millbank Mem. Fund. Quart.*, **44,** Suppl. p. 231.
Sasmor, R. D. (1966) 'Operant conditioning of a small-scale muscle response.' *J. exp. Anal. Behav.*, **9,** 69.
Scharlock, D. P., Tucker, T. J., Strominger, N. L. (1963) 'Auditory discrimination by the cat after neonatal ablation of temporal cortex.' *Science*, **141,** 1197.
Schenectady County Study. Report of the New York State Joint Legislative Committee to study the problem of cerebral palsy (1949). A Survey of Cerebral Palsy in Schenectady County. New York: Legislative Document 55, Section 2.
Schlegel, R. J., Bellanti, J. A. (1969) 'Increased susceptibility of males to infection.' *Lancet*, **2,** 826.

Scholten, J. M. (1965) 'The Babinski reflex.' *Psychiat. Neurol. Neurochir.*, **68,** 279.
Schonell, F. J., Schonell, F. E. (1950) Diagnostic and Attainment Testing. Edinburgh: Oliver and Boyd.
Schulman, J. L., Reisman, J. M. (1959) 'An objective measure of hyperactivity.' *Amer. J. ment. Defic.*, **64,** 455.
—— Kaspar, J. C., Throne, F. M. (1965) Brain Damage and Behaviour: A Clinical-Experimental Study. Springfield, Ill.: C. C. Thomas.
Schulte, F. J. (1966) 'Neonatal convulsions and their relation to epilepsy in early childhood.' *Develop. Med. Child Neurol.*, **8,** 381.
—— Filipp, E., Michaelis, R. (1965) 'Neurologie des Neugeborenen. II. Die Prognose von Funktionsstörungen des zentralen Nervensystems beim Neugeborenen.' *Z. Kinderheiik.*, **93,** 264.
Scottish Council for Research in Education (1967) The Scottish Standardization of WISC. London: University of London Press.
Shaffer, D. (1969) 'Some observations on activity, impulsivity, and attention in groups of boys with and without a conduct disorder and with and without neurological disease.' Unpublished D.P.M. Dissertation, University of London.
Shapiro, M. B. (1951) 'An experimental approach to diagnostic psychological testing.' *J. ment. Sci.*, **97,** 748.
—— (1957) 'Experimental method in the psychological description of the individual psychiatric patient.' *Int. J. soc. Psychiat.*, **3,** 89.
—— (1961) 'The single case in fundamental psychological research.' *Brit. J. med. Psychol.*, **34,** 255.
Shepherd, M., Oppenheim, A. N., Mitchell, S. (1966*a*) 'Childhood behaviour disorders and the child-guidance clinic: an epidemiological study.' *J. Child. Psychol. Psychiat.*, **7,** 39.
—— —— —— (1966*b*) 'The definition and outcome of deviant behaviour in childhood.' *Proc. roy. Soc. Med.*, **59,** 379.
Silverstein, A. B. (1967) 'Estimating full scale IQs from WISC short forms.' *Psychol. Rep.*, **20,** 1264.
Sloan, W. (1955) 'The Lincoln-Oseretsky motor development scale.' *Genet. Psychol. monogr.*, **51,** 183.
Small, J. G. (1962) 'A psychiatric survey of brain-injured children.' *Arch. gen. Psychiat.*, **7,** 120.
—— Milstein, V., Stevens, J. R. (1962) 'Are psychomotor epileptics different? A controlled study. *Arch. Neurol. (Chic.)*, **7,** 187.
—— Small, I. F., Hayden, M. P. (1966) 'Further psychiatric investigations of patients with temporal lobe and non-temporal lobe epilepsy.' *Amer. J. Psychiat.*, **123,** 303.
Smallwood, A. L. (1953) *in* Ministry of Health Memorandum No. 26. London: H.M.S.O. Cited by Henderson (1961).
Smith, J. R. (1941) 'The frequency growth of the human alpha rhythms during normal infancy and childhood.' *J. Psychol.*, **11,** 177.
Soldwedel, B., Terrill, I. (1957) 'Physically handicapped and non-handicapped children in the same elementary school.' *Except. Child*, **23,** 371.
Solomons, G., Holden, R. H., Denhoff, E. (1963) 'The changing picture of cerebral dysfunction in early childhood.' *J. Pediat.*, **63,** 113.
Sperry, W. M. (1962) 'The biochemical maturation of the brain.' *Res. Publ. Ass. nerv. ment. Dis.*, **39,** 47.
Spitz, R. A. (1945) 'Hospitalism: an inquiry into the genesis of psychiatric conditions in early childhood.' *Psychoanal. Stud. Child*, **1,** 53; **2,** 113.
Stamm, J. S., Pribram, K. H. (1960) 'Effects of epileptogenic lesions in frontal cortex on learning and retention in monkeys.' *J. Neurophysiol.*, **23,** 552.
—— —— (1961) 'Effects of epileptogenic lesions of infero-temporal cortex on learning and retention in monkeys.' *J. comp. physiol. Psychol.*, **54,** 614.
Stemmer, C. J. (1964) 'Choreatiforme Bewegungsonrust.' University of Gröningen doctoral thesis.
Stevens, J. R., Sachdev, K., Milstein, V. (1968) 'Behaviour disorders of childhood and the electroencephelogram.' *Arch. Neurol. (Chic.)*, **18,** 160.
Stewart, M. A., Pitts, F. N., Craig, A. G., Dieruf, W. (1966) 'The hyperactive child syndrome.' *Amer. J. Orthopsychiat.*, **36,** 861.
Still, G. F. (1902) 'Some abnormal psychical conditions in children.' *Lancet*, **i,** 1008, 1077, 1163.
Stone, F. H. (1960) 'Psychodynamics of brain-damaged children: a preliminary report.' *J. Child Psychol. Psychiat.*, **1,** 203.
Storey, P. B. (1966) 'Lumbar air encephelopathy in chronic schizophrenia.' *Brit. J. Psychiat.*, **112,** 135.
Stott, D. H. (1966) 'A general test of motor impairment for children.' *Develop. Med. Child Neurol.*, **8,** 523.
Strauss, A. A., Kephart, N. C. (1940) 'Behaviour differences in mentally retarded children measured by a new behaviour rating scale.' *Amer. J. Psychiat.*, **96,** 1117.
—— —— (1955) Psychopathology and Education of the Brain Injured Child, Vol. II. New York: Grune & Stratton.
—— Lehtinen, L. E. (1947) Psychopathology and Education of the Brain Injured Child, Vol. I. New York: Grune & Stratton.
Swinyard, C. A., Swensen, J., Greenspan, L. (1963) 'An institutional survey of 143 cases of acquired cerebral palsy.' *Develop. Med. Child Neurol.*, **5,** 615.

Teuber, H-L. (1962) 'Effects of brain wounds implicating right or left hemispheres in man: hemisphere differences and hemisphere interaction in vision, audition and somesthesis.' *in* Mountcastle, V. B. (Ed.) Interhemispheric Relations and Cerebral Dominance. Baltimore: Johns Hopkins.
—— Rudel, R. G. (1962) 'Behavior after cerebral lesions in children and adults.' *Develop. Med. Child Neurol.*, **4,** 3.
Tizard, B. (1962) 'The personality of epileptics: a discussion of the evidence.' *Psychol. Bull.*, **59,** 196.
—— Margerison, J. H. (1963) 'Psychological functions during wave-spike discharge.' *Brit. J. soc. clin. Psychol.*, **3,** 6.
Tizard, J. (1964) Community Services for the Mentally Handicapped. London: Oxford University Press.
—— (1965) 'Educational research with the cerebral palsied.' Paper presented at a study group at Grey College, University of Durham, April.
—— (1966) 'Epidemiology of mental retardation.' *Int. J. Psychiat.*, **2,** 131.
—— Grad, J. (1961) The Mentally Handicapped and Their Families. Maudsley Monograph No. 7. London: Oxford University Press.
Tizard, J. P. M., Paine, R. S., Crothers, B. (1954) 'Disturbances of sensation in children with hemiplegia.' *J. Amer. med. Ass.*, **155,** 628.
Tuuteri, L., Donner, M., Eklund, J., Leisti, L., Rinne, A-L., Strandström, C., Ylppo, L. (1967) 'Incidence of cerebral palsy in Finland.' *Ann. paediat. Fenn.*, **13,** 41, 45.
Ullman, C. A. (1952) Identification of Maladjusted School Children. Public Health Monograph No. 7. Washington: U.S. Public Health Service.
Vandenberg, S. G. (1964) 'Factor analytical studies of the Lincoln-Oseretsky Test of motor proficiency.' *Percept. mot. Skills*, **19,** 23.
Vygotsky, L. S. (1962) Thought and Language. London: Wiley.
Walton, J. N., Ellis, E., Court, S. D. M. (1962) 'Clumsy children: a study of developmental apraxia and agnosia.' *Brain*, **85,** 603.
Washburn, T. C., Medearis, D. N., Childs, B. (1965) 'Sex differences in susceptibility to infections.' *Pediatrics*, **35,** 57.
Wechsler, D. (1949) 'Wechsler Intelligence Scale for Children Manual. New York: Psychological Corporation.
—— (1958) The Measurement and Appraisal of Adult Intelligence. Baltimore: Williams and Wilkins.
—— (1967) The Wechsler Pre-School and Primary Scale of Intelligence. New York: Psychological Corporation.
Wedell, K. (1960) 'Variations in perceptual ability among types of cerebral palsy.' *Cerebr. Palsy Bull.*, **2,** 149.
Weinberger, H. A., van der Woude, R., Maier, H. C. (1962) 'Prognosis of cortical blindness following cardiac arrest in children.' *J. Amer. med. Ass.*, **179,** 126.
Wepman. J. M. (1958) Auditory Discrimination Test. Chicago: Language Research Associates.
Werry, J. S. (1968) 'The diagnosis, etiology and treatment of hyperactivity in children.' *in* Hellmuth, J. (Ed.) Learning Disorders, Vol. 3. Seattle: Special Child Publications.
—— Weiss, G., Douglas, V. (1964) 'Studies on the hyperactive child. I. Some preliminary findings.' *Canad. psychiat. Ass. J.*, **9,** 120.
Whildin, O. A. (1947) 'The epileptic child and the public school.' *Nerv. Child*, **6,** 99.
Whitmore, K. (1969) 'An assessment service for handicapped children.' *Med. Offr.* **cxxii,** 263.
Williams, M., Jambor, K. (1964) 'Disorders of topographical and right-left orientation in adults compared with its acquisition in children.' *Neuropsychologia*, **2,** 55.
Wilson, W. P., Harris, B. S. H. (1966) 'Psychiatric problems in children with frontal, central and temporal lobe epilepsy.' *Sth. med. J.*, **59,** 49.
Witts, L. J. (Ed.) (1959) Medical Surveys and Clinical Trials. London: Oxford University Press.
Wolff, O., Smallwood, W. C. (1952) 'The effects of meningococcal meningitis on the intelligence and the hearing.' *Arch. Dis. Childh.*, **27,** 302.
Wood, J. W., Keehn, R. J., Kawamoto, S., Johnson, K. C. (1967) 'The growth and development of children exposed *in utero* to the atomic bomb in Hiroshima and Nagasaki.' *Amer. J. publ. Hlth.*, **57,** 1374.
Woods, F. J., Carrow, M. A. (1959) 'The choice-rejection status of speech-defective children.' *Except. Child*, **25,** 279.
Woods, G. E. (1957) Cerebral Palsy in Childhood. Bristol: John Wright.
—— (1963) 'A lowered incidence of infantile cerebral palsy.' *Develop. Med. Child Neurol.*, **5,** 449.
Wootton, B. (1959) Social Science and Social Pathology. London: Allen & Unwin.
Worster-Drought, C. (1964) 'An unusual form of acquired aphasia in children.' *Folia Phoniat.*, **16,** 223.
—— Allen, I. M. (1929) 'Congenital auditory imperception (congenital word deafness) with report of a case.' *J. Neurol. Psychopathol.*, **9,** 193.
Wortis, J. (1956) 'A note on the concept of the 'brain injured' child.' *Amer. J. ment. Defic.*, **61,** 204.
Wright, P. R., Carey, A., Barter, R. W. (1966) 'Cerebral palsy: report of a survey in East Kent.' *Ann. phys. Med.*, **8,** 175.
Yankauer, A., Lawrence, R. A. (1955) 'A study of periodic school medical examinations. I. Methodology and initial findings.' *Amer. J. publ. Hlth.*, **45,** 71.

—— Frantz, R., Drislane, A., Katz, S. (1962) 'A study of case-finding methods in elementary schools. I. Methodology and initial results.' *Amer. J. publ. Hlth.*, **52,** 656.

Yarrow, L. J. (1961) 'Maternal deprivation; toward an empirical and conceptual re-evaluation.' *Psychol. Bull.*, **58,** 459.

—— (1964) 'Separation from parents during early childhood.' *in* Hoffman, M. L., Hoffman, L. W. (Eds.) Review of Child Development Research. New York: Russell Sage Foundation.

Yates, A. J. (1954) 'The validity of some psychological tests of brain damage.' *Psychol. Bull.*, **51,** 359.

Young, F. M., Pitts, V. A. (1951) 'The performance of congenital syphilitics on the WISC.' *J. consult. Psychol.*, **15,** 239.

Yule, W. (1967) 'Predicting reading ages on Neale's Analysis of Reading Ability.' *Brit. J. educ. Psychol.*, **37,** 252.

—— Berger, M., Butler, S., Newham, V., Tizard, J. (1969) 'The WPPSI: an empirical evaluation with a British sample.' *Brit. J. educ. Psychol.*, **39,** 1.

Zangwill, O. L. (1962) 'Dyslexia in relation to cerebral dominance.' *in* Money, J. (Ed.) Reading Disability. Progress and Research Needs in Dyslexia. Baltimore: Johns Hopkins Press.

Zdanska-Brincken, M., Walanski, N. (1969) A graph method for the evaluation of motor development in infants.' *Develop. Med. Child Neurol.*, **11,** 228.

Zigler, E., Phillips, L. (1961) 'Psychiatric diagnosis: a critique.' *J. abnorm. Soc. Psychol.*, **63,** 607.

Zubin, J., Eron, L. D., Schumer, F. (1965) An Experimental Approach to Projective Techniques. London: John Wiley.

Zutt, J. (1950) 'Uber die Unfahigkeit, die Augen geschlossen zu halten. Apraxie des Lidschlusses oder Zwangsblicken?' *Nervenarzt*, **21,** 339.

Authors

HERBERT BIRCH	Research Professor, Albert Einstein College of Medicine, Yeshiva University, New York 70461, U.S.A.
PHILIP GRAHAM	Consultant Physician and Director of the Department of Psychological Medicine. Hospital for Sick Children, London.
MICHAEL RUTTER	Reader in Child Psychiatry, Institute of Psychiatry London; Consultant Physician, Maudsley Hospital, London.
WILLIAM YULE	Lecturer in Child Development, Institute of Education, London (now Lecturer in Psychology, Institute of Psychiatry, London).

Author Index

H

I

J

K

L

M

N

O

P

Q

R

S

T

U

V

Subject Index

Q

R

S